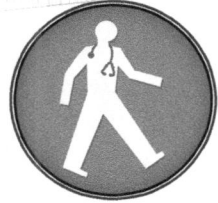

Resident Readiness®
Emergency Medicine

Notice

Medicine is an ever-changing science. As new research and clinical experience broaden our knowledge, changes in treatment and drug therapy are required. The authors and the publisher of this work have checked with sources believed to be reliable in their efforts to provide information that is complete and generally in accord with the standards accepted at the time of publication. However, in view of the possibility of human error or changes in medical sciences, neither the authors nor the publisher nor any other party who has been involved in the preparation or publication of this work warrants that the information contained herein is in every respect accurate or complete, and they disclaim all responsibility for any errors or omissions or for the results obtained from use of the information contained in this work. Readers are encouraged to confirm the information contained herein with other sources. For example and in particular, readers are advised to check the product information sheet included in the package of each drug they plan to administer to be certain that the information contained in this work is accurate and that changes have not been made in the recommended dose or in the contraindications for administration. This recommendation is of particular importance in connection with new or infrequently used drugs.

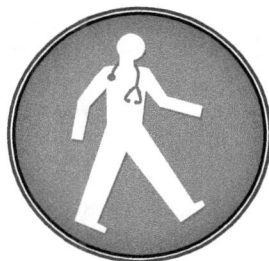

Resident Readiness®
Emergency Medicine

Debra L. Klamen, MD, MHPE

Associate Dean for Education
  and Curriculum
Professor and Chair
Department of Medical Education
Southern Illinois University School
  of Medicine
Springfield, Illinois

Christopher M. McDowell, MD, MEd

Assistant Professor
Residency Director
Division of Emergency Medicine
Southern Illinois University School
  of Medicine
Springfield, Illinois

Ted R. Clark, MD, MPP

Assistant Clinical Professor
Division of Emergency Medicine
Southern Illinois University School
  of Medicine
Springfield, Illinois

Mc Graw Hill Education | Medical

New York   Chicago   San Francisco   Athens   London   Madrid
Mexico City   Milan   New Delhi   Singapore   Sydney   Toronto

1 2 3 4 5 6 7 8 9 0   DOC/DOC   19 18 17 16 15 14

ISBN 978-0-07-178039-1
MHID 0-07-178039-4

This book was set in Minion Pro by Thomson Digital.
The editors were Catherine A. Johnson and Cindy Yoo.
The production supervisor was Richard Ruzycka.
Project management was provided by Shaminder Pal Singh, Thomson Digital.
The designer was Eve Siegel; the cover designer was Anthony Landi.
RR Donnelley was the printer and binder.

This book is printed on acid-free paper.

Library of Congress Cataloging-in-Publication Data

   Resident readiness. Emergency medicine / [edited by] Debra L. Klamen, Ted R. Clark, Christopher M. McDowell.
      p. ; cm.
   Emergency medicine
   Includes bibliographical references and index.
   ISBN-13: 978-0-07-178039-1 (pbk. : alk. paper)
   ISBN-10: 0-07-178039-4 (pbk. : alk. paper)
   I. Klamen, Debra L., editor of compilation. II. Clark, Ted R., editor of compilation. III. McDowell, Christopher M., editor of compilation. IV. Title: Emergency medicine.
   [DNLM: 1. Emergency Medical Services—methods—Case Reports. 2. Emergency Medicine—methods—Case Reports. 3. Intensive Care—methods—Case Reports. 4. Internship and Residency—Case Reports. WX 215]
   RC86.8
   616.02'5—dc23
                                                                              2014001996

McGraw-Hill Education books are available at special quantity discounts to use as premiums and sales promotions or for use in corporate training programs. To contact a representative, please visit the Contact Us pages at www.mhprofessional.com.

To my wonderful husband Phil, who loves me and supports me in all things, especially my crazy passion for horses! To my mother, Bonnie Klamen, and to my late father, Sam Klamen, who were, and are, always there. To my extended family, for their love and understanding. To my students, for keeping me motivated and inspired.—DLK

To the SIU Emergency Medicine Residents, whose insights into the transition from medical school to residency have been vital to the development of this book.—TRC and CMM

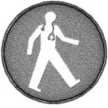

CONTENTS

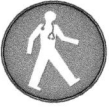

CONTRIBUTORS

Erica J. Cacioppo, MD
Emergency Medicine Resident
Division of Emergency Medicine
Southern Illinois University School of Medicine
Springfield, Illinois
Chapters 16, 17

Ted R. Clark, MD, MPP
Assistant Clinical Professor
Division of Emergency Medicine
Southern Illinois University School of Medicine
Springfield, Illinois
Chapters 1, 2, 3, 4, 5, 6, 8, 10, 11, 12, 13, 15, 21, 23, 24, 25

Antonio Cummings, MD
Assistant Clinical Professor
Division of Emergency Medicine
Southern Illinois University School of Medicine
Carbondale, Illinois
Chapter 6

Jonathan dela Cruz, MD, RDMS
Assistant Professor
Director of Ultrasound
Division of Emergency Medicine
Southern Illinois University School of Medicine
Springfield, Illinois
Chapters 37, 38, 39, 40

Myto Duong, MB, BCh, BAO
Assistant Professor
Director of Pediatric Emergency Medicine
Division of Emergency Medicine
Southern Illinois University School of Medicine
Springfield, Illinois
Chapters 16, 17, 18, 19

Julie Fultz, MD, MDiv
Emergency Medicine Resident
Division of Emergency Medicine
Southern Illinois University School of Medicine
Springfield, Illinois
Chapters 18, 19

Richard Jeisy, MD
Assistant Clinical Professor
Division of Emergency Medicine
Southern Illinois University School of Medicine
Springfield, Illinois
Chapters 8, 9

Ryan N. Joshi, DO, EMT-P
Emergency Medicine Resident
Division of Emergency Medicine
Southern Illinois University School of Medicine
Springfield, Illinois
Chapters 10, 41

Jason A. Kegg, MD, FAAEM
Assistant Professor
Director of Simulation
Division of Emergency Medicine
Southern Illinois University School of Medicine
Springfield, Illinois
Chapters 42, 43

Christi M. Lindorfer, MD
Emergency Medicine Resident
Division of Emergency Medicine
Southern Illinois University School of Medicine
Springfield, Illinois
Chapter 22

Rebecka R. Lopez, MD
Emergency Medicine Resident
Division of Emergency Medicine
Southern Illinois University School of Medicine
Springfield, Illinois
Chapters 41, 42, 43

Christopher M. McDowell, MD, MEd
Assistant Professor
Residency Director
Division of Emergency Medicine
Southern Illinois University School of Medicine
Springfield, Illinois
Chapters 2, 20, 21, 22, 23

Nicholas M. Mohr, MD
Clinical Assistant Professor
Department of Emergency Medicine
Department of Anesthesia, Division of Critical Care
University of Iowa Carver College of Medicine
Iowa City, Iowa
Chapters 26, 27, 28, 29, 30, 31, 32, 33, 34, 35, 36

Quoc V. Pham, MD
Emergency Medicine Resident
Division of Emergency Medicine
Southern Illinois University School of Medicine
Springfield, Illinois
Chapters 11, 15

Charles Reeve, DO
Assistant Clinical Professor
Division of Emergency Medicine
Southern Illinois University School of Medicine
Springfield, Illinois
Chapters 12, 13

Joshua D. Stilley, MD
Clinical Assistant Professor
Department of Emergency Medicine
University of Iowa Carver College of Medicine
Iowa City, Iowa
Chapters 26, 27, 30, 31, 34

Amy Walsh, MD
Global Emergency Medicine Fellow
Department of Emergency Medicine
Regions Hospital
St. Paul, Minnesota
Chapters 26, 29, 33

James R. Waymack, MD
Assistant Professor
Assistant Program Director
Division of Emergency Medicine
Southern Illinois University School of Medicine
Springfield, Illinois
Chapters 7, 14, 24, 25

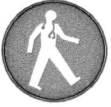

ACKNOWLEDGMENTS

The resident readiness series evolved from ideas that a talented educator and surgeon, David Rogers, had about preparing senior students interested in going into surgery through a resident readiness course. This course was so successful at Southern Illinois University School of Medicine that it spread to other clerkships, and resident readiness senior electives now exist throughout them. The idea for this book series was born by watching the success of these courses, and the interest the senior students having them. It has been a great joy working with Chris McDowell and Ted Clark, completely devoted physicians who retain their humanity for others and passion for education, as well as with the other contributors to this book. We are grateful to the Dean, Dr. Kevin Dorsey, whose dedication to education and innovation allowed us to carve out time in our work to be creative. I (DLK) am greatly indebted to Catherine Johnson from McGraw-Hill, who helped me make the vision of a resident readiness series a reality. Her support and enthusiasm for the project have been unwavering. Likewise, the production manager on the emergency medicine resident readiness book, Shaminder Pal Singh, has been completely dedicated to the task and is deserving of much thanks. We would also like to thank the many contributors to this book, whose commitment to medical education undoubtedly led to long nights writing and editing in its service. Lastly we appreciate our spouses' forbearance for the hours we spent in front of the computer at home; their patience and understanding are without match.

Debra L. Klamen

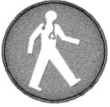

INTRODUCTION

Facing the prospect of an internship is an exciting, and undoubtedly anxiety-provoking, prospect. Four years of medical school, after graduation, culminate in a rapid transition to someone calling you "Doctor" and asking you to give orders and perform procedures without, in many cases, a supervisor standing directly over your shoulder.

This book is organized to help senior medical students dip their toes safely in the water of responsibility and action from the safety of reading cases, without real patients, nurses, families, and supervisors expecting decisive action. The chapters are short, easy to read, and "to the point." Short vignettes pose an organizing context to valuable issues vital to the function of the new intern. Emphasis on the discussion of these cases is not on extensive basic science background or a review of the literature; it is on practical knowledge that the intern will need to function well in the hospital and "hit the ground running." Many of the cases include questions at the end of them to stimulate further thinking and clinical reasoning in the topic area discussed. References at the end of the cases are resources for further reading as desired.

HOW TO GET THE MOST OUT OF THIS BOOK

Each case is designed to simulate a patient encounter and is followed by a set of open-ended questions. Open-ended questions are used purposely, since the cued nature of multiple-choice questions will certainly not be available in a clinical setting with real patient involvement. Each case is divided into four parts.

Part 1

1. **Answers** to the questions posed. The student should try to answer the questions after the case vignette before going on to read the case review or other answers, in order to improve his or her clinical acumen, which, after all, is what resident readiness is all about.

2. A **Case Review:** A brief discussion of the case in the vignette will be presented, helping the student understand how an expert would think about, and handle, the specific issues at hand with the particular patient presented.

Part 2

Topic Title followed by **Diagnostic Reasoning, Workup,** and **Management** discussions: The Diagnostic Reasoning section uses the patient's chief complaint as a launching pad for a discussion of efficient differential diagnosis building and sorting. The Workup and Management sections provide a more generalized, though still focused and brief, discussion of the general issues brought forward in the case presented. For example, in the case of a patient presenting with coma and a significantly elevated glucose, the case review might discuss the exact treatment of the patient presented, while this part of the book will discuss, in general, the diagnosis and treatment of DKA. Of note, not all of the cases in the book will fit entirely in this model, so variations do occur as necessary.

Part 3

Tips to Remember: These are brief, bullet-pointed notes that are reiterated as a summary of the text, allowing for easy and rapid review, such as when preparing a case presentation to the faculty in rounds.

Part 4

Comprehension Questions: Most cases have several multiple-choice questions that follow at the very end. These serve to reinforce the material presented, and provide a self-assessment mechanism for the student.

Section I.
Approach to the Patient in the Emergency Department

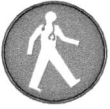

A New Resident Begins the First Day of Emergency Medicine Residency

Ted R. Clark, MD, MPP

CASE DESCRIPTION

You present for your first day in the emergency department (ED) as an emergency medicine (EM) resident. You are armed with the knowledge you accrued through at least 8 years of higher education. You have rotated in EDs and have successfully matched into an EM residency. You feel great and you are ready to work hard.

Your vitals are temperature 37.1 (98.8), blood pressure 130/80 mm Hg, pulse 105 beats/min, respiratory rate 20 breaths/min, and oxygen saturation of 99% on room air.

On examination, your pupils are slightly dilated and you are breathing deeply. You are focused, slightly anxious, but confident in your abilities.

1. Are you prepared?
2. What resources are available to prepare you for this day?
3. How do you use this book?

Answers

1. Yes. Your training has prepared you, but there are additional resources to help you prepare for your first day.

2. There are many types of resources available: comprehensive texts, board review books, clerkship study books, and myriad online resources. There is value in each of these types of books. The comprehensive text is difficult to complete prior to beginning residency. Board review books are geared toward answering test questions. Clerkship study books are designed to help you succeed as a *student*. The EM Residency Readiness book is designed to help you succeed as a new *resident*. This book focuses on how to approach the most common EM patients and is filled with practical advice for the new resident. Additionally, this book addresses the typical off-service rotations that an EM resident will complete during the first year. By completing this book prior to beginning your EM residency, you are specifically addressing the question "am I ready to be an EM resident?"

3. EM Residency Readiness is a case-based book that provides a foundation for each of the major rotations an EM resident will experience during the first year of residency. Specifically, the book addresses ED rotations, ICU rotations, and trauma rotations. Additionally, the book provides a foundation in the important

areas of diagnostic reasoning in the ED, emergency medical services (EMS), ultrasound (US) and teamwork. This book is designed to be read in its entirety prior to starting an EM residency. Specific cases and sections can be subsequently referenced during the corresponding rotation.

DIAGNOSTIC REASONING IN THE ED

The ED Patient

The EM physician sees the largest number of *undifferentiated* patients of any specialty. Furthermore, ED patients display a wide range of acuity from simple colds to cardiac arrest. The typical ED patient will present with a new symptom, also known as a *chief complaint*. The patient cannot necessarily describe whether the problem is medical, surgical, cardiac, gynecologic, neurological, psychiatric, or gastrointestinal. The patient may not be able to provide any information due to a depressed level of consciousness. The diversity of patient presentations in the ED creates a tremendous challenge for EM physicians.

The EM Physician

The EM physician must triage, diagnose, treat, and provide disposition for these *undifferentiated* patients. Furthermore, the EM physician must balance the competing demands of speed and accuracy in the care of patients, a skill most often described as *efficiency*. The most *efficient* emergency physicians employ a systematic approach to the workup of an *undifferentiated* patient.

Systematic Approach to Undifferentiated Patients

The approach to an *undifferentiated* patient typically starts with the development of a *differential diagnosis*, a process we all initially learned in medical school. The natural tendency when developing a *differential diagnosis* is to list the most common diagnoses first. In the outpatient clinic setting or on the inpatient wards in which there is a longitudinal relationship with the patient, this is often the most *efficient* approach. However, in the ED, we must reasonably rule out emergent or life-threatening diagnoses, also known as *critical diagnoses*. An EM physician has about 4 hours to address the *chief complaint(s)* of the patient, stabilize the patient as needed, determine if a *critical diagnosis* exists, determine the existence of subacute or chronic diagnoses, and arrange inpatient or outpatient care. Therefore, an EM physician should develop a broad differential diagnosis based on the patient's *chief complaint(s)* that is organized from most dangerous to least dangerous. Table 1-1 provides an example of an EM physician's *differential diagnosis* for the *chief complaint* of chest pain. How do we sort through this large differential diagnosis? How can we possibly *rule out* all of these diagnoses?

Table 1-1. Emergency Physician Differential Diagnosis for "Chest Pain"

Critical diagnoses

Acute coronary syndrome (STEMI, NSTEMI, unstable angina)

Pulmonary embolism

Aortic dissection

Pneumothorax (tension or stable)

Esophageal rupture (mediastinitis)

Penetrating chest trauma

Blunt chest trauma

Pancreatitis

Subacute diagnoses

Pericarditis

Pneumonia

Stable angina

Bronchitis

Anxiety attack

Nonacute diagnoses

Costochondritis

Muscular strain/pain

GERD

Gastritis

Herpes zoster

The EM physician uses 4 tools to sort among the possible diagnoses and to *rule out* potentially life-threatening diagnoses. The tools are *history, physical examination, testing,* and *observation.*

History and physical examination

The H&P is the first clinical skill learned in medical school, and it is still the most important. Typically, a medical student will learn to perform a detailed H&P in a structured format. In clinical practice, and particularly in the ED, the H&P is honed into a goal-directed process. The *differential diagnosis* will dictate the questions asked during the history and the physical examination maneuvers performed. To put it another way, every question asked and every physical examination maneuver performed provide information that helps the EM physician sort among or rule out the considered diagnoses. Two important points should be made: first, this approach requires an intimate knowledge of the diagnoses being considered; if the EM physician does not understand the diagnosis being considered, inappropriate consideration may be given to certain aspects of the history or physical examination. Second, a particular diagnosis must be considered in the *differential diagnosis* or it will certainly be missed. History and physical examination findings that significantly increase the likelihood of a *critical diagnosis* are termed *red flags*. For instance, in every patient with chest pain, the EM physician should ask about pulmonary embolism (PE) risk factors and should examine the patient's calves for evidence of deep vein thrombosis (DVT). A history of cancer and a swollen left calf would significantly increase the likelihood of PE. Without this information, the EM physician is making inaccurate risk–benefit calculations. Table 1-2 gives an example of the *red flags* for a chief complaint of *low back pain*.

Table 1-2. Critical Diagnoses and Red Flags for a Chief Complaint of Low Back Pain

Critical Diagnosis	History Red Flags	Physical Examination Red Flags
Cauda equina syndrome	Urinary retention, bowel incontinence, saddle anesthesia	Poor rectal tone, significant postvoid residual, saddle anesthesia
Spinal epidural abscess	Fever, IV drug abuse, immunocompromised state, recent LP/epidural	Spinal point tenderness, warmth, erythema, swelling
Ruptured abdominal aortic aneurysm	Known AAA, prior AAA surgery, PVD history, radiation to abdomen	Hypotension, abdominal tenderness, no specific back tenderness, pulsating mass, positive FAST examination
Spinal metastases	History of cancer	Point tenderness over spine, focal neurological changes in lower extremities
Spinal fracture	Trauma, osteoporosis	Point tenderness over spine, step-offs or deformity, neurological deficit
Disc disease with significant nerve root impingement	Pain radiating down legs, specific weakness reported	Neurological deficits

The true strength of the H&P, however, lies in the fact that the majority of *critical diagnoses* can be reasonably *ruled out* with H&P alone. It is worth noting that *ruling out* a diagnosis is not the same as saying there is a 0% chance a diagnosis exists; rather, it is a careful consideration of the risks of additional testing against the likelihood that a given diagnosis may exist. Even our most sensitive tests can rarely *guarantee* that a given diagnosis does not exist.

Testing

The modern ED has thousands of diagnostic tests available for use in the workup of patients. Laboratory tests, plain radiography, advanced imaging, and bedside diagnostics are typically available 24/7 and with relatively little delay. With so many resources available and nearly every external force pushing us toward utilization of these resources, it is often difficult to proceed judiciously. The most important consideration for the use of testing in the ED is the risk/benefit trade-off for our patients. Every test has a certain intrinsic risk. For example, CT scans expose the patients to ionizing radiation, potentially nephrotoxic contrast dye, and the risk of finding "incidentalomas" that require invasive (and potentially harmful) workup. Furthermore, "screening" tests such as the D-dimer may be falsely positive and demand additional, potentially harmful testing. An intimate knowledge of the sensitivity, specificity, and risks for diagnostic tests is required to use them appropriately.

Observation

Occasionally, patients will have medical problems that fall into a gray area between inpatient and outpatient therapy. These patients may require a period of observation to determine if their symptoms are improving or worsening with therapy. Examples include COPD exacerbations, allergic reactions, mild CHF, and dehydration. Once appropriate therapy has been instituted, reassessment can be used to determine the ultimate disposition of such patients.

Example Approach to an ED Patient

Chief complaint

The chief complaint is often listed on the chart or the electronic medical record prior to seeing the patient. The chief complaint should serve as the jumping-off point for your differential diagnosis. Early in your training, you should try making a list of 10 possible diagnoses just based on the chief complaint. Additionally, you can use that list to guide you in your case-based reading and the development of the intimate knowledge of your diagnoses. Beware, however, the chief complaint ascertained at triage can also mislead you. For example, "chest pain" can actually be "epigastric pain" and vice versa; "altered mental status" can be "vertigo" or "focal neurological change."

Vital signs

Typically taken at triage or en route by ambulance, the vital signs are your first indication that a patient may be very sick. The vital signs should be reviewed at the same time as the chief complaint. It is also important to ensure that you have a *complete* set of vital signs including blood pressure, heart rate, respiratory rate, temperature, and pulse oximetry. The vital signs can help you determine which patient you need to see next. Additionally, the vital signs can help you determine how much time you have to gather information before you must provide stabilizing medical intervention.

The ABCs
Airway, breathing, and circulation are the fundamentals of life; therefore, they should be assessed immediately on encountering a patient. The majority of your patient encounters in the ED will start with an introduction and perhaps a handshake. In most instances, the introduction, a glance at the patient's general appearance, and a quick check of the vitals will satisfy the assessment of the ABCs. However, critically ill patients require a more thorough investigation of the fundamentals of life. When assessing the airway, you should look for signs of obstruction, assess for protective reflexes, and intervene by securing an airway if needed. When assessing breathing, you should observe the rate and degree of effort and auscultate for bilateral breath sounds. When assessing circulation, you should check blood pressure, pulses in all 4 extremities, and capillary refill. Any critical issues discovered during the assessment of the ABCs should receive the appropriate intervention before proceeding with the assessment. The clinical cases in this book will cover many such situations.

The safety net
"Two large-bore IVs, O_2, continuous pulse ox, and cardiac monitor!" When you encounter a critically ill patient, it is important to establish what is referred to by EM physicians as the "safety net." Most commonly, experienced EM and ICU nurses will already be working on this by the time you walk into the room; it is still important, however, to verbalize and perform a mental check to ensure these measures are in place.

Using the electronic health record (EHR)
The EHR is a valuable tool in the ED. With few exceptions, you will be meeting your patients for the first time when they present to the ED. Your patients will have variable ability to accurately explain their medical conditions during the interview. If time allows, it is prudent to find a recent History and Physical document in the EHR. It is also a good idea to find documents that are pertinent to the patient's current chief complaint. For instance, if the patient has a chief complaint that may have a cardiac cause, you should attempt to find old EKGs and cardiac catheterization reports. The volume of information available in the EHR can sometimes be overwhelming and learning to sift through the record for information pertinent to the current chief complaint is a valuable skill.

History
As previously discussed, the history is directed by your differential diagnosis. In a busy ED, you typically have about 5 to 7 minutes to establish rapport and

collect the required information. The amount of time you have to collect historical information from a patient in the ED depends on several factors. The acuity
of the patient, the patient's ability to accurately recall medical information, and
the current workload in the ED all influence the time you can dedicate to the
history. It is important to note, however, that it is far more efficient to collect the
required information on the initial contact with the patient, rather than having
to return later for required information that you missed. For this reason, early in
your training, you may need to spend more initial time with your patient. Avoid
trying to impress your attending physician with your *speed* to the detriment of
your *accuracy*. Remember, *efficiency* is a function of both *speed* and *accuracy*, and
it takes time to develop. Initially, you may need to write down certain aspects of
the history. Over time, as you develop mental templates for the history you collect for given chief complaints, you will likely be able to transition away from the
use of notes.

Physical examination

As previously discussed, the physical examination is directed toward the sorting
of your differential diagnosis. The physical examination starts with an assessment
of the vital signs and the ABCs. The same factors that influence the time you have
to perform the history also influence the physical examination. You may have to
perform history and physical examination simultaneously to improve your efficiency. For instance, a common practice among EM physicians is to ask PE and
DVT risk factors while palpating the calves of a patient with chest pain or dyspnea. With few exceptions, you should give every ED patient a basic examination
that includes general appearance, cardiopulmonary examination, and abdominal
examination. Additional examination maneuvers are based on the differential
diagnosis. Developing a standardized examination for common chief complaints
will improve your efficiency.

Testing and interventions

After the completion of your history and physical examination and mental sorting
of your differential diagnosis based on your findings, a diagnostic and management plan will need to be developed. Early in residency, this plan will be developed after discussing the patient with your attending physician. It is good practice
to discuss your differential diagnosis, planned interventions, diagnostic workup,
and projected course of care with the patient, as well. The plan should also be
communicated to the ED team (nurses and technicians), especially if your plan
includes time-sensitive interventions such as a head CT in a potential stroke
patient.

Procedures

A number of emergent and urgent bedside procedures are performed in the ED.
All procedures performed in the ED require a discussion of risks and benefits with
the patient. Most EDs require a signed informed consent form. Exceptions are

made for emergent procedure where the patient is critically ill and unable to consent. There is some variance among hospitals and residencies regarding resident supervision of procedures. There is significant variation in the types of kits and setups utilized to perform ED procedures among hospitals. You should familiarize yourself with the rules and equipment at each of your residency hospitals.

Making difficult decisions

The decision density in the ED is staggering. You will have to decide the patient to see next, questions to ask, tests to order, and which consultants to call. In addition, you will have to interpret the tests, decide upon the interventions and medications, and determine the ultimate disposition of the patient. Every decision carries with it a degree of uncertainty. Some decisions are easy and reflexive (low uncertainty), whereas some patients fall into a "gray area" and the workup and disposition decision can be very difficult (high uncertainty). For example, a healthy patient with an ankle inversion, pain, and swelling can typically be easily worked up with history, physical examination, and perhaps an x-ray. If no injury requiring immediate intervention is identified, the patient can be discharged home quickly and safely. Low-uncertainty decisions are not limited to the less critical patients; for instance, a patient with chest pain and EKG evidence of a STEMI is assessed for other problems (such as dissection), protocolized medications are started, and the patient is immediately referred for cardiac catheterization. Conversely, however, a patient with multiple chronic medical conditions, stable vital signs, and a chief complaint of "light-headedness" could have a number of critical diagnoses. Due to the presence of multiple medical comorbidities the decision to discharge this patient carries a high degree of uncertainty. If a thorough history, physical examination, and ED workup reveals no acute cause of the patient's symptoms, the patient can be discharged. This type of patient is difficult to discharge because they can have a decompensation of a chronic medical condition at any time; however, it is important to remind the patient that there are inherent risks associated with admission to the hospital, and if no indication for admission exists, the patient is better off at home. It is important not only to reassure the patient but also to provide a thorough discussion of the *red flag* symptoms that require immediate return.

To ensure accuracy in your decisions, you should collect the appropriate information and be intimately familiar with the considered diagnoses as well as the diagnostic tests you are performing. It may also improve your efficiency to make a few key decisions soon after the history and physical examination.

An important initial determination is *sick versus not sick*. This decision means essentially determining whether this patient needs an immediate intervention to prevent death or significant deterioration. The vital signs will frequently offer clues for *sick* patients; however, the presence of normal vital signs does not always mean *not sick*. For example, a patient with focal neurological signs and a history of warfarin use may have normal vital signs, but would be classified as *sick*. Additionally, a patient with abdominal pain and a history of abdominal aortic aneurysm may have normal vital signs, but should also be considered *sick* until proven otherwise.

A second decision that should be made is whether the patient will require admission, will be discharged, or will require intervention and reassessment. Many patients can be identified early as requiring admission. Although a considerable amount of workup and intervention may still need to be done in the ED, you can begin the process of admitting the patient to the hospital once the decision has been made. If a patient is identified as someone who will be discharged and does not require workup or intervention, the steps involved in discharging the patient should be immediately completed. Completing all of the required work for this patient during a single block of time will improve your overall efficiency. If the patient requires workup or intervention (a wrist x-ray and splint, eg), however, steps toward discharge should be completed and the patient discharged on completion of the workup and intervention. It is important to note that the care of lower-acuity patients who are to be discharged may need to be interrupted in the face of the requirements of higher-acuity patients.

Staffing your patients

During residency you will staff (or discuss) your patients with your EM attending or upper level residents. There is considerable variability in the staffing preference among EM attendings. It is good practice as a new resident to ask your attendings how they would like the staffing process to work. Typically, early on, you will discuss the patient completely with the attending prior to initiating the plan. As you progress through residency and the EM attendings become more comfortable with you, you will be given more autonomy. You should try to keep your EM presentation to less than 2 minutes; you should emphasize the considered diagnoses and plan.

Admitting a patient

The process of admitting a patient varies dramatically from institution to institution. Some sites have a 1-call medical admission setup, whereas some sites have several possible admitting services. In general, you are required to contact the admitting team and give a presentation of the patient. In addition to the admitting team, all emergent consultations should be contacted from the ED.

Discharging a patient

The majority of patients who present to the ED will be discharged. When you decide to discharge a patient, you have reasonably ruled out by way of history, physical examination, testing, and possibly observation that the patient has an emergent condition that has not been discovered or treated. Additionally, you have decided that any problems you identified have been addressed by your ED intervention, outpatient treatment, follow-up plan, and patient education. You are also responsible for the follow-up and interpretation of any lab or imaging studies. Finally, you are responsible for the education, side effects, and interactions of any medications or therapies you prescribe.

In general, all abnormal vital signs or laboratory values should be corrected or explained prior to discharge. Additionally, a repeat assessment of the patient's symptoms should be completed and documented.

Common Issues in the Care of ED Patients

Patient-centered care

Modern medicine has changed dramatically from the autocratic model of the past in which the physician makes a recommendation and the patient accepts it. In most instances, the management plan, including testing, therapy, and procedures, will be decided upon after a discussion of the risks and benefits with the patient. As described above, every test and procedure performed in the ED carry with it an inherent risk. An example of this type of discussion occurs when talking to a 28-year-old patient with right lower quadrant abdominal pain, no fever, and a normal WBC count. Appendicitis must be considered in this patient (among other diagnoses), but the decision to obtain a CT scan must occur with a discussion of the risks and benefits to the patient. If a CT scan is not obtained, the patient must be informed of the *red flag* symptoms that warrant immediate return to the ED (fever, worsening pain, intractable vomiting, failure of pain resolution in 12-24 hours). Some patients may prefer to have the CT scan after this discussion and some may prefer the wait-and-see approach. The same *patient-centered* approach can be applied to most ED presentations with the notable exception of the critically ill patient or the patient with an altered mental status who cannot participate in their care. In these instances, it is prudent to involve the immediate family or power of attorney in risk–benefit discussions.

DNRs and living wills

When a critically ill patient arrives to the ED, there is often not much time to make intervention decisions. While preparing to intubate or perform advanced cardiac life support (ACLS) on a critically ill patient, it is reasonable to do a quick record check for a signed and valid do not resuscitate (DNR) order. A valid DNR provides the evidence needed to withhold ACLS and intubation. A living will, on the other hand, provides general guidelines for the power of attorney (if available) or the EM physician (in emergent situations) to base end-of-life care decision on. Most living wills read "do not perform artificial or advanced life-saving techniques if there is no hope for meaningful recovery." This phrase is difficult to interpret in the ED because we are often unaware of the cause of the patient's decline on arrival. In such instances, it is better to err on the side of lifesaving intervention. The living will can then be interpreted once the patient is stabilized and the nature of the underlying medical problem is fully discovered. There is considerable variance among states and hospitals regarding the application of DNRs and living wills; therefore, it is prudent to develop an understanding of their use at your respective institution.

Difficult consultant or admission

Occasionally, your plan for care for a patient in the ED will differ from the opinion of your consultant. It is important to remember that regardless of what a consultant may say over the phone, you are ultimately responsible for deciding the disposition of the patient. There is, however, tremendous value in your consultants' opinions; they may have a longitudinal knowledge of the patient, and they have a greater depth of knowledge in their specialty. You must learn to balance your clinical opinion with the opinions of your consultants. Admission and consultation can occasionally become a negotiation with you serving as the advocate for what you feel is right for the patient. The most effective way to enter this process is to have a strong sense of what you feel the patient needs prior to calling your consultant. For instance, if you feel that a patient needs to be admitted, you should enter the call with that idea in mind. It is also reasonable, however, to consider whether you could agree to close outpatient management with 24-hour follow-up. If you are certain that a patient must be managed as an inpatient, you have the ability to "insist" that the consultant either admits the patient or personally evaluates the patient in the ED. Physicians who are on-call for the ED are required to comply in accordance with nearly all hospital system bylaws. You should make every effort to avoid this "standoff" scenario, however. If you effectively build your case and describe your concerns, very rarely will you need to resort to "insisting" that a consultant admits a patient.

Documentation

Documentation in medicine has changed considerably in the last 20 years. Most teaching sites and community EDs have adopted some form of EHR. Some are integrated with the entire hospital, hospital system, or even region. Most sites use hand-written charts, dictation, typed entry, or scribes. Regardless of the data entry method, your ED chart serves 4 main purposes: (1) provides an accurate record of the care given in the ED, (2) provides a data pool for clinical research, (3) provides sufficiently structured information for billing, and (4) provides information in the event of legal proceedings. Items 1 and 2 contribute to the quality and continuity of your patient's care. Items 3 and 4 are simply a reality of our current health care system. Most residencies provide some formal instruction on appropriate documentation. You should also talk to your attending physicians about how to fulfill each of these 4 purposes in your documentation.

Common Pitfalls in Decision Making

Decision making in the ED

Due to the high decision density in the ED, both inexperienced and experienced ED physicians will make errors in judgment. Rapid decisions sometimes require the use of mental *heuristics*, which are typically adaptive, but can lend themselves to decision error. Pat Croskerry, MD, PhD, has written extensively about decision making in the ED. The remainder of this section summarizes some of the most common pitfalls. Additionally, we will discuss some of these issues in greater depth during the cases in this book. The purpose of discussing common pitfalls in decision making in the ED is to make the reader aware and to have the understanding to avoid these pitfalls when faced with similar situations.

Diagnosis momentum

Patients will often get labeled with a diagnosis prior to or early in their ED workup. For example, if a patient checks in and informs triage that he has "chest pain that feels like heartburn," the patient may be labeled as "GERD." Unless the ED physician steps back and considers other possibilities, the patient may not receive an adequate workup or diagnosis. Other examples of this occur when patients arrive by ambulance and EMS reports a "CHF flare" or when a patient is labeled a "pain medication seeker." Such instances also occur during changeover from other ED physicians. The astute ED physician should recognize a premature diagnosis and step back to ensure a complete H&P that encompasses a broad differential diagnosis.

Triage cueing

"Geography is destiny." Modern EDs are often divided into areas based on acuity, as well as being assigned a numerical triage level. The decision to place a patient in a certain area or triage category is a very quick decision made on presentation to the ED. An astute ED physician should realize that just because a patient is in the low-acuity area (or even the waiting room) and has a low-acuity triage level, it does not automatically rule out critical diagnoses. Additionally, it should be recognized that symptoms change, and patients who did not at first seem particularly sick may, in fact, get very sick during their ED stay.

Visceral bias

There will be patients who "annoy" you and patients toward whom you develop positive feelings. Both of these affective states can influence the care decisions that you make. If you recognize that you have a negative affective bias toward a patient, you should make an effort to spend additional time with the patient to ensure that you are providing an adequate workup. Instances may also arise in which positive feelings toward a patient can compromise care. For instance, if a patient reminds you of your mother, you may be subconsciously less inclined to perform invasive procedures even if they are indicated. Again, recognition of such feelings is the most effective method of counteracting their effect.

Search satisfying

This is the tendency to call off the search once something is found. For instance, what is the most commonly missed fracture on x-ray? *The second fracture.* Many will truncate their search after finding 1 fracture. Another example is attributing an elderly patient's alteration of mental status to a mild urinary tract infection. Although the infection may be part or all of the cause of the patient's symptoms, it does not inherently rule out other causes. The best way to combat this error in cognition is to always ask yourself after finding an abnormality: *is there anything else to be found?*

Anchoring

In an effort to save time, an ED physician may fixate on certain features of a presentation, collect confirming evidence, and inappropriately discount conflicting evidence. This approach will increase speed but may sacrifice accuracy. The most effective way to prevent anchoring is to create and explore a broad differential diagnosis, pay close attention to conflicting evidence, and always ask yourself the question *what else could this be?* There are many more types of cognitive errors committed in medical decision making. In addition to those addressed later in the book, consult the section "Suggested Reading" for additional reading.

SUMMARY

This chapter is an introduction to the principles of seeing, diagnosing, and making critical decisions on patients in the ED. Development of true *efficiency* takes patience and repetition. The cases in this book will introduce you to several common types of patients you will encounter during residency both in the ED and on your off-service rotations. Continue to apply the principles discussed in this chapter to both practice cases and your ED patients as you progress through residency. Over time, you will develop both the speed and accuracy to care for patients in the ED environment.

SUGGESTED READING

Croskerry P. The importance of cognitive errors in diagnosis and strategies to minimize them. *Acad Med.* 2003;78:775–780.

Section II.
The ED Rotation—Cases You Will Definitely See

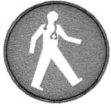

A 67-year-old Male With Severe Chest Pain

Ted R. Clark, MD, MPP and Christopher M. McDowell, MD, MEd

CASE DESCRIPTION

Richard Buffet is a 67-year-old male who presents to the emergency department with severe chest pain. He describes it as "an elephant sitting on my chest." The pain started 1 hour ago while he was raking leaves at home. The pain does not radiate and has no associated nausea or dyspnea. He has no history of similar pain. His past medical history is significant for hypertension and hyperlipidemia. His father had coronary artery disease (CAD) and his brother has a stent. The patient has no prior surgery, cardiac stents, or cardiac testing. He appears to be in moderate distress due to pain.

His vitals are temperature 37.1 (98.8), blood pressure 174/98 mm Hg, pulse 94 beats/min, respiratory rate 20 breaths/min, and oxygen saturation of 94% on room air.

On examination, you note significant diaphoresis. His lungs are clear. His pulse is regular and equal in upper extremities. He has no cardiac murmur. His legs are not swollen and his calves are nontender.

1. What is your differential diagnosis?

2. What are the red flags in Mr Buffet's history and physical examination?

3. What test must be ordered immediately?

Answers

1. The differential diagnosis for chest pain is broad and should include critical, emergent, and nonemergent diagnoses. Table 2-1 provides a broad but not exhaustive differential diagnosis.

2. Mr Buffet has some very concerning features in his history and physical examination as described. Red flags are features in the history and physical examination that lead the physician toward a critical diagnosis. Importantly, critical diagnoses may present without the classic red flag symptoms, but the presence of red flag symptoms urges a workup for a given diagnosis. Many critical diagnoses will cause vital sign changes such as hypotension, tachycardia, bradycardia, tachypnea, hypoxemia, or fever; significant vital sign changes always require careful consideration and an explanation. Table 2-2 provides a summary of the red flags for the common critical diagnoses associated with a chief complaint of chest pain. The features that Mr Buffet has are bolded.

Table 2-1. Emergency Physician Differential Diagnosis for Chest Pain

Critical Diagnoses	Emergent Diagnoses	Nonemergent Diagnoses
Acute coronary syndrome (STEMI, NSTEMI, unstable angina)	Pericarditis	Costochondritis
	Pneumonia	Muscular strain/pain
	Stable angina	GERD
Pulmonary embolism	Bronchitis	Gastritis/PUD
Aortic dissection	Anxiety attack	Herpes zoster
Pneumothorax (tension or stable)	Coronary spasm	Rib contusion/fracture
	Cholecystitis	Spinal root compression
Esophageal rupture (mediastinitis)	Pancreatitis	
Cardiac tamponade		

3. An EKG. There are very few patients who present to the ED with chest pain, who will not receive an EKG. An EKG should be done as soon as possible because early acute myocardial infarction (AMI) intervention or the identification of potentially lethal arrhythmia will have a significant impact on morbidity and mortality. Figure 2-1 shows Mr Buffet's EKG.

CASE REVIEW

Mr Buffet is having an inferior MI. The general principles of management for ST-segment elevation myocardial infarction (STEMI) are improving oxygen delivery, decreasing myocardial demand, limiting progression of clot, and achieving reperfusion as soon as possible. In addition to oxygen and the safety net, Mr Buffet should receive aspirin, nitroglycerin (unless right ventricular infarct is suspected), beta-blocker (unless contraindicated), heparin, and in most cases clopidogrel or a glycoprotein IIb/IIIa inhibitor. Current goals for door to balloon time are <90 minutes, although many sites are much faster than this. If you are at a site that does not have a cardiac catheterization lab and if one is not available by transfer within 120 minutes, thrombolytics are indicated.

CHEST PAIN

Diagnostic Reasoning

Chest pain is a frequently encountered chief complaint in the ED. In addition to the standard chest pain complaint, there are many patients who seek to be evaluated for chest pain "equivalents" such as arm pain and neck pain. Most

Table 2-2. Critical Diagnoses and Red Flags for Chest Pain

Critical Diagnosis	History Red Flags	Physical Examination Red Flags
Acute coronary syndrome	"Crushing" or **pressure in nature, substernal** or left chest in location, onset **with exertion**, radiation to arm, shoulder, or jaw. CAD risk factors	**Diaphoresis**, new murmur, new pulmonary rales
Pulmonary embolism	Sharp or pleuritic chest pain, dyspnea, sudden onset, hemoptysis, syncope, unilateral leg swelling. PE risk factors	Respiratory distress (tachypnea), hypoxia, low-grade fever, clear lungs, signs of deep vein thrombosis
Aortic dissection	"Tearing" pain, maximal at onset, radiating to back, syncope, neurological changes. History of uncontrolled hypertension or connective tissue disorder	Unequal upper extremity BPs or pulses, new murmur, new focal neurological changes, hypertension on presentation, marfanoid features
Pneumothorax	Sharp or pleuritic chest pain, sudden onset, dyspnea, trauma history, COPD or asthma history	Unilateral diminished or absent breath sounds, chest wound, subcutaneous air, tachypnea, hypoxemia. Tension pneumothorax—hypotension, tracheal deviation, JVD
Esophageal rupture	"Burning" central chest pain, preceded by forceful vomiting or foreign body sensation, bright red blood in vomit, history of recent instrumentation of esophagus or nasogastric tube	Subcutaneous emphysema (neck), audible "Hamman crunch" on cardiac auscultation, epigastric tenderness
Cardiac tamponade	Most commonly in the context of acute kidney injury, viral pericarditis, or penetrating trauma. Pericarditis—sharp, worse with lying back, improved with sitting up, history of recent URI	Hypotension, muffled heart tones, JVD, friction rub, effusion and RV collapse on bedside US

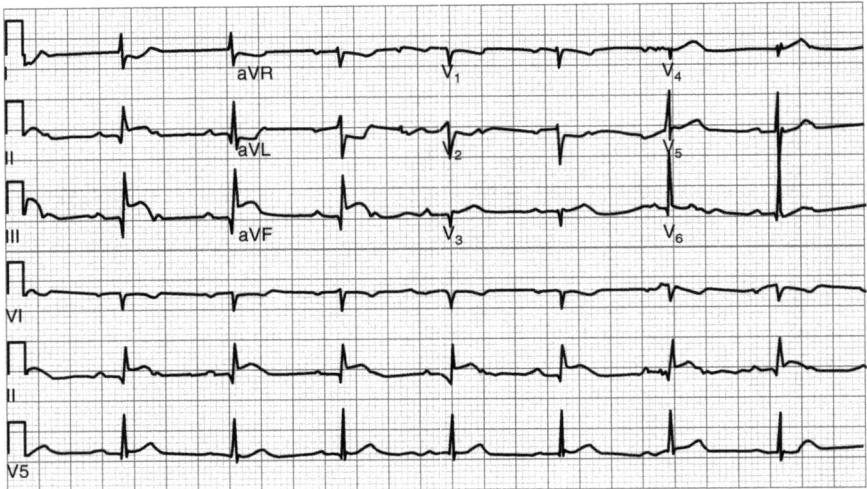

Figure 2-1. Mr Buffet's EKG shows classic ST elevation consistent with an inferior STEMI. EKG interpretation is a crucial skill for an EM physician. For more detailed analysis of EKG interpretation, please see the recommended readings. (Courtesy of David M. Cline, MD, Wake Forest University.)

emergency physicians would agree there are 6 life-threatening etiologies that cannot be missed. Sometimes this is referred to as "the rule of 2's": 2 cardiac, 2 pulmonary, and 2 tubes. Acute coronary syndrome (ACS), cardiac tamponade, pulmonary embolus (PE), pneumothorax, aortic dissection, and Boerhaave syndrome (esophageal rupture) must be considered in every chest pain patient. Table 2-1 lists several common emergent and nonemergent causes of chest pain that must also be considered.

The EM physician must be intimately familiar with the common and uncommon presentations of critical and emergent diagnoses. The common history and physical examination findings found with critical diagnoses for chest pain are listed in Table 2-2. The EM physician should make it a habit to search for these findings by asking questions and performing indicated examination maneuvers on each patient who presents with chest pain or a chest pain equivalent.

Risk factors are an important part of the history in a patient with chest pain. Risk factors for critical diagnoses are an important part of appropriate risk stratification. There are also several clinical decision rules that help assess a patient's risk for a critical diagnosis. Risk factors and decision rules are most clearly laid out for ACS and PE. Table 2-3 summarizes the most commonly considered risk factors and clinical decision rules for ACS and PE. Mental cues such as always asking about pulmonary embolism risk factors while examining the calves, asking about aortic dissection risk factors while palpating bilateral pulses, and asking

Table 2-3. Risk Factors and Decision Rules for a Chief Complaint of Chest Pain

Critical Diagnosis	Risk Factors	Decision Rules
Acute coronary syndrome	Age, male sex, hypertension, hypercholesterolemia, diabetes, current smoker, family history of CAD, and known CAD	**TIMI risk Score for UA/NSTEMI**
Pulmonary embolism	Age >50, exogenous estrogen, cancer, recent hospitalization, recent surgery (especially lower extremity orthopedic), recent long-distance travel, recent extremity trauma, indwelling venous catheter (upper or lower extremity), immobility, current DVT, and prior PE or DVT	**PERC rule for PE** **Wells criteria for PE**

cardiac risk factors before auscultating the heart may help ensure the appropriate information is obtained for risk stratification.

Another critically important step in diagnostic reasoning for patients with chest pain is a review of prior records. Old cardiac catheterization reports, stress test results, and consultation notes are very important for determining the best course of action for the patient. A final step that may be helpful, if available, is discussion with the patient's cardiologist. The patient's primary cardiologist often has useful knowledge about the nature and extent of the patient's cardiac disease; this information is extremely useful for making disposition decisions.

Diagnostic Workup and Management

The extent of the workup for a chief complaint of chest pain is highly dependent on the details of the patient presentation, the patient's risk factors, and the patient's desires. As discussed previously, all potentially sick patients in the ED need the "safety net" established. IV–O_2–pulse ox–monitor is the mantra repeated over and over. Each of these components is necessary for the chest pain patient. IV access allows for quick therapeutic interventions while the pulse oximeter and cardiac monitor are attached. Oxygen helps treat potential ischemia while the ED physician is arriving at a diagnosis. Most patients presenting with chest pain will receive aspirin and an EKG very shortly after arrival to the ED. Some patients may even be triaged based on their EKG and vital signs.

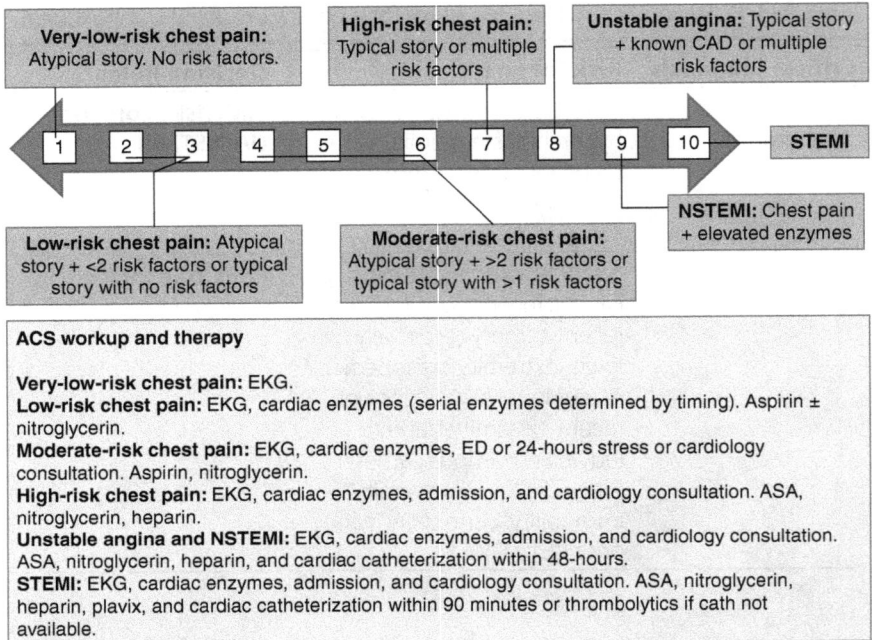

Figure 2-2. The ACS risk spectrum can help determine appropriate therapy and disposition in patients who present with chest pain.

The extent of the workup required for a consideration of ACS can range from EKG only to immediate cardiac catheterization. Mr Buffet has clear evidence of an acute STEMI and should be taken for immediate cardiac catheterization. His case represents the highest level on the *ACS risk spectrum*. Figure 2-2 summarizes possible ACS workups for different patient presentations of chest pain.

The timing of the cardiac enzymes for the low- and moderate-risk groups is important, since these may be going home after completion of the ED workup. In general, an EKG (or serial EKGs) can rule out STEMI and appropriately timed cardiac enzymes can rule out NSTEMI. Troponin I is most commonly used. The ED is a common site for a "2-set AMI rule-out." There are several different protocols ranging from a 2-hour repeat set to a 6-hour repeat set. If the chest pain has been *unremitting* and *unchanging* for >8 hours, a "1-set AMI rule-out" can be utilized. If the chest pain has a duration <8 hours or has materially changed, 2-set AMI rule-out should be obtained. Again, there is variation among EDs in this practice and you should investigate the practice at your training site.

Although careful consideration and workup of ACS is a large component of the overall workup for a patient with a chief complaint of chest pain, workup for other critical and emergent diagnoses must be carefully considered.

Pulmonary embolism is another critical diagnosis that can be notoriously difficult to diagnose. After assessing the signs, symptoms, and risk factors, the patient is typically classified into very-low-risk, low-risk, moderate-risk, or high-risk categories. In general, very-low-risk patients require no further testing, low- and moderate-risk patients may be screened with a D-dimer, and high-risk patients require a CT or V/Q scan. The workup of PE is discussed in more detail later in this book. A PE is managed with anticoagulation and supportive care. Hemodynamically unstable patients should be considered for thrombolytics or thrombectomy.

Aortic dissection should be worked up if the history, physical examination, and risk factors as described above point toward its presence. In particular, chest pain radiating to the back in the presence of significant hypertension, neurological symptoms, or history of connective tissue disorder likely demands workup. The test of choice for dissection is the CT chest/abdomen/pelvis with IV contrast. There is some consideration for the use of D-dimer as a screening tool for dissection. Although some studies have shown promise, the D-dimer lacks sufficient sensitivity to be used to "rule out" aortic dissection. In the ED, a patient with aortic dissection needs aggressive blood pressure control (labetalol drip or esmolol + nitroprusside drip) to a systolic blood pressure <120 mm Hg and perhaps even lower depending on the patient. The cardiothoracic surgeon should be immediately consulted. Depending on the type of dissection, the patient will be managed primarily medically or surgically.

Pneumothorax is initially assessed by history and lung auscultation. If signs of tension pneumothorax are present (hypotension, tracheal deviation, JVD, progressive dyspnea), immediate needle decompression should be undertaken before additional workup is completed. If the patient is stable, the chest x-ray and the bedside ultrasound may be reliably used to assess for pneumothorax. Chest CT is the most sensitive test, but is not necessarily indicated for the detection of pneumothorax. The patient may require observation, a small percutaneous chest tube, or a large-bore tube thoracostomy depending on the size and cause of the pneumothorax.

Esophageal rupture (Boerhaave syndrome) is most commonly related to a history of forceful vomiting or esophageal instrumentation. It may present acutely after a tearing pain and bleeding with vomiting or subacutely with burning chest pain and a history of forceful vomiting. The diagnostic test of choice is a chest CT. A water-soluble contrast swallow may also be indicated. Barium swallow should be avoided. Additional testing should include CBC, CMP, and blood cultures. Antibiotics and urgent GI and cardiothoracic surgery consultation are mandatory.

Cardiac tamponade, like tension pneumothorax, must be detected and treated immediately without much time for diagnostic workup. In addition to a history and physical examination consistent with cardiac tamponade, the EM physician may perform a bedside ultrasound to detect pericardial fluid and evidence of diastolic ventricular collapse. The ultrasound may also be used to guide emergent pericardiocentesis if the patient is unstable. Additional workup after stabilization is directed at finding the cause of the pericardial effusion. Lab work may include renal function testing, coagulation profile, viral titers, and tuberculosis workup. If the effusion is traumatic, CT imaging is necessary.

TIPS TO REMEMBER

- ACS presentations in females can be notoriously atypical, but typical presentations are still more common.
- ACS presentations in the elderly may manifest as nausea or generalized weakness.
- ACS should be considered in patients with epigastric pain.
- Serial EKGs (repeated every 10 minutes) may reveal an evolving STEMI or dynamic NSTEMI EKG changes; consider serial EKGs in high-risk patients.
- Upper extremity DVT can occur with indwelling central lines; this should be considered when considering PE.
- Esophageal rupture can be difficult to diagnose early on if it is not complete; CT scan, water-soluble contrast swallow, and direct endoscopy may be indicated.

COMPREHENSION QUESTIONS

1. Sharp, sudden-onset chest pain and dyspnea after a coughing episode in a patient with moderate COPD is most consistent with which critical diagnosis?

    A. ACS
    B. PE
    C. Pneumothorax
    D. Esophageal rupture
    E. Aortic dissection

2. With regard to the ACS workup, a patient with atypical chest pain and no CAD risk factors should have which of the following workups?

    A. Nothing
    B. EKG
    C. EKG, cardiac enzymes
    D. EKG, cardiac enzymes, stress test
    E. Immediate cardiac catheterization

3. A patient who presents with chest pain, hypotension, JVD, and tracheal deviation most likely needs which of the following interventions?

A. Cardiac catheterization
B. Pericardiocentesis
C. Upper endoscopy
D. Needle decompression
E. Thrombolytics

Answers

1. C. The red flag clues of the history of COPD and the preceding coughing spell make pneumothorax the most likely choice.

2. B. This patient would be considered very-low-risk for ACS. The EKG is a low-cost, noninvasive test and can prevent significant morbidity and mortality by the rapid detection of ischemia and malignant dysrhythmia. Nearly all patients who present to the ED with chest pain, even if considered very-low-risk, will receive an EKG.

3. D. The patient presentation is most consistent with a tension pneumothorax and immediate needle decompression is indicated.

SUGGESTED READINGS

Marx JA, Hockberger RS, Walls RM, eds. *Rosen's Emergency Medicine: Concepts and Clinical Practice*. 7th ed. Philadelphia: Mosby-Elsevier; 2010 [chapter 21] <http://www.mdconsult.com>.
Tintinalli JE, Kelen GD, Stapczynski JS, Ma OJ, Cline DM, eds. *Tintinalli's Emergency Medicine*. 7th ed. New York: McGraw-Hill Education; 2011 [chapters 52–64].

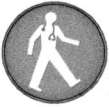

A 35-year-old Female With Left-sided Chest Pain

Ted R. Clark, MD, MPP

CASE DESCRIPTION

Ms Cake is a 35-year-old female who presents to the emergency department with a chief complaint of left-sided chest pain. The pain has been present off and on for the past 2 days. The pain initially started at rest, and it does not appear to be related to exertion. The pain lasts for about 1 to 2 minutes and is sharp in nature. It seems to be exacerbated by movement of the left arm and pressing on the left chest. There are no clear relieving factors. She has no fever, dyspnea, leg swelling, or diaphoresis. She has no chronic medical problems. Specifically, she denies hypertension, high cholesterol, diabetes, and prior DVT or PE. She takes no medications. She has given birth to 2 children vaginally. She has had no surgeries. She does not smoke. Her family history is negative for premature coronary artery disease and clotting disorders.

Her vitals are temperature 37.1 (98.8), blood pressure 122/78 mm Hg, pulse 86 beats/min, respiratory rate 14 breaths/min, and oxygen saturation of 98% on room air.

On physical examination, you note a regular heart rate with no murmur. Her lungs are clear. She has reproducible chest pain with palpation of the left chest wall. She has no calf tenderness or swelling. No deformity or bruising is noted. Her neurological examination is normal.

1. Review the critical diagnoses and red flags for a chief complaint of "chest pain." What red flags does this patient have?

2. Review the risk factors for ACS and PE. What risk factors does this patient have?

3. Where is this patient on the ACS risk spectrum?

4. What emergent and nonemergent diagnoses should be considered?

Answers

1. Ms Cake has chest pain, which is always concerning. She does, however, have very few red flags in her history. The "sharp" nature of the pain could lead one to pursue a diagnosis of PE or pneumothorax, but she has no other history or physical examination findings to suggest these diagnoses. Her history and physical examination are also not consistent with aortic dissection, esophageal rupture, or cardiac tamponade. With regard to ACS, her history and physical examination are very atypical for cardiac ischemia; however, this does not rule

29

out ischemia. Remember: *chest pain that is reproducible with palpation does not rule out ACS*. Further consideration should be given to ACS by considering the patient's risk factors and considering the ACS risk spectrum.

2. Ms Cake has no significant risk factors for ACS or PE. Both the PERC and Wells criteria can be applied to this patient. She is both PERC and Wells negative.

3. Ms Cake is considered *very low risk*. She has an atypical story and no risk factors for ACS.

4. Although there still may be some directed workup for critical diagnoses in Ms Cake, her lack of red flags should lead us to more fully explore emergent and nonemergent causes of her symptoms. Among emergent diagnoses, pericarditis would be a consideration in this patient. Pericarditis typically presents with a sharp or burning-type chest pain, change in the nature of the pain with laying back, relief with NSAIDs, and possibly a preceding viral infection. Among non-emergent diagnoses, Ms Cake's presentation is most consistent with costochondritis, muscular strain, or rib contusion. All 3 of these conditions can present with chest pain that is insidious in onset, long in duration, sharp in character, and worse with movement and palpation.

CASE REVIEW

Ms Cake has a normal EKG. She does not appear to have a critical or emergent diagnosis. The most likely cause of her symptoms is costochondritis, muscle strain, or simply "chest wall pain." The treatment of choice for her symptoms is NSAIDs and topical muscle creams. More important than the over-the-counter therapy you recommend is the reassurance and discussion of critical diagnoses. The EM physician should reassure the patient that based on the history, physical examination, and EKG, there is very little chance of a life-threatening diagnosis. The red flags for life-threatening diagnoses should be reviewed with the patient. The patient can then be safely discharged home.

CHEST PAIN WITHOUT RED FLAGS

Diagnostic Reasoning

Although she has the same chief complaint as Mr Buffet, Ms Cake is a very different patient. She has no red flags in the history and physical examination. She has no major risk factors for ACS or PE. She is *very low risk* on the ACS risk spectrum. While the EM physician is considering the appropriate workup for the critical diagnoses, consideration is also given to emergent and nonemergent diagnoses. Tables 3-1 and 3-2 list common history and physical examination characteristics of select emergent and nonemergent diagnoses for the chief complaint of chest pain.

Table 3-1. Common Emergent Diagnoses for Chief Complaint of Chest Pain

Emergent Diagnosis	Typical History	Typical Physical Examination
Pericarditis	Dull with or without episodes of sharp pain. May be worse with laying back, improves with sitting up. Often with preceding viral illness	Half of patients have a friction rub. EKG usually shows diffuse ST-segment elevation, sinus tachycardia, or nonspecific changes
Pneumonia	Cough, sputum, fever, may have pleuritic-type chest pain	Focal auscultated changes or scattered rhonchi noted
Anxiety attack	Chest pain described as pressure, shortness of breath, tingling in the hands and face. A feeling of anxiety. May have come on in stressful situation or at rest. A history of similar prior is helpful. Symptoms should resolve with relaxation or anxiolytic medication	Patient may be breathing rapidly, but lung examination should be clear and oxygen saturation should be normal. May be mildly tachycardic but should resolve as patient calms down. No red flags for critical diagnoses should be present
Stable angina	Difficult diagnosis to make in the ED. It requires previously diagnosed stable angina of >2 weeks' duration. No symptoms at rest, symptoms resolve after stopping exertion	No new murmur, no red flags for critical diagnoses. Unchanged EKG. No enzyme changes
Pancreatitis	Considered a critical diagnosis for a chief complaint of abdominal pain. Should be considered when the chief complaint is chest pain. Acute onset of severe epigastric pain. Commonly radiates to the back. History of alcohol use or cholelithiasis	Tender in epigastric region. Low-grade fever. Flank or periumbilical ecchymosis indicates hemorrhagic pancreatitis
Cholecystitis	RUQ pain. May have a long history of crampy pain that is exacerbated by eating, but it becomes more severe and constant with cholecystitis. May radiate to right subscapular area	Will often have a fever, RUQ tenderness, and positive Murphy sign. Jaundice is less common

Table 3-2. Common Nonemergent Diagnoses for a Chief Complaint of Chest Pain

Nonemergent Diagnosis	Typical History	Typical Physical Examination
Costochondritis	Sharp, localized, pain reproduced with light palpation. Can be of long duration with short exacerbations of pain	Easily and completely reproducible. No red flags for critical diagnoses. Normal vital signs
Muscle strain	Pain with use or movement of a particular muscle body or group. May have story of preceding overuse or strenuous use	Pain reproducible with use of muscle body or palpation of muscle body. No red flags for critical diagnoses. Normal vital signs
GERD	Burning or gnawing pain. Usually lower half of the chest. Worse with laying back. May have acid taste in mouth. Prior history of similar symptoms or a diagnosis of GERD is helpful. May improve with antacids (not diagnostic)	No red flags for critical diagnoses. Will likely require at least EKG
Gastritis/peptic ulcer disease	Dull, burning, epigastric pain. Often worse at night. May be relieved with antacids (not diagnostic)	No red flags for critical diagnoses. Mild epigastric tenderness without peritoneal signs
Herpes zoster	Sharp, tingling, shooting, or burning pain in a dermatomal distribution precedes rash by 1-10 days. Prior history of shingles or chicken pox	Skin is usually hyperesthetic both before and after presence of the dermatomal rash. No red flags for critical diagnoses
Rib contusion/ fracture	Localized pain, dull to sharp. Pain worse with movement, palpation, or inspiration. History of trauma	Pain to palpation, visible bruising, crepitus, or deformity. Look for signs of pneumothorax. No red flags for critical diagnoses

Diagnostic Workup and Management

Based on the patient history and physical examination, there is a very low suspicion for the presence of a critical diagnosis in this patient. It is still reasonable, however, to order an EKG on Ms Cake. Although there will be variation among EDs, it is unlikely that this patient will need the "safety net" or continuous monitoring. Despite the unlikely presence of a critical diagnosis, if there is evidence in the history and physical examination of an emergent or nonemergent diagnosis, additional workup may be indicated.

Pericarditis may not be immediately life threatening, but it can progress to serious illness and should be identified in the ED. If a patient has a history and physical examination concerning for pericarditis, the EM physician should order an EKG and cardiac enzymes, and perform a bedside US to assess for effusion. The treatment of choice is NSAIDs. If cardiac enzymes are elevated or there is evidence of effusion, congestive heart failure, or arrhythmia, cardiology consultation is necessary. The vast majority of patients with simple pericarditis will be managed as outpatients.

Pneumonia is very common and patients can present from well appearing to critically ill. If there is clinical suspicion for pneumonia, chest x-ray is the diagnostic test of choice. Additional workup should include a CBC. If the patient is to be admitted, blood cultures are required. Ideally, antibiotics should be started on a patient within 4 hours of presentation to the ED when diagnosed with pneumonia. Antibiotic coverage varies depending on etiology (community, nosocomial, ventilator associated, and aspiration) and patient status (immunocompromised, septic, and comorbidities).

Anxiety attack is unlikely to be life threatening, but it does require emergent therapy to alleviate suffering and prevent hyperventilation. Important aspects of the history include prior episodes, prior workup, and current therapy for anxiety. The mainstay of therapy is anxiolysis with benzodiazepines, a thorough history and physical examination for critical diagnoses, directed workup, and reassurance.

Stable angina is a very difficult diagnosis to make in the ED. It is defined as exertional chest pain for >2 weeks, constant in duration and relief, and without new associated symptoms. For the purposes of the ED, it requires a prior diagnosis of stable angina that is being managed medically. It is a diagnosis of exclusion, and the assumption should be made that the nature of the patient's angina has in some way changed to prompt a presentation to the ED. Because the patient has known coronary artery disease, a careful ACS workup should be undertaken and the ED physician should consult the patient's cardiologist.

TIPS TO REMEMBER

- Chest pain that is reproducible on palpation does not rule out critical diagnoses.
- Chest pain that resolves with antacids does not rule out critical diagnoses.

- The EM physician should explore red flags and risk factors for all presentations of chest pain.
- Epigastric pain may be an atypical presentation of ACS or other chest pain critical diagnosis.

COMPREHENSION QUESTIONS

1. A 65-year-old male presents with sharp left-sided chest pain that lasts 1 to 2 minutes and is reproducible with chest wall palpation. It has been occurring for about 3 days. He has no fever, cough, dyspnea, or DVT symptoms. He denies similar prior episodes. He does not remember injuring himself. He has hypertension, diabetes, and high cholesterol. He has no known coronary artery disease. He smokes. His brother had a heart attack at age 60. The patient is currently pain free. Vital signs are stable and examination has no red flags. Which is the most appropriate ACS workup for this patient?
   - A. EKG
   - B. EKG and cardiac enzymes
   - C. EKG, cardiac enzymes, and inpatient or ED stress test
   - D. EKG, cardiac enzymes, and admission for cardiac catheterization within 24 hours
   - E. Immediate cardiac catheterization

2. A 35-year-old female patient presents with a dull anterior chest pain of 2 days' duration. The pain is worse with lying back, but it does not radiate. The patient has no dyspnea. There is no fever and no cough. There are no other red flags present in the history. Her vitals are T 37.2, BP 122/78, P 108, RR 14, and O_2 saturation 98% on room air. The presentation is most consistent with which diagnosis?
   - A. Pneumonia
   - B. ACS
   - C. PE
   - D. Pericarditis
   - E. Costochondritis

Answers

1. C. This patient has a very atypical story, but he has considerable risk factors. On the ACS spectrum, he is moderate to high risk. An atypical story and reproducible chest wall pain are not adequate to rule out ACS in a patient with this many risk factors. He does not require urgent catheterization (STEMI) or even catheterization within 24 hours (NSTEMI/UA) as long as his EKGs and enzymes are normal. He does, however, need a cardiac stress test to help determine if his symptoms are due to ischemic heart disease.

2. **D.** The patient's presentation is most consistent with pericarditis. Her story is not consistent with pneumonia or costochondritis. She has no red flags for PE or ACS. She will need an EKG, bedside ultrasound, and cardiac enzymes.

SUGGESTED READINGS

Marx JA, Hockberger RS, Walls RM, eds. *Rosen's Emergency Medicine: Concepts and Clinical Practice.* 7th ed. Philadelphia: Mosby-Elsevier; 2010 [chapter 18] <http://www.mdconsult.com>.
Tintinalli JE, Kelen GD, Stapczynski JS, Ma OJ, Cline DM, eds. *Tintinalli's Emergency Medicine.* 7th ed. New York: McGraw-Hill; 2011 [chapters 52–64] <http://www.accessmedicine.com>.

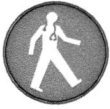

A 15-year-old Female With Acute Abdominal Pain

Ted R. Clark, MD, MPP

CASE DESCRIPTION

Ms Murphy is a 15-year-old female who presents to the ED with a chief complaint of abdominal pain. The pain started about 10 hours ago as a generalized ache but is now more severe and in the lower abdomen. The pain is worse with walking or moving and is relieved with laying still. She has nausea, has vomited twice, and has not felt like eating all day. She is not sure if she has a fever. She denies dysuria, vaginal discharge, or diarrhea. She denies being sexually active. She denies sick contacts. She has no prior medical history and she has never had a surgery.

Her vitals are temperature of 38.5°C (101°F), blood pressure 114/70 mm Hg, pulse 110 beats/min, respiratory rate 20 breaths/min, and oxygen saturation of 100% on room air.

On physical examination, the patient appears uncomfortable. The abdominal examination reveals tenderness to palpation in the right lower quadrant. Percussing the abdomen exacerbates the pain. The abdomen is soft and there are no masses felt. There is no tenderness to percussion over the kidneys. The pelvic examination reveals no discharge, no cervicitis, no mass, and no cervical motion tenderness. The rectal examination reveals no blood and no evidence of perirectal abscess. The heart and lung examination is normal.

1. What is your differential diagnosis for a chief complaint of abdominal pain?

2. What are the red flags in Ms Murphy's history and physical examination?

3. What laboratory test is imperative in this patient?

Answers

1. There is a broad differential diagnosis for the chief complaint of abdominal pain. Figure 4-1 demonstrates an effective way to organize the differential diagnosis by location.

2. Ms Murphy gives a classic history for appendicitis. The presence of right lower quadrant pain, tenderness, fever, nausea, and poor appetite (anorexia) can all be considered red flags. In addition, the history of generalized abdominal pain progressing to right lower quadrant pain over 6 to 24 hours is classic for appendicitis. Importantly, patients only rarely present with all the classic symptoms of a critical diagnosis; any single red flag should prompt further consideration of a critical diagnosis such as appendicitis. Table 4-1 lists critical diagnoses and red flags for a chief complaint of abdominal pain.

Diffuse Pain

Aortic aneurysm (leaking, ruptured)	Mesenteric ischemia
Aortic dissection	Metabolic disorder
Appendicitis (early)	(Addisonian crisis, AKA,
Bowel obstruction	DKA, porphyria, uremia)
Diabetic gastric paresis	Narcotic withdrawal
Familial Mediterranean Fever	Pancreatitis
Gastroenteritis	Perforated bowel
Heavy metal poisoning	Peritonitis (of any cause)
Hereditary angioedema	Sickle cell crisis
Malaria	Volvulus

Right Upper Quadrant Pain
Appendicitis (retrocecal)
Biliary colic
Cholangitis
Cholecystitis
Fitz-Hugh-Curtis Syndrome
Hepatitis
Hepatic abscess
Hepatic congestion
Herpes zoster
Myocardial ischemia
Perforated duodenal ulcer
Pneumonia (RLL)
Pulmonary embolism

Left Upper Quadrant Pain
Gastric ulcer
Gastritis
Herpes zoster
Myocardial ischemia
Pancreatitis
Pneumonia (LLL)
Pulmonary embolism
Splenic rupture/distension

Right Lower Quadrant Pain
Aortic aneurysm (leaking, ruptured)
Appendicitis
Crohn disease (terminal ileitis)
Diverticulitis (cecal)
Ectopic pregnancy
Endometriosis
Epiploic appendagitis
Herpes zoster
Inguinal hernia
(incarcerated, strangulated)
Ischemic colitis
Meckel diverticulum
Mittelschmerz
Ovarian cyst (ruptured)
Ovarian torsion
Pelvic inflammatory disease
Psoas abscess
Regional enteritis
Testicular torsion
Ureteral calculi

Left Lower Quadrant Pain
Aortic aneurysm (leaking, ruptured)
Diverticulitis (sigmoid)
Ectopic pregnancy
Endometriosis
Epiploic appendagitis
Herpes zoster
Inguinal hernia
(incarcerated, strangulated)
Ischemic colitis
Mittelschmerz
Ovarian cyst (ruptured)
Ovarian torsion
Pelvic inflammatory disease
Psoas abscess
Regional enteritis
Testicular torsion
Ureteral calculi

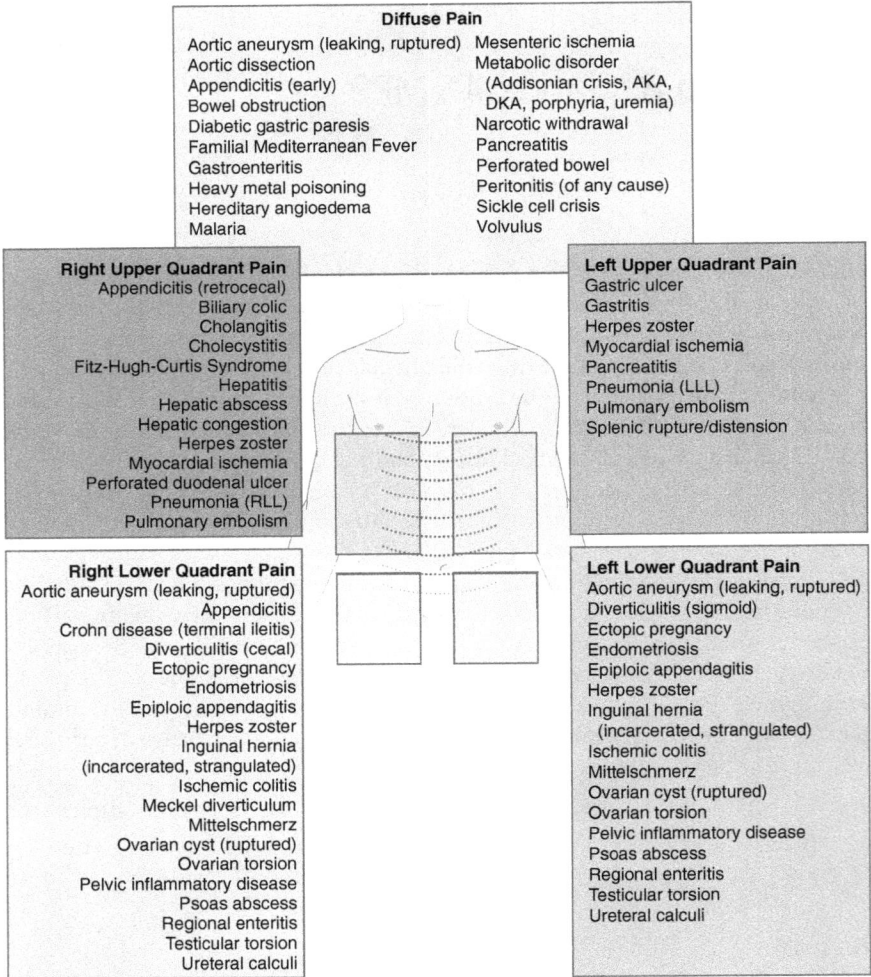

Figure 4-1. Differential diagnosis for abdominal pain by location. (Reproduced, with permission, from Cline DM, Ma OJ, Cydulka RK, et al. *Tintinalli's Emergency Medicine Manual.* 7th ed. Copyright © The McGraw-Hill Companies, Inc. 2011. All rights reserved.)

3. A urine pregnancy test should be ordered on all women of childbearing age who present with abdominal pain unless the uterus is absent. History of tubal ligation, an intrauterine device, birth control medications, or an adamant history of no sexual activity are not sufficient to rule out pregnancy. For any other presentation, women of childbearing age should have a urine pregnancy test if any potentially harmful medications or testing is to be performed.

Table 4-1. Critical Diagnoses and Red Flags for Abdominal Pain

Critical Diagnosis	History Red Flags/ Risk Factors	Physical Red Flags
Acute appendicitis	Diffuse pain progressing to **RLQ pain** over 8-12 h. Low-grade fever, nausea, **anorexia**, mild vomiting. Most common ages 11-20, but can occur at any age	**RLQ tenderness.** Guarding. Rebound tenderness. Fever
Ectopic pregnancy	Severe, **sharp**, constant lower abdominal pain. Pain may be more diffuse with rupture. **Usually right or left sided.** Risk factors include nonwhite race, older age, **history of STD or PID, infertility, IUD, previous ectopic, or prior tubal ligation**	Signs of peritonitis or shock may be present with rupture. **Adnexal mass** or tenderness on pelvic examination. Vaginal bleeding may or may not be present
Ruptured or leaking AAA	Acute **epigastric or back pain**. May be associated with syncope or signs of shock. Pain may radiate to back or groin. Risk factors include advanced age, **known vascular disease**, HTN, DM, and smoking	Patient may be in shock. **Pulsatile mass** on abdominal examination. Bedside FAST examination may show free fluid. **Bedside ultrasound may confirm presence of AAA**
Mesenteric ischemia	Diffuse, very painful. May have history of **intestinal angina after meals**. Risk factors include **atrial fibrillation, known vascular disease, hypercoagulable states, valvular heart disease**	**"Pain out of proportion to examination."** Rectal examination may be positive for occult blood
Intestinal obstruction	**Crampy**, diffuse abdominal pain. Often associated with **vomiting and/or obstipation**. Risk factors include young age or old age, **prior abdominal surgeries, known hernias, prior bowel obstructions**	Abdominal distention, **hyperactive bowel sounds**, and diffuse tenderness. May have peritoneal signs if strangulation exists

(continued)

Table 4-1. Critical Diagnoses and Red Flags for Abdominal Pain (*Continued*)

Critical Diagnosis	History Red Flags/ Risk Factors	Physical Red Flags
Perforated viscus	Acute onset of constant pain. Commonly epigastric due to ruptured peptic ulcer. May be diffuse if peritonitis exists. Risk factors include **known PUD, recent instrumentation, and prior diverticulitis**	Epigastric pain, low-grade fever, decreased bowel sounds. **"Rigid abdomen" if peritonitis exists**
Acute pancreatitis	Sharp or burning epigastric pain often **radiating to the back**. Nausea and vomiting are common. Risk factors include **alcohol, gallstones,** hyperlipidemia, hypercalcemia, or **recent ERCP**	Low-grade fever is common. Epigastric tenderness. May be tachycardic or hypotensive. **Cullen or Grey-Turner sign** if hemorrhagic
Acute cholecystitis/ cholangitis	Crampy or constant **RUQ pain**. May **radiate to right scapular area**. Prior history of similar but less severe pain. **Duration >2 h** more common with cholecystitis or cholangitis versus biliary colic. **More common in multiparous, obese women.** Peak age 35-60 years	Fever commonly present. RUQ tenderness. **Positive Murphy sign.** Jaundice may be present. **Charcot triad:** RUQ pain, jaundice, and fever. **Reynolds pentad:** also with shock and altered mental status
Hepatic abscess	**Insidious** course of fever, **RUQ pain**, anorexia, and malaise. Risk factors include recent biliary tract infection or instrumentation, ruptured appendicitis, PID, penetrating liver trauma, and travel to Africa, South America, India, or Southeast Asia	Fever, RUQ tenderness, and hepatomegaly. Jaundice may be present
Hepatitis	**Insidious** course of fever, **RUQ pain**, jaundice, nausea. Risk factors include heavy alcohol use, injection drug use, travel to hepatitis A endemic regions, heavy Tylenol use	Low-grade fever. **RUQ tenderness.** Hepatomegaly. **Jaundice**

(continued)

Table 4-1. Critical Diagnoses and Red Flags for Abdominal Pain (*Continued*)

Critical Diagnosis	History Red Flags/ Risk Factors	Physical Red Flags
Diverticulitis	Acute onset of typically **LLQ pain**. May have diarrhea. Nausea. Risk factors include age >65, prior history of diverticulitis or diverticulosis	Fever. LLQ tenderness. May have signs of peritonitis with rupture
Pelvic inflammatory disease	**Vaginal discharge, gradual onset** of lower abdominal pain. Pain typically bilateral, but may be unilateral with tubo-ovarian abscess. Risk factors include prior STD or PID	Fever, bilateral adnexal tenderness, **purulent vaginal discharge**. **Cervical motion tenderness** is present on pelvic examination. Adnexal mass may be present with tubo-ovarian abscess
Ovarian torsion	**Sudden, unilateral, lower abdominal or pelvic pain.** May radiate to the groin, back, or flank. Usually constant, but may be crampy and intermittent. Risk factors include known ovarian cysts or masses	Afebrile. Unilateral lower abdominal tenderness. Adnexal mass may be present. Pelvic examination usually without discharge or cervical motion tenderness
Testicular torsion	**Sudden onset of unilateral testicle or abdominal pain.** May be crampy and intermittent. Usually without other symptoms. May occur during physical or sexual activity	**Testicle pain, abnormal lie, loss of cremasteric reflex.** Afebrile. May have some lower abdominal pain. No penis discharge
Splenic rupture	**LUQ pain.** Typically in the setting of **trauma**. May be present in the setting of illnesses that cause splenomegaly, such as **mononucleosis**	Tender LUQ. May have splenomegaly. May have bruising from trauma. May have shock if significant bleeding exists. **Bedside FAST** may reveal peritoneal fluid

(continued)

Table 4-1. Critical Diagnoses and Red Flags for Abdominal Pain (*Continued*)

Critical Diagnosis	History Red Flags/ Risk Factors	Physical Red Flags
Spontaneous bacterial peritonitis	Diffuse abdominal pain. Gradual onset. May have altered mental state. Typically presents in the context of **ascites** or **peritoneal dialysis**	Fever often present. **Peritoneal signs** often present. Typically without focal tenderness. May have signs of sepsis
Incarcerated hernia	**Acute abdominal pain** at known or unknown hernia site. May have symptoms of bowel obstruction	**Firm, tender, nonreducible hernia.** May have peritoneal signs and fever if ischemia is present
Nephrolithiasis	**Right or left flank pain radiating to the lower abdomen.** Pain is severe, sharp, and crampy. May have dysuria or hematuria. Risk factors include prior ureteral stones	Patient is in obvious discomfort. **"Writhing" in pain** is characteristic. May be mildly tender in the lower abdomen. May have CVA tenderness. **Usually afebrile** unless stone is infected
Pyelonephritis	**Dysuria, unilateral or bilateral flank pain.** Often report fever and chills. May have history of recent UTI	**CVA tenderness.** Usually febrile. Nausea is common
Acute coronary syndrome	**Vague nausea or upper abdominal pain.** Sometimes described as **"gas"** or **"indigestion."** More common atypical presentation in females or elderly. Risk factors include known CAD or common CAD risk factors	There may be no abdominal tenderness. The patient may have diaphoresis, increased work of breathing, or tachycardia

CASE REVIEW

Ms Murphy has signs and symptoms consistent with acute appendicitis. A pregnancy test, CBC, BMP, and urinalysis should be ordered. An abdominal CT or RLQ ultrasound can be used to confirm the diagnosis. The patient should be kept NPO, pain and nausea medication should be administered, and maintenance IV fluids should be started. On confirmation of the diagnosis, antibiotics (most commonly ampicillin–sulbactam) should be administered. A general or pediatric surgeon should be consulted for urgent removal of the appendix.

ABDOMINAL PAIN

Diagnostic Reasoning

Acute abdominal pain accounts for up to 10% of all ED visits. The differential diagnosis is very broad and is most often considered in the context of the location of the pain. Patients with abdominal pain are diagnostically challenging due to the diversity of clinical presentations, the high number of critical diagnoses to be considered, and a high proportion of presentations (up to 40%) that do not result in a definitive diagnosis. Additionally, there are several groups of patients that deserve special consideration when presenting with abdominal pain: the elderly, the immunocompromised, and women. Finally, the EM physician must also consider abdominal pain as a potential atypical presentation of cardiopulmonary, metabolic, or endocrine disease.

Careful consideration of the patient with acute abdominal pain starts by considering the most common critical diagnoses as listed in Table 4-1. As with any patient presentation, the EM physician must first establish the safety net and address any immediate problems identified by a quick survey of airway, breathing, and circulation (ABCs). The patient's vital signs may provide the first clue that a critical diagnosis may exist. For example, a 65-year-old male with known vascular disease, abrupt onset of abdominal pain, and a low blood pressure should raise immediate suspicion for ruptured abdominal aortic aneurysm. Although the differential in this patient includes several other entities, the ruptured AAA is the most immediately life threatening and rapid steps must be taken to confirm or deny the diagnosis. It should be noted, however, that many critical diagnoses for abdominal pain present with normal vital signs and a normal survey of the ABCs.

The patient history should contain a standard HPI, but should also include the red flag questions summarized in Table 4-1. For example, a patient with a history of prior abdominal surgery or known hernias has a much higher risk of bowel obstruction. An experienced EM physician typically develops a mental "script" that addresses the most important aspects of the history for any given chief complaint.

The physical examination can further focus the broad differential diagnosis in a patient with acute abdominal pain. In addition to noting the location of the abdominal tenderness, the EM physician must quickly identify the "surgical abdomen." Importantly, if the patient displays rigidity, significant distention, or clear peritoneal signs, the surgical consultant should be contacted prior to the completion of labs and imaging. Another valuable tool for the diagnostician is the serial examination. It is important to complete and document a repeat examination on all acute abdominal pain patients, particularly those who will be discharged.

Diagnostic Workup and Management

In contrast with patients with a chief complaint of "chest pain," "dyspnea," or "altered mental status," only a small percentage of patients with acute abdominal pain will be truly unstable. There are, however, a large number of surgical emergencies that require efficient workup and surgical consultation. Also, it is still important to first establish the "safety net" and address any issues that arise on a survey of the ABCs. After this is completed, the EM physician can proceed with diagnostic workup and management.

The extent of the workup for a patient with acute abdominal pain can range from a urine pregnancy test only to extensive lab testing and advanced imaging. In general, patients over 65, patients with prior bariatric surgery, and immunocompromised patients will require more workup. After the initial assessment, the EM physician should be able to place the patient in a basic workup category: (1) symptomatic treatment and repeat examination only; (2) symptomatic treatment, laboratory testing (often urinalysis, urine pregnancy test, CBC, and basic or complete metabolic panel), repeat examination, and the decision to image based on results; (3) symptomatic treatment, laboratory testing, and immediate imaging; (4) resuscitation and immediate surgical consultation (concurrent with further workup).

There are several useful laboratory tests when working up abdominal pain. Some tests, such as a serum lipase, can essentially confirm a diagnosis. Other tests, such as WBC count and venous lactate, are used to provide information in support of the presence or absence of a diagnosis. Importantly, the low sensitivity and specificity of such tests preclude their ability to "confirm" or "rule out" a diagnosis. A common error among inexperienced clinicians is placing too much emphasis on such tests.

The most common imaging tests performed on patients with acute abdominal pain are the bedside ultrasound, the formal ultrasound, the abdominal plain film, and the abdominal CT. The bedside ultrasound (performed by the EM physician) is typically used to answer a specific clinical question. For instance, bedside ultrasound can "confirm" a suspected diagnosis such as AAA or cholecystitis, or it can be used to "confirm" the presence of an intrauterine pregnancy when ectopic pregnancy is considered. Importantly, formal ultrasound (performed by radiology) or CT imaging is often needed if the EM physician cannot obtain a clear answer to the clinical question. Formal ultrasound is most commonly used for suspected diagnoses of cholecystitis, ectopic pregnancy, ovarian torsion, testicular torsion, and less commonly appendicitis. The abdominal CT scan gives the most general information and is utilized in most other suspected diagnoses. The abdominal plain film should be utilized when high-grade bowel obstruction or perforation is suspected.

Symptomatic management is usually directed at controlling pain and nausea. If the patient has evidence of dehydration, it may also be beneficial to provide IV fluid. There are several antiemetic options, but ondansetron is currently the most broadly used. It is available in IV form and oral dissolvable tablets. Although there has been some controversy in the past, it is now generally agreed upon that opioid analgesia is acceptable in acute abdominal pain and does not significantly alter the findings in serial abdominal examinations. IV ketorolac is also widely used and is particularly efficacious for the "colicky" pain associated with gallbladder disease and urolithiasis.

Final management is dictated by the diagnosis. A summary of the management for the most common critical and emergent diagnoses is listed below.

Acute appendicitis is usually confirmed on abdominal CT. More frequently in pediatric patients, the diagnosis is confirmed with ultrasound. Rarely, a patient with a classic presentation will be taken to the OR without prior imaging. The patient may also have an elevated WBC count. Management includes making the patient NPO, starting maintenance IV fluids, administering antibiotics such as ampicillin–sulbactam, and consulting a general surgeon. The patient requires urgent surgery to prevent rupture, peritonitis, and possibly sepsis.

Acute cholecystitis is most commonly diagnosed with ultrasound but is frequently diagnosed on CT. The patient may also have elevated WBC count and mildly elevated liver enzymes. Patients with confirmed cholecystitis require NPO status, maintenance IV fluids, antibiotics such as ampicillin–sulbactam, and a general surgery consultation. Most patients receive urgent surgery, but some may be observed for a period of time prior to surgery if there are no signs of systemic infection.

Bowel obstruction can be diagnosed on plain abdominal x-rays or abdominal CT scan. The patient may also have an elevated WBC count, elevated amylase, or, if ischemia is present, an elevated serum lactate. Patients with low-grade obstructions require NPO status, NG tube to suction, maintenance IV fluids, and a general surgery consult. Many low-grade obstructions resolve spontaneously over a few days. Patients with high-grade obstructions, closed-loop obstructions, or obstructions with evidence of ischemia require urgent surgery.

Acute pancreatitis is typically diagnosed with an elevated lipase in the right clinical context. The patient may also have elevated amylase, WBC count, low calcium, or hyperglycemia. Acute pancreatitis can be quite severe and result in shock, respiratory failure, and multisystem organ failure. General management includes NPO status, IV fluid resuscitation, pain and nausea control, blood cultures if the patient is febrile, electrolyte monitoring, and admission to a medicine team or GI specialist. If pancreatitis is due to a stone in the common duct, the patient may need urgent endoscopic retrograde pancreatography with stone removal. Complications such as hemorrhage, abscess, and pseudocyst formation can be further assessed on abdominal CT.

Diverticulitis is typically diagnosed on abdominal CT, but may be treated empirically based on the clinical information without CT confirmation if the clinical presentation is classic and the patient has had prior episodes of diverticulitis. The patient may also have an elevated WBC count. If the patient has no signs of sepsis, abscess, or perforation, diverticulitis can be treated at home with a clear liquid diet and antibiotics such as ciprofloxacin and metronidazole. An alternative antibiotic regimen is amoxicillin–clavulanic acid. The patient should receive instructions to return for worsening pain, fever, or inability to obtain or take the antibiotics. If the patient has signs of sepsis, abscess, or perforation, IV antibiotics, surgical consultation, and admission are required.

TIPS TO REMEMBER

- A patient with a "surgical abdomen" requires immediate stabilization and consultation with a general surgeon.
- A pelvic examination is indicated in any female with lower abdominal pain, even in the absence of vaginal discharge or pregnancy.
- The threshold for abdominal imaging should be much lower in patients who are immunocompromised, older than 65, or have had prior bariatric surgery.

COMPREHENSION QUESTIONS

1. A 15-year-old female patient presents with RLQ pain that is sudden and sharp. The patient denies fever, vomiting, or anorexia. She denies vaginal discharge or dysuria. The patient is writhing in pain and tender to palpation in the RLQ. There are no peritoneal signs. The patient is afebrile. WBC count is normal and urine pregnancy test is negative. Which of the following is the most appropriate initial imaging?

    A. Pelvic ultrasound
    B. Abdominal CT with IV and PO contrast
    C. Abdominal CT without contrast
    D. Abdominal plain film x-ray

2. A 65-year-old male presents with epigastric pain that has suddenly worsened to generalized abdominal pain. The patient is febrile. Vital signs are otherwise stable. The abdominal examination reveals rigidity and rebound tenderness diffusely. Which of the following is the next best step in the workup and management?

    A. Administration of IV antibiotics

    B. Plain film x-ray of the abdomen

    C. Surgery consultation prior to additional workup

    D. Abdominal CT with IV contrast

Answers

1. A. The patient's presentation is most concerning for ovarian torsion. Appendicitis, tubo-ovarian abscess, urolithiasis, and ectopic pregnancy are all concerns, but there is no additional evidence to support these diagnoses. An abdominal CT may be indicated if the ultrasound is negative.

2. C. This patient is presenting with a "surgical abdomen" on examination. In such cases, it is best to alert the surgery consultant prior to completing the workup. The patient presentation is consistent with a perforated ulcer, and the abdominal x-ray to assess for free air would be indicated after the surgical consultation is performed. An abdominal CT with IV contrast could be performed instead if the patient is otherwise stable, but PO contrast should be deferred due to the resulting delay in diagnosis.

SUGGESTED READINGS

Marx JA, Hockberger RS, Walls RM, eds. *Rosen's Emergency Medicine: Concepts and Clinical Practice.* 7th ed. Philadelphia: Mosby-Elsevier; 2010 [chapter 18] <http://www.mdconsult.com>.

Tintinalli JE, Kelen GD, Stapczynski JS, Ma OJ, Cline DM, eds. *Tintinalli's Emergency Medicine.* 7th ed. New York: McGraw-Hill; 2011 [chapters 74, 84] <http://www.accessmedicine.com>.

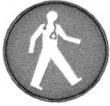

A 50-year-old Male With Upper Abdominal Pain

Ted R. Clark, MD, MPP

CASE DESCRIPTION

Mr Coffee is a 50-year-old male who presents to the ED with a complaint of upper abdominal pain. The pain has been present for about 3 days. He states the pain is fairly constant and burning in nature. There is no radiation. The pain is somewhat relieved with antacids. The pain does not seem to be exacerbated by eating. The patient states he has had similar pain in the past, but it usually resolves on its own. The patient denies fever, vomiting, diarrhea, dark stools, chest pain, and dyspnea. He reports daily NSAID use for his chronic knee pain. Mr Coffee has a past medical history of hyperlipidemia and osteoarthritis. He has had no prior surgeries. He reports occasional ETOH use. He denies smoking. He has no family history of CAD.

His vitals are temperature of 37 (98.6), blood pressure 140/70 mm Hg, pulse 80 beats/min, respiratory rate 18 breaths/min, and oxygen saturation of 100% on room air.

On examination, the patient is noted to have mild tenderness in the epigastric region. There are no rebound and no peritoneal signs. There is no pain in the RUQ or the lower abdomen. Bowel sounds are normal. There is no distention or mass. There are no ascites, no caput medusae, and no spider angiomata. There is no bruising noted on the abdomen or flank. The rectal examination reveals no dark stool, no gross blood, and the stool is hemoccult negative. The cardiac and pulmonary examinations are normal.

1. What is your differential diagnosis for Mr Coffee?

2. What are the red flags in Mr Coffee's history and physical examination?

3. What 2 bedside diagnostic tests should be considered in this patient?

Answers

1. By referencing Figure 4-1, a very broad differential diagnosis for upper abdominal pain can be developed. The patient's pain is most correctly described as epigastric pain. When considering a patient with epigastric pain, the EM physician should consider possibilities in the RUQ and LUQ, as well as atypical presentations of chest pain and lower abdominal pain. The critical diagnoses that should be carefully considered in this patient are acute pancreatitis, acute cholecystitis, AAA, perforated viscus (related to peptic ulcer disease [PUD]), mesenteric ischemia, splenic rupture, and acute coronary syndrome (ACS).

There are several diagnoses on this list, as well as other critical diagnoses not listed, that are considered, but are effectively ruled out due to the lack of red flags in the history and physical examination. For instance, it would be extremely unlikely to have cholecystitis with no RUQ tenderness, no fever, and 3 days of constant pain; thus, a RUQ ultrasound or a CT scan is not indicated for the pursuit of this diagnosis. Similarly, it would be unlikely that Mr Coffee would have a perforated viscus without peritoneal signs and fever; thus, the EM physician may prefer serial examinations to abdominal imaging. In contrast, Mr Coffee has the risk factors of hyperlipidemia and male sex for ACS. Although this would be an atypical presentation for ACS, it should be considered.

Although EM physicians always consider critical diagnoses first, most patients do not have a critical diagnosis. In addition to the diagnoses discussed above, the EM physician should consider many emergent and nonemergent diagnoses. Mr Coffee's presentation is most consistent with gastritis, uncomplicated PUD, early acute or chronic pancreatitis, GERD, or biliary colic.

2. Mr Coffee has no red flags for critical diagnoses. The pertinent negatives in his history and physical examination should be noted. He is afebrile, his vital signs are normal, and he has no peritoneal signs on examination. These 3 pertinent negatives make a critical diagnosis much less likely, although far from impossible. Mr Coffee does have 2 noteworthy risk factors, however. His daily NSAID use puts him at risk for gastritis and PUD. Additionally, his history of alcohol use should be further explored as it may increase his likelihood of developing pancreatitis.

3. Gastritis and PUD are at the top of the list of possible diagnoses for Mr Coffee. The history, physical examination, and risk factor of NSAID use support these as possible diagnoses. The most common complication of PUD is bleeding. For this reason, it is important to check a stool hemoccult in this patient. Additionally, an EKG would be a reasonable test due to its noninvasive nature and the potential harm of missing an acute MI.

CASE REVIEW

Mr Coffee has epigastric abdominal pain and no significant red flags. His history, physical examination, and risk factors are most consistent with gastritis or PUD. A stool hemoccult should be performed. It is reasonable to check a lipase to assess for pancreatitis. It is also reasonable to check an EKG for acute MI. A CBC will be helpful if you are concerned about blood loss with PUD or have a continuing suspicion for infection (in this case cholecystitis/cholangitis would be the primary concern). Liver function tests (LFTs) may also be considered if there is suspicion for cholecystitis/cholangitis, although these are not necessarily elevated. For consideration, Mr Coffee's hemoccult, lipase, EKG, CBC, and LFTs are normal.

No imaging is indicated at this time. It is not possible to differentiate between gastritis and PUD in the ED; an endoscopy is required to make that distinction. The empiric treatment, however, is the same. The patient can be started on an H_2 blocker such as ranitidine (or on a proton-pump inhibitor if already on an H_2 blocker) and given a gastric protectant such as sucralfate. The patient should be instructed to avoid NSAIDs and alcohol, and should be informed of the potential complications of PUD. Primary care follow-up within 1 week is reasonable. Finally, a repeat abdominal examination, a documented discussion of the critical diagnoses, and good verbal and written instructions for follow-up and immediate return are required.

ABDOMINAL PAIN WITHOUT RED FLAGS

Diagnostic Reasoning

Although this patient has the same chief complaint as Ms Murphy, the absence of red flags in the history and physical examination will change the workup and management. After the EM physician performs the complete history and physical examination and determines the likelihood of a critical diagnosis is very low, attention should then be turned to emergent and nonemergent diagnoses. Table 5-1 presents a description of the most common emergent and nonemergent causes of abdominal pain. The list is not exhaustive, and, often, no definitive diagnosis can be made.

Importantly, the absence of red flags in the history and physical examination does not mean that the search for dangerous diagnoses is over. It is imperative that EM physicians discuss the critical diagnoses with the patient, discuss the absence of findings that point to a dangerous cause, and discuss the risks and benefits of possible testing. By verbally expressing your reasoning to the patient, you are both providing good patient education and giving yourself an additional opportunity to pick up clues that may lead you to a critical diagnosis.

Diagnostic Workup and Management

Patients with abdominal pain, no significant red flags, and a reasonable explanation for their symptoms may not require additional workup. Mr Coffee has a reasonable story for gastritis/PUD and has no additional acute findings on history and examination. As described above, a CBC, CMP, lipase, and EKG are reasonable tests with his presentation. Additionally, the management for gastritis/PUD in the ED is described above. Workup and management of additional selected emergent and nonemergent diagnoses for the chief complaint of abdominal pain are described below.

Biliary colic is typically diagnosed clinically; however, care must be taken to consider the entire spectrum of biliary disease including cholecystitis and

Table 5-1. Common Noncritical Diagnoses for Chief Complaint of Abdominal Pain

Noncritical Diagnosis	Typical History	Typical Physical Examination
Gastritis/PUD	Epigastric pain. Typically burning. May have nausea without vomiting. Gradual onset. May be affected by eating. May be worse with supine position. Risk factors include NSAID use and prior gastritis	Epigastric tenderness. No peritoneal signs. No fever. Assess for stool hemoccult
Gastroenteritis	Vomiting and diarrhea must be present. Pain is diffuse, crampy, intermittent, and nonlocalizing. Nausea and vomiting occur before pain. May have fever and body aches. May have sick contacts or seasonal exposure. Typically viral	No localizing tenderness. No peritoneal signs. May have signs of dehydration. Diarrhea is watery and nonbloody
Biliary colic	RUQ pain. Worse after eating. Afebrile. Radiation to right shoulder. Duration <1-2 h	May have RUQ tenderness. No peritoneal signs
Chronic pancreatitis	Epigastric pain. Nausea or vomiting. Similar prior episodes. Alcohol use. Not as severe as acute pancreatitis	Epigastric tenderness. Nausea. Vomiting
Ovarian cyst	Sharp, unilateral, lower pelvic pain. May have had similar prior symptoms.	Tenderness to palpation in the adnexal region. Mass may be felt if large. Pelvic usually normal—contrast these findings with those of a tubo-ovarian abscess or PID
Epiploic appendagitis	Sharp, stabbing pain. May be rapid onset. Pain can be localized to any region of the abdomen. May have nausea and vomiting. No fever history. Mimics appendicitis	Focal tenderness in any abdominal quadrant, but usually RLQ, LLQ, or periumbilical. No peritoneal signs

(continued)

Table 5-1. Common Noncritical Diagnoses for Chief Complaint
of Abdominal Pain (*Continued*)

Noncritical Diagnosis	Typical History	Typical Physical Examination
Menstrual cramping	Lower abdominal or pelvic cramping pain. Associated with menstruation. No fever. No nausea and vomiting	May have lower abdominal or pelvic tenderness. Pelvic examination with blood in vault but no other abnormalities. Pregnancy test is mandatory to differentiate from ectopic pregnancy or miscarriage
Endometriosis	Cramping pelvic pain. Diverse symptoms. Associated with menstruation. May radiate to lower back or rectal area. May have dyspareunia or dysuria. No fever	Diffuse pelvic tenderness. Should have normal vital signs and no peritoneal signs. Pelvic examination can be normal or elicit pain
Normal pregnancy	All abdominal pain in pregnancy must be carefully considered. Round ligament pain is most common in the second trimester. It is sharp, pelvic pain that is more common on the right side. Duration is <1 min but may have multiple occurrences. Exercise or rapid movement may cause the pain. No nausea, vomiting, or diarrhea	No fever. No vaginal bleeding. No change in vaginal discharge. Often the pain is not reproducible with palpation. Pelvic examination should be normal. May be elicited with jumping up and down
Constipation	Diffuse abdominal pain and distention. Afebrile. Decreased stool output. Still passing gas. No vomiting. May be elderly or have history of opioid use or iron supplements	Diffuse fullness. No focal tenderness. Rectal examination may reveal fecal impaction. A diagnosis of exclusion

(*continued*)

Table 5-1. Common Noncritical Diagnoses for Chief Complaint
of Abdominal Pain (*Continued*)

Noncritical Diagnosis	Typical History	Typical Physical Examination
Inflammatory bowel disease	Cramping abdominal pain. Insidious onset. Diarrhea streaked with blood and/or mucous. May have weight loss if long duration. May have other autoimmune diseases	Diffuse or localized tenderness. May have fever. Rectal examination may show fissures. May be hemoccult positive
Irritable bowel syndrome	Clinical diagnosis based on chronic abdominal pain, bloating, alternating diarrhea and constipation. Diagnosis of exclusion. More common among patients with chronic headaches, fibromyalgia, and depression	No fever. Normal vitals. Diffuse tenderness. No blood in stool. No blood in vomit

cholangitis. Biliary colic pain should be limited in duration (<1-2 hours), related to eating, and not associated with fever. If an ultrasound is performed, gallstones may be visualized. CBC and CMP should be normal; elevated WBC count or liver enzymes should raise suspicion for infection or obstruction, respectively. Management of biliary colic includes pain control (ketorolac is particularly effective), nausea medication, diet modification (avoid high-fat foods), and referral to a surgeon for scheduled cholecystectomy. Equally important are clear patient instructions on the red flag symptoms of cholecystitis and cholangitis.

Gastroenteritis is very common, but it is also one of the most common misdiagnoses given for critical diagnoses such as appendicitis and cholecystitis. For this reason, the EM physician must remain vigilant. The diagnosis of gastroenteritis is clinical. To make the diagnosis, the patient must have both vomiting and diarrhea. Additionally, the patient will commonly have systemic features such as body aches, fever, or chills. It helps to have a history of sick contacts or for it to be gastroenteritis "season." The abdominal examination may have diffuse tenderness, but localizing tenderness is uncommon and warrants additional consideration of critical diagnoses. A CMP may show mild dehydration. A CBC may show an elevation of the WBC count. If a CT scan is performed, it is likely to be normal or show diffuse inflammation or mesenteric adenitis. Management includes hydration, symptom control, and repeat abdominal examination. The EM physician should discuss the risks and benefits of abdominal CT scan to help the patient understand why it may not be helpful in his or her case. A discussion of the red flags for immediate return is mandatory.

Chronic pancreatitis is most common in conjunction with chronic alcohol use, but may be due to recurrent stones, ductal abnormalities, or tumors. It presents similarly to acute pancreatitis, but is typically less severe. The patient will typically have epigastric tenderness and usually has a history of similar symptoms. Laboratory testing may reveal an elevated WBC count and mildly elevated lipase. Elevated liver enzymes and bilirubin should raise suspicion for choledocolithiasis. An abdominal CT typically shows inflammation and chronic degeneration of the pancreas, but may show pseudocysts or dilated pancreatic ducts. Chronic pancreatitis can usually be managed in the outpatient setting, but depending on the severity of symptoms may require hospitalization. Contrast this with acute pancreatitis, which almost always requires admission. Management includes hydration, symptom control, and clear liquid diet.

Ovarian cysts may present as unilateral pelvic pain. Cysts are most common during the childbearing years. Unless complications arise, they are generally benign. Pain typically manifests by compression of adjacent structures, rupture and hemorrhage, or ovarian torsion. The pain associated with compression is generally gradual in onset, whereas the pain from rupture or torsion tends to be severe and sudden in onset. The physical examination typically reveals unilateral tenderness in the pelvic region. An adnexal mass may be appreciated on pelvic examination. The CBC and CMP are usually unremarkable. A pregnancy test is mandatory. An abdominal CT will show ovarian cysts and can usually show hemorrhage, but it is poorly sensitive for torsion. A pelvic ultrasound is required if torsion is suspected. Management of an uncomplicated cyst consists of pain control and careful instructions regarding the red flags for torsion and hemorrhage.

Inflammatory bowel disease typically presents with crampy and diffuse abdominal pain that is gradual in onset. It is usually associated with diarrhea and is very commonly associated with blood and mucous in the stool. Fever, weight loss, and anemia may be present. The abdominal examination typically reveals diffuse tenderness. The rectal examination may reveal fistulas or fissures in advanced disease. CBC may reveal anemia or mildly elevated WBC count. CMP is typically unremarkable unless significant dehydration is present. Abdominal CT is usually indicated to assess for complications such as perforation, bowel obstruction, toxic megacolon, fistula formation, or abscess. Management is based on the presence of complications. If no significant complications are present and the diagnosis is presumed, GI consultation should be sought. The stable patient may follow closely with GI in the outpatient setting for confirmatory testing. Steroids or sulfasalazine may be started in consultation with GI.

TIPS TO REMEMBER

- A patient with abdominal pain and no red flags may not require any additional workup, but a discussion of the risks and benefits of possible testing is mandatory.
- A discussion of possible critical diagnoses with the patient is required.
- A patient with epigastric pain and risk factors for CAD should receive an EKG.
- A patient with a suspected diagnosis of gastritis/PUD should have a hemoccult test.
- Gastroenteritis is very common, but it is also a very common misdiagnosis. Be careful not to anchor and fail to consider critical diagnoses.
- On discharge, the EM physician should discuss the red flags for immediate return.

COMPREHENSION QUESTIONS

1. A 65-year-old male presents with epigastric pressure, shortness of breath, and diaphoresis for about 1 hour. He denies similar prior symptoms. The symptoms came on at rest. He has no other symptoms. He has a history of hypertension, diabetes, hyperlipidemia, and chronic alcoholism. He is tachycardic. The rest of his vital signs are normal. His physical examination reveals no abdominal tenderness, no signs of DVT, and is otherwise unremarkable. Which of the following is the most likely critical diagnosis?
    A. Acute pancreatitis
    B. ACS
    C. Chronic pancreatitis
    D. Pulmonary embolism
    E. Acute cholecystitis

2. A 24-year-old female with no past medical history presents with 1 day of vomiting and chills. She has not felt like eating anything today. She denies fever or body aches. She denies dysuria. She does reports that her child recently recovered from gastroenteritis. She has some pain in the lower portion of the abdomen. She reports the pain was present prior to the vomiting. Her temperature is 100.4. Her vital signs are otherwise normal. Her abdominal examination reveals tenderness in the suprapubic region and RLQ. Her pelvic examination is normal. Her urine pregnancy test is negative. Which of the following is the most likely diagnosis?
    A. Ovarian torsion
    B. Tubo-ovarian abscess
    C. Appendicitis
    D. Gastroenteritis
    E. Urinary tract infection

Answers

1. B. ACS is the most likely critical diagnosis in this patient due to epigastric pressure, associated dyspnea and diaphoresis, absence of abdominal tenderness, and presence of several CAD risk factors. The other diagnoses should be considered, but are less likely. An urgent EKG is mandatory.

2. C. The patient has RLQ tenderness, vomiting, fever, and anorexia. Her symptoms are most consistent with appendicitis. A diagnosis of gastroenteritis cannot be made without diarrhea. An EM physician should be careful not to be drawn to a diagnosis of gastroenteritis based only on sick contacts. Ovarian torsion would not typically have a fever. Tubo-ovarian abscess would likely have significant findings on pelvic examination or a history of STD. Urinary tract infection typically has a history of frequency, urgency, or painful urination.

SUGGESTED READINGS

Marx JA, Hockberger RS, Walls RM, eds. *Rosen's Emergency Medicine: Concepts and Clinical Practice.* 7th ed. Philadelphia: Mosby-Elsevier; 2010 [chapter 18] <http://www.mdconsult.com>.
Tintinalli JE, Kelen GD, Stapczynski JS, Ma OJ, Cline DM, eds. *Tintinalli's Emergency Medicine.* 7th ed. New York: McGraw-Hill; 2011 [chapters 74, 84] <http://www.accessmedicine.com>.

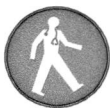

A 23-year-old Female With Dyspnea

Antonio Cummings, MD and Ted R. Clark, MD, MPP

CASE DESCRIPTION

Ms Cava is a 23-year-old female who presents to the emergency department with shortness of breath. She has had shortness of breath for about 6 hours. She states that the shortness of breath came on suddenly at rest. She states it is now worse with exertion and incompletely relieved with rest. She also reports some sharp left-sided chest pain. She denies extremity pain or swelling. She has had no similar prior pain. Past medical history is negative for PE, DVT, cancer, asthma, and heart disease. She takes only a birth control pill. She has had no prior surgeries. The patient denies smoking. She reports a recent 5-hour car trip.

Her vitals are temperature 37.1°C (98.8°F), blood pressure 129/76 mm Hg, pulse 108 beats/min, respiratory rate 22 breaths/min, and oxygen saturation of 93% on room air.

On examination, you note mildly increased respiratory effort, and clear lungs. Heart examination reveals tachycardia, but is otherwise normal. She has some mild tenderness to palpation of the left chest wall. Her left lower extremity is mildly swollen. Her extremities have normal perfusion and neurological function.

1. What is your differential diagnosis?

2. What are the red flags in Ms Cava's history and physical examination?

3. What are the important risk factors for the critical diagnoses you are considering for Ms Cava?

Answers

1. Table 6-1 provides a broad, but not exhaustive list of critical, emergent, and nonemergent diagnoses for the chief complaint of dyspnea.

2. Ms Cava has several red flags that raise suspicion for a critical diagnosis. Sudden-onset dyspnea with pleuritic chest pain raises concern for pulmonary embolism and pneumothorax. Her use of an oral contraceptive pill and recent long-distance travel raise additional concern for pulmonary embolism. Her vital signs show tachycardia, tachypnea, and oxygen saturations that are lower than we would expect in an otherwise healthy patient. These features raise concern for pulmonary embolism, pneumothorax, pericarditis, and pneumonia. Table 6-2 summarizes the classic history and physical red flags for the critical diagnoses in a patient with a chief complaint of dyspnea.

Table 6-1. Emergency Physician Differential Diagnosis for Dyspnea

Critical Diagnoses	Emergent Diagnoses	Nonemergent Diagnoses
Pulmonary	Pneumonia	Mild asthma
Pulmonary embolism	Asthma exacerbation	Mild pneumonia
Airway obstruction	Aspiration	Acute bronchitis
Tension pneumothorax	Pulmonary hypertension	Pleural effusion
Anaphylaxis	Pneumothorax	Chronic COPD
Noncardiogenic pulmonary edema	Acute exacerbation COPD	Stable CHF
	Pericarditis	Chronic restrictive lung disease
Acute coronary syndrome	Anxiety attack	
Congestive heart failure (CHF)	Anemia	
Cardiac tamponade		

3. Table 6-3 summarizes common risk factors and decision rules for selected critical diagnoses in a patient with a chief complaint of dyspnea.

CASE REVIEW

Ms Cava has dyspnea and some red flags for pulmonary embolism. Prior to initiating additional workup, we should make sure the patient has a patent airway, and is oxygenating appropriately. She should be hooked up to continuous pulse oximetry, blood pressure monitoring, and a cardiac monitor. A large-bore peripheral IV should be inserted and blood sent for CBC, BMP, and PT/PTT. An EKG should be ordered, as well as a pregnancy test. Her Wells PE score is 4.5 (based on heart rate and lack of a better explanation of her symptoms), which places her in the moderate pretest probability category. Additionally, she is pulmonary embolism rule-out criteria (PERC) positive due to her heart rate, oxygen saturations, and estrogen use. Due to her moderate pretest probability, she should receive a CT scan of the chest with IV contrast. Ms Cava's CT scan is positive for a segmental PE in the left lung. Bedside echo reveals normal heart function, and her EKG reveals sinus tachycardia.

After the diagnosis of PE is established, the patient should be admitted to a telemetry bed and started on heparin. Since Ms Cava shows no signs of hemodynamic compromise or instability, thrombolytics and thrombectomy are not indicated.

Table 6-2. Critical Diagnoses and Red Flags for Dyspnea

Critical Diagnosis	History Red Flags	Physical Red Flags
Pulmonary embolism	Sudden onset, recent long-distance travel, surgery, or recent immobilization, active malignancy, estrogen use, history of previous DVT or PE, hypercoagulability	Tachycardia, low-grade fever, tachypnea, decreased oxygen saturation
Airway obstruction	Occurrence while eating, no previous lung disease, history of swallowing difficulties	Tachypnea, grabbing at the throat, difficulty bagging patient
Tension pneumothorax	History of COPD or pneumothorax, recent thoracic procedure, sudden onset, pleuritic chest pain	Increased JVD, diminished breath sounds on 1 side of the chest, hypotension
Anaphylaxis	Abrupt onset, previous history of allergic reaction, new medication or IV infusion	Oral swelling, stridor, wheezing, hives
Noncardiogenic edema	Recent dependence on IV fluids, new medication	Crackles on examination, exertional dyspnea, orthopnea
Acute coronary syndrome	"Crushing" or pressure in nature, substernal or left chest in location, onset with exertion, radiation to arm, shoulder, or jaw. CAD risk factors	Diaphoresis, new murmur, new pulmonary rales
Acute pulmonary edema (CHF)	History of MI, new-onset chest pain, hx of PE, dietary or medication noncompliance	JVD, peripheral edema, S3 or S4, now cardiac dysrhythmia
Cardiac tamponade	Trauma to the chest, hx of lung cancer or pericarditis, hx of uremia, exertional dyspnea	Hypotension, distant heart sounds, distended neck veins

Table 6-3. Risk Factors and Decision Rules for a Chief Complaint of Dyspnea

Critical Diagnosis	Risk Factors	Decision Rules
Pulmonary embolism	Age >50, exogenous estrogen, cancer, recent hospitalization, recent surgery (especially lower extremity orthopedic), recent long-distance travel, recent extremity trauma, indwelling venous catheter (upper or lower extremity), immobility, current DVT, and prior PE or DVT	**PERC rule for PE** **Wells criteria for PE**
Severe asthma/COPD	Prior intubation, prior ICU admission, currently on steroids, no relief with nebulizers	
CHF	History of myocardial infarction, coronary artery disease, or ischemic or nonischemia cardiomyopathy. Poorly controlled hypertension. Prior CHF admissions	**CHF 30-day and 1-year mortality rules**

DYSPNEA

Diagnostic Reasoning

The differential diagnosis for a chief complaint of dyspnea is broad and has several critical diagnoses. In addition, there is significant overlap with the differential diagnosis for chest pain. Cardiopulmonary causes make up the vast majority of critical and emergent diagnoses for the chief complaint of dyspnea. Importantly, many emergent diagnoses can become critical diagnoses if they present in their most severe form. Table 6-1, although fairly comprehensive, does not include dyspnea from secondary sources such as overdose, acidosis, or neuromuscular dysfunction (such as Guillain-Barré syndrome). As with most ED presentations, the EM physician will start with the ABCs, the safety net, and an exploration of red flags in the vital signs, the history, and the physical examination.

In a patient with dyspnea, lung auscultation is very important. Rapid intervention in life-threatening situations is often based only on physical examination. An effective EM physician should be able to distinguish acute exacerbations of COPD and CHF with auscultation by differentiating between wheezes and fine crackles (rales). Also, it is important to recognize the unilateral diminished breath sounds that accompany pneumothorax and the focal changes that occur with consolidative pneumonia. Waiting for further testing prior to initiating treatment or treating the patient inappropriately can result in significant morbidity and mortality.

In addition to a history and physical examination focusing on red flags, risk factors are important both in assessing the possibility of a given diagnosis and in considering the potential severity of a presentation. Ms Cava has the risk factors of oral contraceptive pill use and recent long-distance travel that raise suspicion for pulmonary embolism. Importantly, in patients with acute exacerbations of chronic diseases such as CHF and COPD, risk factors can help the EM physician determine the degree of management required. For instance, a patient who presents with a COPD exacerbation and is already on steroids, albuterol, and antibiotics at home will be much more likely to require admission.

In addition to using risk factors to guide the workup, several useful *clinical decision rules* can be applied to a patient with a chief complaint of dyspnea. Pulmonary embolism is a notoriously difficult diagnosis that has been studied extensively in the ED. The 2 most commonly applied *clinical decision rules* for pulmonary embolism are the *Wells criteria for pulmonary embolism* and the *PERC*.

Wells criteria for pulmonary embolism are used to determine the *pretest probability* of a PE. Table 6-4 demonstrates the scored values of the Wells criteria. The pretest probability of PE is high (78.4%) if the patient has >6 points, moderate (27.8%) if the patient has 2 to 6 points, and low (3.4%) if the patient has <2 points. A pretest probability is a clinician's determination of the likelihood of a given diagnosis being present prior to obtaining the results of diagnostic testing. The clinician bases the pretest probability on history, physical examination, and risk factors. The pretest probability can be calculated based on decision rules or *clinical gestalt*.

Table 6-4. Wells Criteria for PE

Factor	Points
Suspected DVT	3
Alternative diagnosis less likely than PE	33
Heart rate >100 beats/min	1.5
Prior venous thromboembolism	1.5
Immobilization within the prior 4 weeks	11.5
Active malignancy	1
Hemoptysis	1
Total points	

Table 6-5. Pulmonary Embolism Rule-out Criteria

Age <50
Heart rate <100
SaO_2 >94% on room air
No history of prior DVT or PE
No recent surgery or trauma
No hemoptysis
No exogenous estrogen
Yes to all = PERC negative

Once the EM physician has determined a preprobability of PE, difficult decisions must be made regarding the extent of the diagnostic workup. The PERC clinical decision rule can be applied to patients with a low pretest probability. The criteria are listed in Table 6-5. A patient must meet all 8 criteria to be deemed *PERC negative.*

If a patient is *PERC negative,* the risk of a PE is believed to be less than the risk of continued testing. Importantly, PERC can only be applied to patients with low pretest probability. Also, just because a patient is PERC positive does not necessarily mean there is a need for additional testing for PE. If the EM physician has concern for PE and neither Wells nor PERC provide reassuring results, diagnostic testing is necessary. The diagnostic workup and management for pulmonary embolism as well as for other critical diagnoses for dyspnea are discussed below.

Diagnostic Workup and Management

As with a presentation of chest pain, most patients who present with dyspnea should be placed on a cardiac monitor and pulse oximetry. Any immediate threats to life noted in the ABCs should be addressed. For example, a patient with dyspnea, respiratory distress, absence of left-sided breath sounds, and hypotension should receive immediate needle decompression. Similarly, if a patient presents with dyspnea, hypoxia, hypertension, and rales on pulmonary examination, nitroglycerin and BiPAP or intubation should be provided.

Most patients with a chief complaint of dyspnea will receive a laboratory workup including CBC, BMP, EKG, and chest x-ray. If ACS or CHF is suspected, a BNP and cardiac enzymes should be added. If early respiratory distress is suspected, a venous or arterial blood gas can aid in decision making. If significant distress is present, intubation or adjuncts such as BiPAP should be considered. If pneumonia is suspected, blood cultures should also be added. Additional supportive care may include fluid resuscitation, oxygen, and pain control. A chest CT can be considered if the workup does not reveal a cause for the patient's symptoms. A chest CT is more sensitive for pneumonia, pneumothorax, and pleural effusion. Ultrasound (bedside or formal) can also be used for the detection of pericardial effusion and pneumothorax.

As discussed above, the decision to workup a patient for PE is based on clinical decision rules. More specifically, if the EM physician determines that the patient has moderate or high pretest probability and the application of the PERC rule does not support exclusion of PE, then additional diagnostic testing is needed. There are 4 important tests to consider: D-dimer, chest CT with IV contrast, ventilation–perfusion (V/Q) scan, and lower extremity venous Doppler study for DVT.

The D-dimer is a blood test that is most commonly used as a screening test for PE. The D-dimer has a high sensitivity (93%-95%) but a low specificity (50%). If the pretest probability is low, then a negative D-dimer has a sensitivity of 99%. The poor specificity of the D-dimer is due to the fact that many inflammatory and infectious processes can elevate the D-dimer, including malignancy, trauma, pregnancy, recent surgery, pneumonia, viral infection, and advanced age. Unfortunately, due to its poor specificity, false-positive D-dimer tests frequently result in additional testing that can potentially cause harm. Thus, it is important to avoid the temptation to "roll the dice" and order a D-dimer on a patient who is considered *very low risk*.

Chest CT with IV contrast is the test of choice for detection of a PE. Although not perfectly sensitive, the chest CT is currently the most available and accepted method for evaluating for PE. The risks of the test include radiation exposure and IV contrast exposure. The risk of allergic reaction, kidney damage, and slightly increased long-term cancer risk should be explained to the patient. The chest CT should be ordered in patients with a moderate or high pretest probability for PE.

The V/Q scan is most commonly used as a backup to chest CT in patients with a contrast allergy or acute kidney injury. The sensitivity is similar; however, the results can be nondiagnostic if underlying lung disease such as COPD or pneumonia exists. The test is also much more technically difficult to read. The patient is still subjected to the risk of radiation exposure, although it is lower than CT.

The lower extremity Doppler is used to assess for the presence of DVT. It is estimated that 90% of PEs come from lower extremity DVTs. For this reason, lower extremity Doppler studies may be used as an adjunct in patients who cannot receive CT or V/Q for various reasons. The absence of a DVT, unfortunately, does not rule out PE, but a positive DVT scan in a patient with moderate or high pretest probability is an indication for PE treatment.

Although careful consideration and workup of PE is a large component of the overall workup for the patient with a chief complaint of dyspnea, workup for other critical and emergent diagnoses must be carefully considered. ACS and several other cardiac diagnoses are discussed in the preceding cases; however, a brief discussion of the diagnostic workup and management of other diagnoses is warranted.

Airway obstruction should be considered in young children, elderly patients, intoxicated patients, patients who began having dyspnea while eating, patients with neck masses, patient with oropharyngeal swelling, and patients with a transport dysphagia (such as a stroke victim). Management depends on the degree of the obstruction. If the patient has evidence of obstruction such as stridor but is otherwise oxygenating and ventilating well, the patient should be moved to a more controlled environment such as the operating room prior to attempts to relieve the obstruction. It is also prudent to involve ENT in the event that a surgical airway is needed. If the patient has a complete obstruction, hypoxia, or is unconscious, then the obstruction must be addressed immediately. Infants with airway obstruction should receive back blows and, if time allows, direct observation with a laryngoscope or fiber-optic scope and forceps removal. If the obstruction cannot be relieved, then a needle cricothyrotomy should be performed in children up to age 8. The Heimlich maneuver may be attempted in conscious adults. If unsuccessful, direct visualization and removal should be performed. If the obstruction cannot be relieved, then cricothyrotomy is indicated. The "blind sweep" should be avoided as it may result in a worsening of the obstruction.

Anaphylaxis should be considered in a patient with acute dyspnea, especially if associated with facial swelling, rash, hives, or recent exposure to common allergens (bee stings, peanuts, etc). In these cases, it is essential to deliver IM epinephrine (0.3 mg IM at a 1:1000 concentration) to the patient to counteract the vasogenic edema and cardiovascular collapse that can accompany anaphylaxis. An IV epinephrine drip may be needed to prevent rebound. Diphenhydramine (H_1 blocker), an H_2 blocker, and IM steroids should also be given to avoid a late reaction. True anaphylaxis should be admitted to a monitored bed for further evaluation.

Acute CHF can be rapidly fatal if not diagnosed and treated appropriately. CHF should be suspected in any patient with SOB, rales on pulmonary auscultation, a chest x-ray showing pulmonary edema, a history of recent MI, or a patient with increasing peripheral edema. Mainstays of treatment are to lower myocardial oxygen demand, decrease preload, and to ensure oxygenation. This can be done with either BiPAP or intubation, followed by preload reduction with nitroglycerin and afterload reduction with an ACE inhibitor. After acute stabilization loop diuretics such as furosemide can help eliminate excess fluid. In a patient with renal failure and fluid overload, emergent dialysis is indicated. Severe CHF exacerbations should be admitted to the ICU with a cardiology consult.

Tension pneumothorax can be immediately life threatening. It occurs most commonly in the setting of trauma, but it can occur as a result of a spontaneous pneumothorax or after central line placement. This is a clinical diagnosis and the standard teaching is that it should not be discovered on a chest x-ray because it should have been discovered and corrected without delay. While the classic case of diminished breath sounds, hypotension, jugular distention, and tracheal deviation *away* from the affected lung may be present, the presentation of tension pneumothorax seldom has *all* classic signs. Once identified, the EM physician should perform needle decompression with a 16- or 18-gauge needle in the second intercostal space at the midclavicular line. Proper placement will result in a "woosh" of air and temporary decompression of the tension pneumothorax. The procedure may need to be repeated. A tube thoracostomy should be quickly placed on the affected side for definitive decompression. The patient should be admitted for further monitoring.

The management of a diagnosed PE is dependent on the degree of clot burden and its physiological effect on the patient. If a PE is discovered and the patient is otherwise stable, anticoagulation with heparin is indicated. If the patient is significantly hypoxic (oxygen saturations <90%), hypotensive, or there is evidence of right heart strain on EKG or cardiac ultrasound, systemic thrombolytics, intra-arterial thrombolytics, or thrombectomy should be considered. In general, if a patient is hypotensive and has a large saddle embolus, then open thrombectomy is indicated and a cardiothoracic surgeon should be consulted. The indications for intra-arterial thrombolytics or intra-arterial thrombectomy are still debated, but, in general, these therapies are indicated for patients with PE and right heart strain on cardiac ultrasound. Systemic thrombolytics are typically used in patients with a PE and extensive right heart strain who may be too unstable for or are otherwise not amenable to open or intra-arterial techniques.

TIPS TO REMEMBER

- The D-dimer is only appropriate for patients with whom there is a low pretest probability but clinical suspicion.
- Clinical decision rules will help you remember risk factors and avoid unnecessary and potentially harmful testing.
- In cases of cardiopulmonary collapse, right ventricular strain, or saddle embolism thrombolytics or thrombectomy should be considered.
- Pregnant patients require careful consideration in the workup for PE because the D-dimer is more likely to be falsely positive and radiation exposure to the fetus should be avoided if possible.

COMPREHENSION QUESTIONS

1. A 25-year-old male presents with dyspnea and pleuritic chest pain. He recently had a cast on his right leg and now has a swollen, tender calf. Based on Wells criteria for PE, what is his pretest probability of having a PE?

    A. <2% (very low)
    B. 3.4% (low)
    C. 27.8% (moderate)
    D. 78.4% (high)

2. The next best diagnostic step for the patient in question 1 is which of the following?
- A. A D-dimer
- B. A chest CT with IV contrast
- C. A chest x-ray
- D. A venous Doppler study of the right leg

3. What conditions can lead to a falsely elevated D-dimer?
- A. Infection
- B. Pregnancy
- C. Recent surgery (<2 weeks)
- D. All of the above

4. The patient in question 1 is found to have a large saddle embolus and subsequently develops hypoxia, hypotension, and evidence of right ventricle strain on bedside ultrasound. How should the patient be managed?
- A. Oxygen, IV fluids, heparin, and admission to the ICU
- B. Oxygen, IV fluids, and systemic thrombolytics
- C. Oxygen, IV fluids, and cardiothoracic surgery consultation for possible thrombectomy or systemic thrombolytics
- D. Oxygen, IV fluids, heparin, admission to ICU, and intra-arterial thrombolytics within 12 hours

Answers

1. D. The patient has a Wells score of 9 based on clinical suspicion of DVT (3), no alternative diagnosis (3), tachycardia (1.5), and recent immobilization (1.5). Thus, he has a high (78.4%) pretest probability.

2. B. Since the patient has a high pretest probability for PE based on the Wells score, the patient should receive a chest CT with IV contrast or a V/Q scan. The D-dimer is not sufficiently sensitive to rule out PE in a patient with moderate or high pretest probability. A chest x-ray can support alternative diagnoses, but it cannot assess for PE. A venous Doppler can confirm DVT, but assessment for PE is a diagnostic priority in this patient.

3. D. All of the above can cause an elevation of the D-dimer, as can active malignancy, liver disease, or trauma.

4. C. This patient has signs of significant hemodynamic compromise. This clot needs to be extracted either mechanically or using TPA. If it is available immediately, open thrombectomy is preferred for a large central embolus; otherwise, thrombolytics are indicated. Intra-arterial thrombolytics are a good option, but only if immediately available.

SUGGESTED READINGS

Marx JA, Hockberger RS, Walls RM, eds. *Rosen's Emergency Medicine: Concepts and Clinical Practice*. 7th ed. Philadelphia: Mosby-Elsevier; 2010 [chapter 17] <http://www.mdconsult.com>.
Tintinalli JE, Kelen GD, Stapczynski JS, Ma OJ, Cline DM, eds. *Tintinalli's Emergency Medicine*. 7th ed. New York: McGraw-Hill; 2011 [chapter 60] <http://www.accessmedicine.com>.

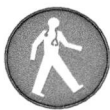

A 72-year-old Male With Dyspnea

James R. Waymack, MD

CASE DESCRIPTION

Mr Blue is a 72-year-old male with a history of chronic obstructive pulmonary disease (COPD) who presents to your emergency department with a chief complaint of increasing shortness of breath over the past 2 days. He has a chronic daily cough productive of white sputum, which has recently developed a yellow tinge. He has not had fever or chills. He has smoked 1 pack per day of cigarettes for the past 50 years. He denies chest pain.

His vitals are temperature 37.1°C (98.8°F), blood pressure 150/76 mm Hg, pulse 110 beats/min, respiratory rate 24 breaths/min, and oxygen saturation of 88% on room air.

On examination, you note moderately increased respiratory effort, equal breath sounds, and tight diffuse wheezes. Heart examination reveals tachycardia, but is otherwise normal. His extremities have no swelling or tenderness. His extremities have normal perfusion and neurological function.

He was last admitted to the hospital 3 months ago for a similar exacerbation. During the previous admission he received a course of corticosteroids and antibiotics. He has required noninvasive positive pressure ventilation (NIPPV) in the past but has never been mechanically ventilated. He denies ever having chest tube thoracostomy performed.

1. What are the main objectives when treating a patient with a COPD exacerbation?

2. What should be included in the differential diagnosis of a patient presenting with a possible COPD exacerbation?

3. What diagnostic studies are indicated in a patient with a possible COPD exacerbation?

4. When are antibiotics indicated in a patient with a possible COPD exacerbation?

5. When does a patient require NIPPV or intubation and mechanical ventilation for a possible COPD exacerbation?

Answers

1. The main objectives regarding treatment of a COPD exacerbation are improving oxygenation, decreasing bronchospasm, and treating underlying causes or concomitant disease processes.

2. The differential diagnosis in a patient with a possible COPD exacerbation includes congestive heart failure, pulmonary embolism, acute coronary syndrome, pneumothorax, and pneumonia. A more complete differential diagnosis is listed in Table 6-1.

3. Diagnostic studies performed in the ED for a patient with a possible COPD exacerbation include continuous pulse oximtery, basic laboratory studies, arterial blood gas, chest radiography, electrocardiogram, and possibly others depending on the patient's presentation.

4. Antibiotics should be administered if there is evidence of infection, such as a change in volume of sputum or increased purulence of sputum.

5. If a patient has respiratory distress or refractory hypoxia on supplemental oxygen, a trial of NIPPV can be undertaken. If NIPPV is contraindicated, if the patient has refractory hypoxia or respiratory acidosis after a trial of NIPPV, or if the patient goes into respiratory failure, then endotracheal intubation and mechanical ventilation are indicated.

CASE REVIEW

Mr Blue has a presentation most consistent with a COPD exacerbation. Although the EM physician cannot immediately exclude other contributing factors to Mr Blue's dyspnea, it is clear that there is at least a significant component that can be attributed to COPD. Thus, after the EM physician establishes the safety net, COPD therapy should be started immediately. The EM physician should give Mr Blue oxygen, albuterol and ipratropium nebulizer therapy, and corticosteroids immediately. Mr Blue may also benefit from NIPPV, but if he does not respond quickly, or further deteriorates, he may require endotracheal intubation and mechanical ventilation. In addition to treating COPD, the EM physician should consider contributing diagnoses. A chest x-ray is indicated to assess for pneumonia, CHF, or pneumothorax. A CT is not immediately indicated, but should be considered if evidence of PE is found on further examination. An EKG is indicated because a cardiac event can both precipitate and be precipitated by respiratory insufficiency. A CBC and CMP are also reasonable to assess for anemia, evidence of infection, or metabolic abnormalities.

COPD

Diagnostic Reasoning

A COPD exacerbation is usually triggered by infection, a respiratory irritant, hypoxia, or cold weather. These questions are key components of the history. If the patient reports a fever, increased production of mucus, or increased purulence of mucous, then viral or bacterial infection may be a possibility. It is also important to recognize in the history the severity of the patient's illness and prior exacerbations. Is the patient on supplemental oxygen or chronic steroids at home? When was the last exacerbation and was the patient treated with antibiotics or corticosteroids? Has the patient ever been hospitalized or required NIPPV or mechanical ventilation? Obtaining this information will allow you to anticipate the clinical course and possible disposition of the patient early during the ED stay. Other components in the history can contribute to the differential diagnosis of dyspnea in the ED patient. It is helpful to elicit a history of coronary artery disease or congestive heart failure if present. Has the patient been having chest pain or experiencing increasing peripheral edema, orthopnea, or paroxsysmal nocturnal dyspnea? If there is a history of or risk factors for thromboembolic disease or a differing presentation from the patient's usual COPD exacerbation, then investigations for pulmonary embolism may also be warranted.

A complete physical examination should be performed on every ED patient, but in regards to a COPD exacerbation attention should be focused on respiratory effort, lung auscultation, and systemic signs of hypoxia. The patient will often be sitting upright in the tripod position in an attempt to improve ventilation or pursing his or her lips to create positive airway pressure. During inspection of the patient attention should be focused on use of accessory muscles for respiration, retractions, and respiratory fatigue. Lung auscultation will often demonstrate diffuse wheezing; however, if bronchospasm is severe, the lung fields may be markedly diminished or even quiet. Attention should also be paid toward the face and extremities for evidence of cyanosis or clubbing.

Routine laboratory studies include a complete blood cell count to assess for leukocytosis and anemia, basic chemistries to evaluate electrolytes, renal function, and blood glucose. These are indicated in every critically ill ED patient. Continuous pulse oximetry will identify hypoxemia, but an arterial blood gas will be needed to evaluate hypercapnia and acid–base disturbances. Cardiac markers and B-type natriuretic peptide may also be obtained to help differentiate between CHF and COPD. While less frequently used today, theophylline levels should be checked if the patient is taking this medication.

A chest x-ray is always indicated in a patient with COPD to evaluate for not only pneumonia but also the possibility of pneumothorax. Patients with COPD form blebs in their lung parenchyma as the disease progresses and these blebs have the propensity to rupture causing pneumothorax. Signs of congestive heart failure may be present on the radiograph. If there is a high suspicion for pulmonary embolism or there is a pneumothorax present, computed tomography of the chest is indicated to assess for thromboembolic disease or blebs, respectively.

An electrocardiogram is also a critical action when evaluating every patient who presents to the ED with dyspnea. The common ECG finding related to chronic COPD is *p pulmonale*, where there are large peaked p waves. This study may also help identify other causes of dyspnea in your differential such as cardiac ischemia, acute myocardial infarction, cor pulmonale, or arrhythmias such as multifocal atrial tachycardia.

Fundamentals of Disease

The underlying cause of dyspnea in a patient experiencing a COPD exacerbation is a release of inflammatory mediators. There is increasing bronchoconstriction, hypersecretion of mucus, and pulmonary vasoconstriction. These processes lead to airway narrowing, increasing V/Q mismatch, and hypoxemia. There is an increased work of breathing due to airway resistance and lung hyperinflation. As the patient works to breathe harder, there is an increase in oxygen demand, which generates more carbon dioxide and worsening hypercapnia. Unlike asthma though, the primary cause of respiratory distress is V/Q mismatch and not airway obstruction.

Diagnostic Workup and Management

When encountering any patient in the ED, it is important to implement the safety net, including intravenous access, supplemental oxygen as needed, continuous pulse oximetry, and cardiac monitoring. The process of improving oxygenation in the patient with a COPD exacerbation is continuously reassessed throughout the patient's stay and may be altered depending on response to therapy, diagnostic testing, or a decline in respiratory status. If the patient has oxygen saturations less than 90%, supplemental nasal cannula oxygen should be started. If the patient is hypoxic on home oxygen, it should be increased to a maximum of 6 L/min. If the patient is persistently hypoxic, a non-rebreather mask can be applied at 15 L/min. If the patient continues to be hypoxic or there is concern for hypercapnia, an arterial blood gas should be obtained to assess for hypoxemia and respiratory acidosis. These values can often be compared with previous results to see if the patient has deviated from baseline. Patients with COPD often have chronic hypercapnia and hypoxemia. Further interventions include NIPPV, if not contraindicated, and mechanical ventilation, if necessary. Indications for mechanical ventilation include respiratory fatigue (paradoxical breathing, accessory muscle use, or respiratory rate >35), severe hypoxemia, altered mental status, failure of noninvasive ventilation, respiratory arrest, or cardiovascular instability.

Pharmacotherapy for a COPD exacerbation includes the short-acting inhaled β_2 agonists and anticholinergics. Depending on the severity of the exacerbation single treatments may be considered or the patient may be placed on continuous therapy. Corticosteroids should be administered to decrease airway inflammation. Oral and parenteral steroids have been shown to have equal efficacy; route of administration should be based on the patient's ability to take oral medications. If the patient is able to tolerate oral medication, 60 mg of prednisone is given. The intravenous alternative is 125 mg of methylprednisolone. Corticosteroid therapy should be continued for 7 to 10 days. Antibiotics should be administered if there is suspicion that infection may have been the precipitating factor of the exacerbation; infection is suggested by an increased amount or change in purulence of sputum. Antibiotic coverage should be directed toward the most common pathogens, including *Streptococcus pneumoniae, Haemophilus influenza, Moraxella catarrhalis,* and *Pseudomonas aeruginosa.* Patients with recent hospitalization or presentation from an extended care facility require coverage for health care–associated pneumonia.

Some patients who have quick improvement of their symptoms may be discharged home with close outpatient follow-up, continued bronchodilator use, and a short course of corticosteroids and antibiotics if indicated. Many patients with an acute COPD exacerbation will require hospitalization for failure to improve, increasing oxygen requirements, need for closer monitoring, or assisted ventilations. Patients requiring mechanical ventilation or closer monitoring will need ICU admission.

Special Considerations

- Historically there has been concern about reducing a COPD patient's respiratory drive by administering supplemental oxygen. However, the patient should not be allowed to have persistent hypoxemia and oxygen should be given to keep oxygen saturations close to 90%. A Venturi mask will allow more precise oxygen administration than a nasal cannula.
- Contraindications to NIPPV include altered mental status, high aspiration risk, inability to maintain an airway, facial trauma, respiratory arrest, or cardiovascular instability.

TIPS TO REMEMBER

- If there is minimal improvement in hypoxemia after starting supplemental oxygen, other diagnoses should be considered including pulmonary embolism or pneumothorax.
- Smoking cessation counseling should be performed with every patient.
- Do not fail to consider disease processes such as pulmonary embolism, pneumothorax, heart failure, or acute coronary syndrome in the dyspneic patient.
- The mainstays of treatment for COPD exacerbations include correction of hypoxemia, the use of a bronchodilator, decreasing airway inflammation, and antibiotic therapy if indicated.
- Patients should be continuously reevaluated to determine if treatment is working or if further intervention or admission is needed.

COMPREHENSION QUESTIONS

1. Common bacteria implicated in acute exacerbations of COPD include *Staphylococcus aureus*, *S. pneumoniae*, and *M. catarrhalis*. Which other organism should be considered in this patient population?
   A. *P. aeruginosa*
   B. *Corynebacterium diphtheriae*
   C. *Klebsiella pneumoniae*
   D. *Mycobacterium tuberculosis*

2. Which intervention has been proven to decrease mortality in patients with COPD?
   A. Supplemental oxygen
   B. Corticosteroids
   C. Antibiotics
   D. Inhaled β-adrenergic agonists

3. A 59-year-old male with a previous history of COPD and exacerbations requiring hospitalization presents with complaints of acute shortness of breath and cough productive of yellow sputum. He has been given 125 mg of methylprednisolone and 3 albuterol nebulizers with minimal improvement in his symptoms. Which of the following interventions may be helpful in preventing endotracheal intubation?
   A. IV antibiotic therapy
   B. Repeat corticosteroid dosing
   C. NIPPV
   D. Heliox

Answers

1. A. *Pseudomonas* is often found as a colonizing organism and may contribute to an acute decline in a patient with COPD. Antibiotics that would provide appropriate coverage include levofloxacin, ceftazidime, cefepime, or piperacillin–tazobactam.

2. A. Of the choices listed supplemental oxygen is the only intervention that has been shown to improve mortality.

3. C. NIPPV may improve oxygenation and decrease the work of breathing. Arterial blood gas measurements should be performed to monitor for worsening of hypercarbia while on NIPPV. If the patient does not improve on NIPPV or it is contraindicated, intubation may be required.

SUGGESTED READING

Tintinalli JE, Kelen GD, Stapczynski JS, Ma OJ, Cline DM, eds. *Tintinalli's Emergency Medicine*. 7th ed. New York: McGraw-Hill Education; 2011 [chapter 73] <http://www.accessmedicine.com>.

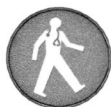

A 64-year-old Female With Vertigo

Richard Jeisy, MD and Ted R. Clark, MD, MPP

CASE DESCRIPTION

Ms Tripp is a 64-year-old female who presents to the emergency department with her husband. She complains of dizziness. On further questioning she states this is a sensation like the room is spinning and she is off-balance when she tries to walk. The dizziness was present on waking, which was 3 hours prior to arrival. She feels nauseated and has some double vision, but has not vomited. Her symptoms are constant and are not changed by movement or rest. She had similar symptoms lasting about 30 minutes last week, but denies other previous occurrences. She denies headache, hearing loss, tinnitus, light-headedness, fevers, or chills.

The patient's past medical history includes hypertension, hyperlipidemia, CAD requiring 2 stents, osteoarthritis, and mild depression. She has had a hysterectomy. She denies alcohol or drug use, and quit smoking 8 years ago. Family history includes hypertension in her mother and an MI in her father at age 72.

Physical examination shows a pulse of 77 bpm, blood pressure of 134/85 mm Hg, respiratory rate of 12, pulse oximetry of 97%, and temperature of 37.3°C. The patient is a female appearing her stated age who looks uncomfortable, but is in no acute distress. HEENT examination shows no nystagmus or tympanic membrane abnormalities. Cardiovascular examination is significant for a left-sided carotid bruit. Respiratory examination and abdominal examination are all unremarkable. Neurological examination finds intact cranial nerves, sensation, motor function, and no pronator drift. On finger-to-nose testing, the patient is able to touch the examiner's finger with difficulty. She is alert and oriented to person, place, and time.

Basic testing shows a finger-stick glucose of 103. CBC, CMP, and EKG are not significant. Orthostatic vital signs are normal.

1. What is the differential diagnosis?

2. What is the most likely diagnosis and what findings support this?

3. What other physical examination elements should be performed? What findings would be concerning?

4. What other tests and imaging are indicated?

5. What are the next steps in the management of this patient?

Answers

1. The differential diagnosis of vertigo is broad and can be best thought of in terms of critical, emergent, and nonemergent diagnoses (Table 8-1). In addition, it is

Table 8-1. Emergency Physician Differential Diagnosis for Vertigo

Critical Diagnoses	Emergent Diagnoses	Nonemergent Diagnoses
Vertebrobasilar syndrome (VBS)	Infection: labyrinthitis, vestibular neuronitis, Ramsay Hunt syndrome, neurosyphilis	Benign positional vertigo (BPV)
Intracerebral or cerebellar hemorrhage	Multiple sclerosis	Ménière disease
Posterior circulation stroke	Epilepsy	Movement disorders: Parkinson, Huntington
Neoplasm	Hematologic: anemia, hyperviscosity syndrome	Complex migraines
	Toxicologic: aminoglycoside toxicity, alcohol, antiepileptic toxicity	

common to consider the differential diagnosis in terms of central and peripheral vertigo.

2. The most likely diagnosis for this patient falls into the category of central vertigo. In general, causes of central vertigo are more concerning than peripheral vertigo. When symptoms are consistent with central vertigo, the differential diagnosis includes the critical and emergent diagnoses of vertebrobasilar syndrome (VBS), cerebellar hemorrhage or infarct, multiple sclerosis, and neoplasm. This patient's history of hypertension, CAD, age, diplopia, and cerebellar signs on the examination point toward VBS, cerebellar infarct or hemorrhage, or cerebellar tumor. The finding of a carotid bruit causes concern for cerebrovascular disease and raises further concern for VBS.

3. This patient should also have gait, tandem gait, Romberg, and visual acuity tested. Concerning findings would include ataxia, inability to perform tandem gait, or an abnormal Romberg test. A Dix-Hallpike test can be helpful in confirming a diagnosis of BPV, but should be avoided if a central cause is suspected.

4. If clinical suspicion exists for a central cause of vertigo, CT or MRA with angiogram should be strongly considered. Indications and contraindications for this testing will be discussed further.

5. If a central cause is suspected, the patient may ultimately require hospitalization and neurology consultation. If a peripheral cause is suspected, symptomatic treatment of vertigo with meclizine or benzodiazepines is warranted. Ondansetron is typically used for the treatment of associated nausea.

CASE REVIEW

Ms Tripp's central vertigo requires admission and expert consultation. All such patients need advanced neuroimaging including MRI and MRA of the neck. Depending on your specific practice environment, this may be done prior to admission in the emergency department, or after admission. Neurology or neurosurgery needs to evaluate the patient for management recommendations as well as establishment of ongoing follow-up. The question of antiplatelet therapy is one that will be addressed by these consultants.

VERTIGO WITH RED FLAGS

Diagnostic Reasoning

The approach to vertigo, as with all complaints in emergency medicine, is ultimately directed toward deciding if a patient has a critical or emergent diagnosis. The chief complaint of vertigo adds a layer of uncertainty to this question because very few patients use the term "vertigo." Most will present with a complaint of "dizziness." Therefore, the first step in diagnosis is to elicit what specific symptoms the patient is having. Light-headedness, which falls into the category of near-syncope, involves a different workup than true vertigo. Ask the patient to describe in detail the first time he or she had this feeling, and use the answer to direct your further history toward syncope or vertigo. A patient with true vertigo will often describe the "room spinning" or feeling "off-balance."

If the patient does have true vertigo, the next step is to classify the vertigo as either central or peripheral. Central vertigo is much more likely to be a critical or emergent diagnosis. The temporal pattern and severity can provide diagnostic clues (Table 8-2). Central vertigo is most commonly characterized by a

Table 8-2. Characteristics of Central and Peripheral Vertigo

Characteristic	Central Vertigo	Peripheral Vertigo
Onset	Gradual, insidious	Sudden
Duration	Constant	Intermittent
Severity	Vague, less intense	"Violent"
Aggravating factors	Variable	Movement
Associated symptoms	Variable, usually nystagmus	Nausea, vomiting, severe nystagmus, tinnitus, hearing loss
Symptom fatigue	No	Yes

persistent, progressive vertigo. It is less likely to be affected by position and is less likely to be accompanied by tinnitus and hearing loss. Central vertigo is also much more likely to be associated with focal neurological changes. Peripheral vertigo is typically more abrupt in onset, more severe, and more likely to be associated with severe nausea and vomiting. It is often episodic and may recur after a long period of dormancy. It also may have been preceded by an upper respiratory infection. Vertigo with a headache may be related to a tumor, hemorrhagic stroke, or sinus disease. Risk factors for cerebrovascular disease must also be considered. A patient with significant coronary artery disease, peripheral vascular disease, or common vascular disease risk factors is much more likely to have significant cerebrovascular disease. Ms Tripp's symptoms are most consistent with central vertigo.

Physical examination can provide further clues and should be focused toward the ear and neurological examinations. Both otitis media and cholesteatomas can cause vertiginous symptoms. Cranial nerve abnormalities, especially paresis or swallowing difficulties, are concerning for central vertigo. Romberg and tandem gait abnormalities are also red flags. Nystagmus is frequently present in patients with both peripheral and central vertigo. Carotid or vertebral bruits confirm the presence of cerebrovascular disease and raise concern for a central cause of the vertigo.

While attempting to classify vertigo as central or peripheral can aid the decision-making process in the emergency department, the clinician must have a high index of suspicion. Serious causes of central vertigo can present without any specific red flags. **Anyone who is elderly or has known hypertension, CAD, previous CVA, or CVA risk factors should be evaluated for specific central vertigo causes.**

Fundamentals of Disease

Coordination, balance, and sense of location are synchronized by the CNS using input from 3 different systems. Visual, vestibular, and proprioceptive inputs are integrated, and a mismatch between any 2 can cause a sense of vertigo. Visual systems provide information about body position and relate this information through higher brain centers. The vestibular system is composed of 3 semi-circular canals bilaterally and sends inputs to the brain that help control head positioning and movement. The proprioceptive system uses information from muscles and joints to determine the location of body parts in relation to each other.

Inputs from all 3 systems from both sides of the body are usually in equilibrium. When 1 of these inputs is disrupted unilaterally, the result is vertigo. Symmetric damage can result in gait instability, but rarely produces vertigo. Many of the neuronal inputs and nuclei associated with these systems are housed in the brainstem and cerebellum. The blood supply of the brainstem and cerebellum arises from vertebral and basilar arteries. Any disruption of the blood flow to these areas will cause interference of these systems, resulting in symptoms. The same risk factors that predispose people to coronary artery disease cause vascular damage to the vertebrobasilar system. The result is TIAs or ischemic CVAs. Similarly, in vertebrobasilar insufficiency, the patient has a blockage that is usually compensated by the contralateral artery. These patients can turn their heads and occlude the patent artery, causing transient brainstem ischemia. This is one of the principal reasons that arterial studies are needed. Essentially, VBS is a TIA of the posterior circulation and is a significant warning sign for an impending, and more severe, ischemic stroke.

Diagnostic Workup and Management

As with all patients, the first step in management is to assess the patient's stability. Causes of vertigo may progress to the point of patient instability and require emergent intervention such as intubation and advanced hemodynamic control measures.

In the stable patient with vertigo, management is directed toward 2 goals, symptomatic relief of the vertigo and its associated nausea. Multiple medications can be helpful in this regard. Medications with anticholinergic properties are first-line treatment. Examples include transdermal scopolamine, and H_1 antihistamines such as meclizine. Astemizole is an antihistamine without anticholinergic properties that works well. Calcium channel blockers (CCBs) have been found to relieve peripheral vertigo. Nimodipine is a CCB that is indicated in patients not responding to anticholinergics or antihistamines. Antidopaminergic agents (neuroleptics) are another class of drugs that can be used as second-line therapy. Promethazine and metoclopramide fall into this category. Ondansetron has been used in specific instances such as brainstem disorders and multiple sclerosis, but its utility in other causes is unknown.

Unfortunately, these medications often do not work well for central vertigo. Benzodiazepines, including diazepam and clonazepam, are indicated in central vertigo and occasionally in severe peripheral vertigo. Their disadvantage is that they can cause sedation and dependence.

A few basic labs should be performed, although they do not frequently aid in the diagnosis. A finger-stick glucose should be checked immediately to rule out hypoglycemia. A basic metabolic panel to screen for electrolyte abnormalities is warranted. If the patient is on any anticoagulation, a PT/INR and PTT should also be checked.

Advanced imaging is indicated in any patient with suspected central vertigo. Head CT is easiest to obtain, but the sensitivity is decreased due to the close proximity of bony structures. Additionally, noncontrast head CT does not evaluate for cerebrovascular disease and VBS. MRI and MRA are the definitive tests and will demonstrate ischemic stroke as well as vertebrobasilar narrowing and blockages.

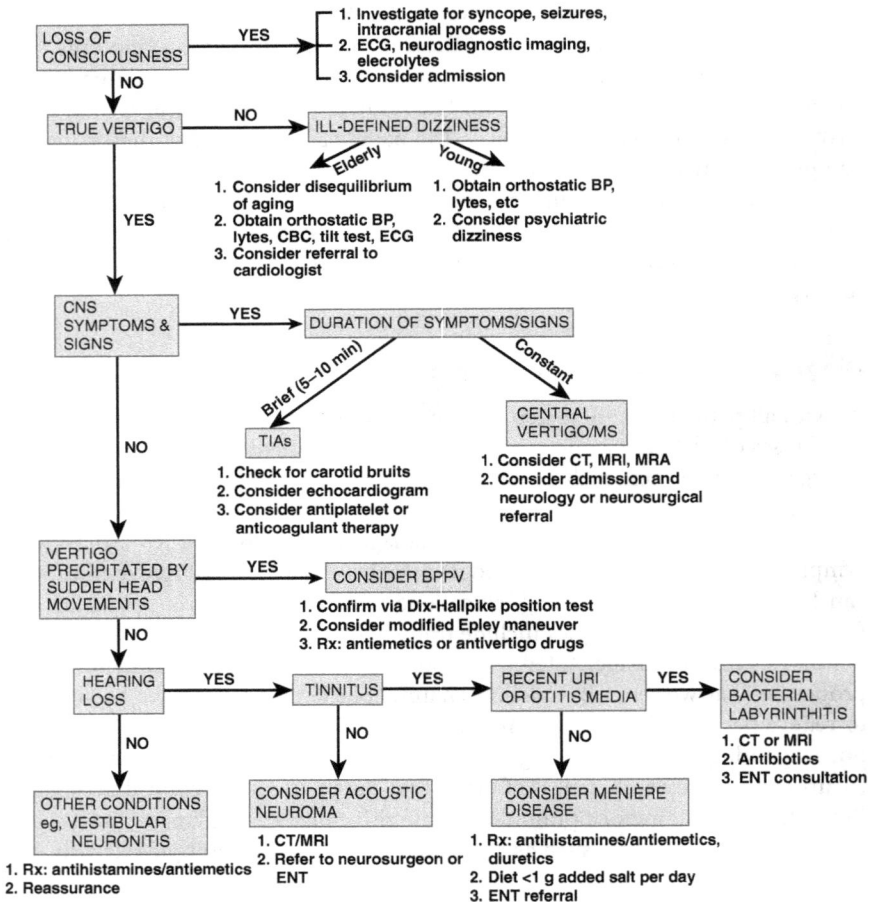

Figure 8-1. Diagnostic algorithm for the chief complaint of vertigo. (Reproduced, with permission, from Tintinalli JE, Stapczynski JS, Ma OJ, et al. *Tintinalli's Emergency Medicine: A Comprehensive Study Guide.* 7th ed. McGraw-Hill Education; 2011 [Figure 164-2].)

Carotid and vertebral artery Doppler studies can be used in place of MRA. Figure 8-1 provides a basic framework for an approach to a patient with vertigo.

TIPS TO REMEMBER

- New-onset vertigo in the elderly and those with CVA risk factors is central vertigo until proven otherwise and must be treated as such.

- MRI/MRA is the imaging of choice in suspected central vertigo.

COMPREHENSION QUESTIONS

1. Which of the following history findings is least concerning for central vertigo?
   A. Mild vertigo
   B. Tinnitus
   C. Patient history of hypertension
   D. Diplopia

2. An elderly patient with vertigo and a normal head CT can be safely discharged.
   A. True
   B. False

3. Which of the following physical findings is concerning for central vertigo?
   A. Decreased hearing
   B. Horizontal nystagmus
   C. Inability to perform tandem gait
   D. Orthostatic hypotension

Answers

1. B. Tinnitus is not associated with central vertigo. Diplopia, CVA risk factors including hypertension, and milder vertigo are all associated with central vertigo.

2. B. False. Many causes of central vertigo, including vertebrobasilar insufficiency and cerebellar ischemic CVA, will not show up on a CT. Patients need an MRI and artery studies such as Doppler studies or an MRA.

3. C. Inability to perform tandem gait is a red flag for central vertigo. Decreased hearing and horizontal nystagmus point toward a peripheral cause. Orthostatic hypotension increases the likelihood that the patient has near-syncope and not a true vertigo.

SUGGESTED READINGS

Marx JA, Hockberger RS, Walls RM, eds. *Rosen's Emergency Medicine: Concepts and Clinical Practice.* 7th ed. Philadelphia: Mosby-Elsevier; 2010 [chapter 12] <http://www.mdconsult.com>.
Tintinalli JE, Kelen GD, Stapczynski JS, Ma OJ, Cline DM, eds. *Tintinalli's Emergency Medicine.* 7th ed. New York: McGraw-Hill; 2011 [chapter 164] <http://www.accessmedicine.com>.

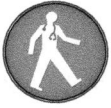

A 32-year-old Male With Vertigo

Richard Jeisy, MD

CASE DESCRIPTION

Mr Spinnaker is a 32-year-old male who presents to the emergency department complaining of dizziness. He feels like the room is spinning and is severely nauseated. He says this began suddenly 30 minutes prior to arrival. He has vomited once and noticed that moving his head makes the dizziness worse. If he keeps his head still, his symptoms are bearable. He has never had similar symptoms and denies headache, vision changes, tinnitus, or recent illness.

The patient's past medical history includes eczema and an appendectomy. He denies tobacco or illicit drug use, and drinks alcohol on occasional weekends. He was adopted and does not know his family history.

Vital signs include a pulse of 85 bpm, BP of 132/77 mm Hg, pulse oximetry of 99%, respirations of 16/min, and a temperature of 36.8°C.

On physical examination, the patient appears younger than his stated age and is in mild distress. He is keeping his head as still as possible and moves it slowly to speak with you. HEENT shows PERRLA, extraocular movements are intact, no nystagmus, and normal tympanic membranes without erythema or fluid collection. His neck is supple, nontender, and without bruits. Cardiovascular, respiratory, and abdominal examinations are normal. Neurological examination includes cranial nerves II to XII intact, normal motor and sensory examinations, no pronator drift, normal finger-to-nose testing, and normal gait and tandem gait. He is alert and oriented to person, place, and time.

1. What is the most likely differential diagnosis for this patient?

2. What other history questions and physical examination steps are needed?

3. What laboratory tests are indicated?

4. Does this patient need imaging? What kind?

5. What are the next treatment and management steps?

Answers

1. This patient's symptoms are most consistent with peripheral vertigo. The differential diagnosis for peripheral vertigo includes benign positional vertigo (BPV), vestibular neuronitis, Ménière disease, bacterial or viral labyrinthitis, traumatic vertigo, and ototoxicity.

2. This patient should be asked specifically about any recent trauma, changes in his hearing, medications, or similar prior episodes. A complete neurological examination, including basic hearing testing, should be performed. Since his

symptoms are most consistent with peripheral disease, the Dix-Hallpike test should also be performed.

3. A finger-stick glucose is indicated. Other labs are not necessary, but a CBC and BMP to look for signs of infection and electrolyte abnormalities are reasonable considerations.

4. With a good history and physical examination for peripheral vertigo and no significant cerebrovascular disease risk factors, imaging is not immediately indicated in this patient. Indications for imaging in peripheral vertigo will be discussed below.

5. Mr Spinnaker needs a trial of medication to get his vertigo and nausea under control. If his symptoms can be controlled, he may be discharged with a prescription and follow-up. More detailed management is discussed below.

CASE REVIEW

Mr Spinnaker has symptoms consistent with peripheral vertigo. The Dix-Hallpike test can be used to help confirm the diagnosis. Due to the classic presentation and the lack of risk factors for more serious disease, no imaging or lab testing is necessary. The focus is on symptomatic treatment.

PERIPHERAL VERTIGO

Diagnostic Reasoning

As discussed in a previous case of vertigo, the first step to diagnosing vertigo is making sure the patient has true vertigo. The next is to look for any red flags for central vertigo. In patients without red flags, the focus is on discerning the most likely cause of a patient's peripheral vertigo and treating it appropriately.

The causes of peripheral vertigo are due to disorders within the ear, vestibular system, or cranial nerve VIII. Table 9-1 provides a summary of causes of peripheral vertigo.

Table 9-1. Causes of Peripheral Vertigo

Ear canal foreign body	Posttraumatic vertigo
Benign positional vertigo (BPV)	Otitis media
Perilymph fistula	Vestibular neuronitis
Vestibular ganglionitis	Labyrinthitis
Ototoxicity/vestibulotoxicity	Cranial nerve VIII lesion

Otitis media and foreign body are easily diagnosed on otoscopic evaluation. Findings of tympanic membrane erythema, retraction, or middle ear fluid are present with otitis media. If the tympanic membrane is in contact with any material, vertigo can be the result. This includes foreign bodies as well as cerumen or hair. These may be removed in the emergency department, but occasionally need ENT consultation.

BPV is suggested when vertigo is caused or exacerbated by sudden head movements. The confirmation of this condition is through the use of the Dix-Hallpike position test, which is only 50% to 80% sensitive, but fairly specific. BPV is caused by free-floating particles in one of the semicircular canals that activate the canals inappropriately. Remember that the Dix-Hallpike test should not be performed on patients with a suspected central vertigo. The patient should be warned that the test might cause more vertigo and it is reasonable to provide symptomatic treatment prior to the test. To perform the Dix-Hallpike test, the patient is asked to sit upright and is instructed to keep his eyes on the physician's nose. For testing of the right posterior canal, the patient's head is turned 30° to 45° to the right, and the head is held there while the patient is rapidly laid down with the head hanging over the edge of the bed until it is 20° below the level of the stretcher. The test is positive if the patient has rotatory nystagmus within 30 seconds. The nystagmus will be toward the affected ear and last less than a minute. The test is then repeated to the left side. In BPV, vertigo improves with repeated head repositioning and can result in symptomatic relief.

Ménière disease usually presents in elderly patients, but may begin at any age. Symptoms usually last 2 to 8 hours and recur several times per week or month. Tinnitus, hearing loss, and occasional unilateral ear fullness accompany the vertigo. The diagnosis is confirmed by ENT via glycerol testing and vestibular-evoked myogenic potentials.

Perilymph fistula is a disorder allowing air pressure changes in the middle ear to be transmitted to the vestibular system. It is caused by infection, trauma, or sudden air pressure changes. It is often associated with straining, air travel, or scuba diving precipitating sudden vertigo, and may be accompanied by hearing loss. Confirmation is via nystagmus resulting from pneumatic otoscopy. ENT referral with possible surgical repair is required.

Vestibular neuronitis is thought to be viral is nature. Sudden vertigo, sometimes preceded by a viral illness, may be so intense that bed rest is required. The vertigo improves with time and does not recur.

Vestibular ganglionitis is also thought to be due to a virus such as varicella zoster. Inflammation in the vestibular ganglion causes vertigo, and the disease is associated with Ramsay Hunt syndrome, which causes deafness, vertigo, and facial nerve palsy. The presentation is often confused with BPV and Ménière disease. The confirmatory finding is grouped vesicles on an erythematous base found in the external auditory canal. Patients are treated with antivirals within 72 hours of vesicle appearance.

Labyrinthitis can be viral or bacterial in nature. Symptoms include vertigo and hearing loss. Viral labyrinthitis resolves with time. Bacterial labyrinthitis has the additional hallmark of middle ear findings, and patients usually appear toxic. This can progress to meningitis and requires antibiotic treatment and admission with ENT consult for possible surgical drainage.

Ototoxicity and *vestibulotoxicity* can be caused by a wide variety of medications. Hearing loss is usually associated with vertigo in these cases. Offending medications include aminoglycosides, erythromycin, fluoroquinolones, NSAIDs (especially aspirin), furosemide, certain chemotherapy agents, and antimalarials. The medication list of patients presenting with vertigo should be reviewed for these medications, and the patient should be asked about recent additions or changes to dosages.

Cranial nerve VIII lesions including acoustic schwannomas can cause mild vertigo. Patient presentations may look like central vertigo with a gradual onset, and hearing loss often precedes the vertigo.

Posttraumatic vertigo is common following head injuries and is due to direct damage to labyrinthine membranes. Vertigo is immediate after the injury and results in vomiting. It can portend a temporal bone fracture. Emergent CT imaging is warranted in patients with this presentation.

Fundamentals of Disease

Visual, vestibular, and proprioceptive systems all contribute to balance and coordination. Peripheral vertigo is caused by disturbances involving the vestibular system. This system is made up of several distinct components. The cupulae senses rotary motion. The semicircular canals are filled with a fluid called endolymph. Movement of the fluid causes the canals to sense head tilting and movement. The information from the vestibular system travels along cranial nerve VIII to the brainstem. Equal input from the bilateral vestibular systems keeps a person in equilibrium. Consequently, unilateral disruption causes vertigo. This disruption can be from any of the previously mentioned disease processes.

Dizziness and vertigo are common chief complaints in the emergency department. It is estimated that over 7.5 million patients present with these complaints to ambulatory settings yearly. BPV is the most common cause of vertigo with an estimated incidence of 107 cases per 100,000 people per year.

Diagnostic Workup and Management

Several medication options exist for the treatment of peripheral vertigo. They include anticholinergics, antihistamines, calcium channel blockers, antiemetics, and benzodiazepines. The most commonly used medications are meclizine, diazepam, and ondansetron.

In patients with BPV, symptoms can be treated without medication as well. Symptoms are fatigable, and vestibular rehabilitation exercises can be taught to patients. Repeated Dix-Hallpike testing can have similar effects. The Epley maneuver may be helpful as well. This maneuver can move the offending semicircular canal particles from the canal into the utricle. It is typically performed in the ENT office.

Patients with peripheral vertigo do not routinely require emergent imaging. However, in patients with findings concerning for bacterial labyrinthitis or post-traumatic vertigo a head CT or MRI in the emergency department is warranted.

After the patient has been medicated, he or she should be reevaluated. If the vertigo is improved and the patient can ambulate, he or she may be safely discharged home. Close follow-up with a PCP or ENT is needed for all new-onset vertigo patients. Occasionally patients cannot be safely discharged due to symptom severity and require admission.

TIPS TO REMEMBER

- Emergent neuroimaging is not necessary in all vertigo patients and should be used based on the suspected etiology of the peripheral vertigo.
- The Dix-Hallpike position test can be used as confirmation for BPV, but should not be used in patients with suspected vertebrobasilar insufficiency.

COMPREHENSION QUESTIONS

1. Which diagnosis requires emergent ENT consultation?
    A. Bacterial labyrinthitis
    B. Benign paroxysmal positional vertigo
    C. Ménière disease
    D. Vestibular neuronitis

2. Which of the following medications is least concerning for ototoxicity and vestibulotoxicity?
    A. Aspirin
    B. Gentamicin
    C. Hydrocodone
    D. Cisplatin

3. Patients with vertigo should not be medicated prior to the Dix-Hallpike because it can mask the results.
    A. True
    B. False

Answers

1. **A.** Bacterial labyrinthitis requires emergent ENT consultation and may require surgical drainage. The other diagnoses may benefit from ENT follow-up, but on a nonemergent basis.

2. **C.** Aspirin, gentamicin (aminoglycoside), and cisplatin all have the well-known side effect of ototoxicity. Hydrocodone does not.

3. **B.** False. Patients should be premedicated so that they can better tolerate the Dix-Hallpike test. This will not change the test results, and will make the patient more comfortable.

SUGGESTED READINGS

Marx JA, Hockberger RS, Walls RM, eds. *Rosen's Emergency Medicine: Concepts and Clinical Practice.* 7th ed. Philadelphia: Mosby-Elsevier; 2010 [chapter 12] <http://www.mdconsult.com>.
Tintinalli JE, Kelen GD, Stapczynski JS, Ma OJ, Cline DM, eds. *Tintinalli's Emergency Medicine.* 7th ed. New York: McGraw-Hill; 2011 [chapter 164] <http://www.accessmedicine.com>.

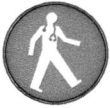

An 82-year-old Female With Altered Mental Status

Ryan N. Joshi, DO, EMT-P and Ted R. Clark, MD, MPP

CASE DESCRIPTION

Ms Brown is an 82-year-old female with reported alteration of mental status (AMS) transferred to the ED by EMS from a nursing home. Nursing home paperwork indicates that the patient has a history of normal mentation, but awoke this morning with confusion. The nursing home records note no falls but do report decreased urine output. Ms Brown rouses to voice but seems confused to place and time. The family is present at the bedside and states that the decreased level of consciousness and confusion are new for the patient. The family denies similar prior events. The family denies that the patient reported any recent fevers, nausea, vomiting, abdominal pain, chest pain, headache, or neurological changes. They saw her yesterday and she was in her normal state of health. The patient will answer questions, but her historical accuracy is in doubt.

A chart review shows that the patient has a history of hypertension, diabetes, and poor gait thought to be due to generalized deconditioning. She has had a hysterectomy, appendectomy, and cholecystectomy in the remote past.

Her vitals are temperature 38.5, blood pressure 122/82 mm Hg, pulse 105 beats/min, respiratory rate 18 breaths/min, and oxygen saturation of 99% on room air.

On examination, the patient has a slightly depressed level of consciousness but is easily arousable to voice. She is oriented to self but not to place or time. Skin is warm and moist. Heart is regular with no murmurs, but she is mildly tachycardic. Abdomen is soft. There is mild tenderness in the suprapubic region. Neurological examination reveals no focal neurological changes. The patient is incontinent of urine.

1. What are 3 large categories for a chief complaint of altered mental status, and how can you differentiate among them?

2. Which of the 3 major categories best describe this patient? What are the major categories and the differential diagnoses for a patient with delirium?

3. What red flags exist in this patient's history and physical examination that point to a possible critical diagnosis?

4. What testing should be ordered immediately in any patient with altered mental status? What is a "coma cocktail?"

Answers

1. AMS is a fairly nonspecific chief complaint. Although it encompasses many presentations, it can be most accurately subdivided into the categories of delirium, dementia, and psychosis. Importantly, dizziness and vertigo should be considered as separate chief complaints. Table 10-1 provides an overview of the 3 broad categories of AMS and how to differentiate among them.

2. Ms Brown has acute confusion, fever, tachycardia, and disorientation. Additionally, she lacks hallucinations, delusions, or a psychiatric history. She is most accurately classified as having delirium. Table 10-2 lists the 5 major categories of causes of delirium and several common diagnoses in each category.

3. This patient has several concerning features. Essentially, delirium is almost always a result of an emergent diagnosis and sometimes a critical diagnosis. The acute confusion, fever, and tachycardia are all red flags for an emergent or critical diagnosis.

4. Any patient who presents with altered mental status should have a finger-stick glucose performed as soon as possible. Hypoglycemia is a very common and easily reversible cause of altered mental status. Some EMS services will administer the "coma cocktail" prior to arrival in the ED. The "coma cocktail" includes dextrose, thiamine, oxygen, and naloxone.

Table 10-1. Major Subcategories of Altered Mental Status

	Delirium	**Dementia**	**Psychosis**
Onset	Sudden	Insidious	Sudden, but may have prior history
Vital signs	Often abnormal	Rarely abnormal	Rarely abnormal unless agitated
Level of consciousness	Often decreased	Usually normal	Usually normal
Attention level	Often decreased	Usually normal	Sometimes distracted
Orientation	Acutely impaired	Poor memory, but usually oriented to self and place	May be impaired
Hallucinations or delusions	Visual hallucinations more common if present. Delusions are rare	Usually absent unless severe dementia	Usually auditory with pervasive delusions

Table 10-2. Differential Diagnosis for Delirium

Infection	Pneumonia, UTI, meningitis, encephalitis, sepsis
Metabolic/endocrine	**Hypoglycemia, DKA, hyperglycemic hyperosmolar nonketotic coma** (HHNKC), electrolyte imbalance, hepatic encephalopathy, uremia, thyroid disorders, adrenal disorders, dehydration, nutritional (Wernicke's), hypothermia/hyperthermia, inborn errors of metabolism
Neurological	Seizure/postictal state, stroke/TIA, SAH, SDH, ICH, CNS mass/abscess, CNS trauma
Cardiopulmonary	Hypoxia, hypercarbia, CHF, AMI, PE, hemorrhagic shock, severe anemia, hypertensive encephalopathy, congenital heart defects
Toxicological/withdrawal	ETOH, methanol, ethylene glycol, opiates, benzos, barbs, anticholinergic, cholinergic, antihistamines, NMS, antiseizure medications, antipsychotics, invenomations, carbon monoxide, ETOH/benzo/barb withdrawal

CASE REVIEW

Ms Brown has symptoms suggestive of an infectious cause of her symptoms. A CMP, CBC, serum lactate, blood cultures, urinalysis, and chest x-ray are obtained. The CMP is essentially normal. CBC shows a normal hemoglobin and a WBC count of 22, predominantly neutrophils. Serum lactate is 2.2. Urinalysis shows 200 WBCs, many bacteria, and is nitrite positive. The chest x-ray is normal. Based on these results, it appears that Ms Brown has a urinary tract infection (UTI) with signs suggestive of sepsis. Due to the fever, tachycardia, and altered mental status, Ms Brown should receive an IV antibiotic such as ceftriaxone, fluid resuscitation, and admission for further care.

ALTERED MENTAL STATUS

Diagnostic Reasoning

Ms Brown presents with a chief complaint of AMS. The first step in the clinical reasoning process is to place the patient into 1 of the 3 large categories. It is crucial that the emergency physician be familiar with the differences between delirium, dementia, and psychosis. Importantly, delirium is nearly always caused by an emergent issue and most of these patients will need to be admitted. A patient with dementia typically only requires a workup for exacerbating causes and outpatient follow-up unless an issue of patient safety exists. Psychosis requires a very careful consideration of masquerading medical causes in addition to a psychiatric consultation for possible admission.

When considering delirium, the history and physical examination may provide important clues as to the cause. History can sometimes be limited by the patient's mental status, but a careful review of nursing home records, the EHR, and family input will provide valuable information. The goal of the history and physical examination is to place the patient into 1 of the 5 categorical causes of delirium. For example, a patient with recent head trauma, focal neurological changes, or seizure activity will most likely have a neurological cause of the delirium. Similarly, a patient with fever and tachycardia will most likely have an infectious cause. An astute emergency physician will gather the information required to launch a directed workup, but care must be taken not to prematurely exclude the often insidious metabolic and toxicological causes of delirium. A complete neurological examination and a survey for toxidromes are mandatory.

Diagnostic Workup and Management

The workup for a patient with delirium is often broad. The first step, as always, is setting up the safety net and performing an assessment of the ABCs. A finger-stick glucose should also be completed. Once the patient is determined to be relatively stable and blood glucose issues are addressed, a workup will be directed toward the suspected categorical cause of the delirium.

> *Infection.* A patient with evidence of infection should receive a CBC, CMP, serum lactate, blood cultures, urinalysis, and chest x-ray. If a CNS infection is suspected, then lumbar puncture should be performed. If the patient has evidence of sepsis—fever (or hypothermia), tachycardia, and hypotension—empiric antibiotics and early goal-directed resuscitation should be initiated prior to the identification of a source.

> *Metabolic/endocrine.* History and physical features such as the smell of ketones or a history of diabetes, a history of liver disease or examination stigmata, a history of thyroid disease or an enlarged thyroid, a history of alcoholism or drug abuse, or chronic steroid use may point the emergency physician toward a metabolic or endocrine cause for delirium. A patient with suspected metabolic or endocrine cause of delirium may require additional testing such as a blood gas, ammonia level, thyroid levels, or random cortisol level. These will often be added to a broader workup that includes other possible causes.

> *Neurological.* A patient with seizures, focal neurological changes, head trauma, or prior intracranial hemorrhage may require additional workup for neurological causes of delirium. A head CT, MRI, lumbar puncture, or EEG may be indicated in these patients.

Cardiopulmonary. The presence of dyspnea, hypoxia, chest pain, DVT symptoms, or a history of COPD, CHF, or MI may require additional workup in the patient with delirium. An EKG, chest x-ray, chest CT, blood gas, and cardiac enzymes may be indicated.

Toxicological/withdrawal. A careful survey of toxidromes, a history of alcoholism, a history of suicide attempts, the use of medications with a narrow therapeutic window, or the addition of new medications may prompt the emergency physician to order additional testing for toxicological contributors to delirium. The patient may need testing for specific medication or toxin levels or treatment for alcohol withdrawal.

Once a cause for the patient's delirium has been identified, supportive therapy should be maintained in combination with therapy directed toward the specific cause. (The discussion of treatment for each of the possible causes of AMS is beyond the scope of this chapter.) Often, a clear cause is not determined and the patient may undergo several therapy modalities until the precise cause becomes clear.

TIPS TO REMEMBER

- UTI is one of the most common causes of AMS in the elderly. A urinalysis should be ordered on all elderly patients with AMS.

- CNS infection is commonly overlooked in febrile patients with altered mental status. If no other infectious source is determined, a lumbar puncture is indicated.

- Always review the medication list and check levels on any potentially toxic medications in the patient with AMS.

COMPREHENSION QUESTIONS

1. Dementia is frequently associated with which of the following findings?
   A. Abnormal vital signs
   B. Normal level of consciousness
   C. Persistent delusions
   D. History of psychiatric illness

2. Patients who present with delirium should have which of the following performed?
   A. Continuous cardiac monitoring
   B. Finger-stick glucose
   C. Continuous pulse oximetry
   D. All of the above

Answers

1. **B.** Patients with dementia often have a normal level of consciousness and can carry on a normal conversation. A physician may not even notice significant issues until questions directed at orientation and memory are asked. Vital signs are typically normal and delusions are rare. There may or may not be a history of psychiatric illness.

2. **D.** Patients with delirium nearly always have an emergent or critical diagnosis. Such patients should be continuously monitored. Finger-stick glucose should always be performed immediately on assessment.

SUGGESTED READINGS

Marx JA, Hockberger RS, Walls RM, eds. *Rosen's Emergency Medicine: Concepts and Clinical Practice.* 7th ed. Philadelphia: Mosby-Elsevier; 2010 [chapter 97] <http://www.mdconsult.com>.
Tintinalli JE, Kelen GD, Stapczynski JS, Ma OJ, Cline DM, eds. *Tintinalli's Emergency Medicine.* 7th ed. New York: McGraw-Hill; 2011 [chapter 94] <http://www.accessmedicine.com>.

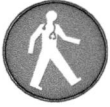

A 30-year-old Female With Altered Mental Status

Quoc V. Pham, MD and
Ted R. Clark, MD, MPP

CASE DESCRIPTION

Ms Pick is a 30-year-old female who presents to the ED with confusion and decreased level of consciousness. The patient will rouse to voice, but is unable to provide much meaningful history. The patient's husband is with her and provides the history. He states the patient has been depressed for the past month after losing her job, but has otherwise been in her normal state of health. When he returned home from work today, he found her sleeping on the bed. She was very difficult to arouse. On waking, she was noted to have slurred speech and confusion. Next to the bed, the husband found an empty bottle of lorazepam and an empty pint of vodka. The patient reports that she "just wants to go to sleep." The patient reports that she took "a handful" of 0.5 mg lorazepam. No other physical complaints.

Past medical history includes a history of depression and anxiety. She has a prescription for citalopram and lorazepam. She has no prior psychiatric hospitalizations or suicide attempts. She does have a counselor that she sees monthly.

Her vitals are temperature 37.0, blood pressure 122/82 mm Hg, pulse 80 beats/min, respiratory rate 10 breaths/min, and oxygen saturation of 99% on room air.

On examination, the patient has a depressed level of consciousness but is rousable to voice. Her GCS is 13. She is oriented to self and time. She knows she is "in the hospital." She appears to be protecting her airway. Her lungs are clear to auscultation bilaterally. Her respiratory rate is slow, but her depth of respiration appears adequate. Heart is regular with no murmurs. She has normal peripheral perfusion. Abdomen is soft, nontender, and nondistended. Neurological examination reveals no focal neurological changes, but the patient is poorly cooperative.

1. Is the patient's symptom complex most consistent with dementia, delirium, or psychosis? What features lead you to this conclusion?

2. What are the 5 major toxidromes (toxic syndromes) and what are their key features?

3. What is the basic treatment for suspected benzodiazepine overdose?

Answers

1. Ms Pick's symptom complex is most consistent with delirium. Table 10-1 describes the typical presentation of each of the major subcategories of AMS. It should be noted that delirium in the ED is a symptom complex, whereas in

Table 11-1. Key Features of Toxidromes

Sympathomimetic	Agitation, diaphoresis, tachycardia, hypertension
Cholinergic	Depressed LOC, confusion, generalized weakness, SLUDGE (salivation, lacrimation, urination, defecation, GI upset, emesis), miosis, bradycardia
Anticholinergic	Agitation, visual hallucinations, dry skin, flushed skin, dilated pupils, urinary retention, decreased bowel sounds (hot as a hare, red as a beet, dry as a bone, mad as a hatter)
Sedative/hypnotic	Depressed LOC, slow respirations, decreased bowel sounds, miosis (opiates)
Serotonergic	Tremor, agitation, elevated temperature, confusion, myoclonus, hyperreflexia, muscle rigidity

psychiatry, it is be used as a diagnosis. Ms Pick's AMS has the typical delirium features of sudden onset, depressed level of consciousness, impaired orientation, and abnormal vital signs (depressed respiratory rate).

2. The 5 major toxidromes and their key features are listed in Table 11-1.

3. A patient with a suspected overdose requires the safety net and a rapid assessment of the ABCs. Alternative causes for the AMS should be actively pursued (infection, hypoglycemia, electrolyte disturbance, neurological injury). A "coma cocktail" (dextrose, naloxone, oxygen, thiamine) may be administered. The major risk with benzodiazepine overdose (like all sedatives/hypnotics) is respiratory depression and failure to protect the airway. The end result may be respiratory arrest/insufficiency resulting in hypoxia or hypercarbia and ultimately death. The risk is especially high when benzodiazepines are mixed with other sedatives such as alcohol or opiates. Basic treatment is supportive. Intubation for respiratory insufficiency or airway protection may be required. Continuous monitoring is required as the patient's status may change depending on the time of ingestion and the exact medication ingested. There is a reversal agent for benzodiazepine overdose (flumazenil). In practice, however, this agent is only used in selected cases such as pediatric exposure and benzodiazepine-naïve patients. The major risk with flumazenil is the precipitation of intractable seizures.

CASE REVIEW

Ms Pick's presentation is consistent with AMS from an overdose of a benzodiazepine and alcohol. The time of the overdose is not immediately known. A review of the ABCs reveals depressed respirations. Intubation is not immediately indicated, but preparations should be made. The patient should be placed on continuous monitoring, including end-tidal CO_2. If evidence of respiratory insufficiency develops, the patient will require intubation. Her depressed LOC is not compatible with BiPAP, and her chronic benzodiazepine use precludes the use of flumazenil. In addition to supportive care for her perceived benzodiazepine overdose, the patient needs additional directed workup for other potential causes of altered mental status. A CBC, CMP, EKG, urinalysis, and urine pregnancy test should be ordered. A head CT should be considered if there are any focal neurological changes, evidence of trauma, history of headache, or uncertainty regarding the cause of the AMS. The patient will require admission to the ICU for close monitoring and subsequent psychiatric evaluation.

ALTERED MENTAL STATUS—OVERDOSE

Diagnostic Reasoning

Overdose is a common cause of AMS. The most common overdose encountered in the ED is alcohol intoxication. Frequently, however, there will be coingestants involved. History is often limited in the cases of overdose, and the EM physician should focus on identifying immediately reversible causes of AMS (hypoglycemia, opiate overdose), identifying critical diagnoses that require specific intervention (intracranial hemorrhage, respiratory failure), providing supportive care, and collecting additional information from available sources (family, police, EMS).

On initial presentation of a patient with suspected overdose, the EM physician should establish the safety net, check the ABCs, and check a blood glucose. The "coma cocktail" (dextrose, naloxone, thiamine, oxygen) can be used without much fear of deleterious effects. If the patient has evidence of opiate ingestion, additional naloxone may be required. If the patient has respiratory insufficiency or failure to protect the airway and there is no immediately reversible cause identified, the patient should be intubated. It should be noted that patients with overdose have a widely variable presentation. The presentation depends on the toxin involved and can present as depressed level of consciousness, agitation, psychosis, or asymptomatically.

It is important that the EM physician does not anchor on alcohol or another ingestion as the cause for AMS. For example, a patient with evidence of alcohol ingestion may get tucked away in a quiet corner of the ED and subsequently die from an undetected expanding epidural hematoma. For this reason, it is imperative for the EM physician to perform a complete history and physical examination even when the cause for the AMS seems "obvious." The EM physician should continue to consider the 5 major categories of delirium—infection, metabolic/endocrine, neurological, cardiopulmonary, and toxicology/withdrawal state.

The EM physician should collect additional information from family, police, and EMS. Particularly in the case of overdose, the patient may be unable or unwilling to provide additional information. The family often has information on the patient's status prior to the overdose, the patient's habits regarding drug or alcohol use, the patient's psychiatric history, and the patient's prescribed medications. Police and EMS can often describe what was observed at the scene, the presence of pill bottles or illicit drugs, and additional history obtained from bystanders at the scene. This additional information can guide further management and workup.

Finally, the EM physician should use toxicology resources such as online poison databases, Poison Control Center, and, if available, the toxicology consultation service to assist with clinical decisions in overdose patients. These resources can help the EM physician identify expected rare complications, as well as determine appropriate observation periods and monitoring.

Diagnostic Workup and Management

The prior AMS case discussed diagnostic workup directed at the 5 major categorical causes of delirium. Toxicology is a subspecialty of emergency medicine, and it requires special consideration with regard to diagnostic workup and management. Important considerations with regard to workup include the recognition of toxidromes, knowledge of the metabolic and cardiac effects of common toxins, and specific testing for certain toxins. Important considerations with regard to the management of overdoses are the use of specific antidotes, expected complications, and the principles of supportive care.

The most common toxidromes are summarized in Table 11-1. It is important to note that all features of a toxidrome may not be present and there is commonly overlap. The basic features of a toxidrome, however, can be used to guide further workup and management. For example, a patient who presents with hypertension, tachycardia, diaphoresis, and agitation raises concern for sympathomimetic overdose. This realization will lead the EM physician to question further regarding drug use, to avoid the use of β-blockers to control blood pressure, to consider cardiac complications, and to use benzodiazepines to control symptoms.

Although many toxins cause an alteration of mental status, many do not cause easily recognizable external effects, but may cause potentially deadly cardiac or metabolic changes. For example, calcium channel blocker and β-blocker overdose can cause refractory hypotension and cardiac conduction blocks, tricyclic antidepressants can cause refractory and fatal arrhythmias, aspirin and NSAIDs can cause a refractory metabolic acidosis, and acetaminophen can cause liver failure after an asymptomatic period.

The entire breadth of possible toxicological presentations is beyond the scope of this book, but from a workup perspective, most overdose patients will require at least several basic tests. A basic starting workup for a suspected overdose is finger-stick glucose, BMP, LFTs, urinalysis, urine drug screen, acetaminophen and aspirin levels, ethanol level, serum osmolality, and EKG. Specific levels for

Table 11-2. Antidotes for Specific Toxins/Toxidromes

Opiates	Naloxone—competitively inhibits the activation of opiate receptors
Benzodiazepines	Flumazenil—competitively inhibits the activation of GABA receptors
Toxic alcohols (methanol, ethylene glycol, isopropyl alcohol)	Fomepizole—competitive inhibitor of alcohol dehydrogenase. Prevents conversion of alcohol to toxic metabolites Ethanol—same as fomepizole
Acetaminophen	N-Acetylcysteine (NAC)—repletes reaction cofactor that speeds conversion of toxic metabolites to nontoxic forms
Digoxin	Digoxin immune fab—binds to digoxin and speeds elimination
Serotonergic toxidrome	Cyproheptadine—competitively inhibits activation of histamine and serotonin receptors
Cholinergic toxidrome	Atropine—competitively inhibits the action of acetylcholine at muscarinic receptors (controls SLUDGE symptoms) Pralidoxime (2-PAM)—"reactivates" acetylcholinesterase that has been "deactivated" by toxins such as organophosphates
Anticholinergic toxidrome	Physostigmine—inhibits acetylcholinesterase, thereby increasing the presence of acetylcholine at nerve junctions. Rarely used for this indication

any medications that the patient takes with a narrow therapeutic window such as lithium, digoxin, theophylline, carbamazepine, phenytoin, and valproic acid should also be obtained. Toxic alcohol levels (methanol, ethylene glycol, and isopropyl alcohol) should also be considered.

One unique aspect of the management of overdoses is the presence of antidotes. Table 11-2 lists some common toxins and their antidotes. Importantly, antidotes vary in their clinical effect. Some will directly reverse the action of a toxin (naloxone, flumazenil); some will prevent the complication of a given toxin (N-acetylcysteine); some will speed the elimination of a given toxin (digoxin immune fab).

Another important feature of the management of patients with suspected overdose is GI decontamination. The mainstay of GI decontamination is activated charcoal. Forced emesis (ipecac) and gastric lavage ("pumping the stomach") are very rarely used. In general, any suspected significant toxic ingestion which absorbs activated charcoal (basically anything except heavy metals, alcohols, corrosives, and hydrocarbons) that presents within 1 hour of ingestion should receive activated charcoal either orally or through an NG tube. Additional techniques such as multidose activated charcoal and whole bowel irrigation can be used in very limited situations. Removal of certain toxins from the intravascular space may require dialysis or forced diuresis. The specific indications for these interventions are beyond the scope of this book.

The disposition of patients with overdose requires an understanding of the pharmacokinetics and expected complications of the toxin. For example, a patient with an overdose of a long-acting opioid such as methadone will require continued monitoring and possibly a naloxone drip. A patient with an overdose of a short-acting benzodiazepine such as alprazolam may only require an observation period in the ED. A patient with a significant aspirin overdose will require continued monitoring of metabolic status and possibly dialysis. Finally, all patients who present with an overdose should be evaluated for suicidal ideation, and may require admission for psychiatric care after being medically cleared.

TIPS TO REMEMBER

- Overdose is an important cause of altered mental status and should always be considered.
- Ethyl alcohol is the most common toxicological cause of depressed level of consciousness, but the EM physician should carefully consider alternative causes (such as trauma, hypoxia, or other toxins).
- Patients with overdose can be lethargic, agitated, psychotic, or asymptomatic.
- Use your online resources and Poison Control Center to help with toxin management.
- Anticipate the required observation period and potential complications of an overdose.
- Consider psychiatric screening for all overdose patients after being medically cleared.

COMPREHENSION QUESTIONS

1. Which of the following is *not* part of the "coma cocktail?"
    A. Flumazenil
    B. Naloxone
    C. Dextrose
    D. Oxygen

2. A patient presents with confusion, agitation, dilated pupils, and dry skin. What is the toxidrome?

 A. Sedative/hypnotic
 B. Sympathomimetic
 C. Cholinergic
 D. Anticholinergic

Answers

1. A. Flumazenil is a benzodiazepine antagonist. It is not part of the coma cocktail, and it is rarely used in the ED due to the risk of withdrawal seizures. One indication for flumazenil is a significant benzodiazepine overdose in a child with no previous benzodiazepine use.

2. D. Confusion, agitation, and dilated pupils are features most consistent with either anticholinergic or sympathomimetic toxidromes. Dry skin is most consistent with the anticholinergic toxidromes. Sympathomimetic toxidromes, in contrast, will demonstrate moist skin. In addition, anticholinergic toxidromes may demonstrate urinary retention.

SUGGESTED READINGS

Marx JA, Hockberger RS, Walls RM, eds. *Rosen's Emergency Medicine: Concepts and Clinical Practice.* 7th ed. Philadelphia: Mosby-Elsevier; 2010 [chapter 146] <http://www.mdconsult.com>.
Tintinalli JE, Kelen GD, Stapczynski JS, Ma OJ, Cline DM, eds. *Tintinalli's Emergency Medicine.* 7th ed. New York: McGraw-Hill; 2011 [chapters 170, 177] <http://www.accessmedicine.com>.

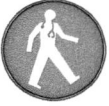

A 72-year-old Female With Low Back Pain

Charles Reeve, DO and Ted R. Clark, MD, MPP

CASE DESCRIPTION

Ms Rivera is a 72-year-old female who presents to the ED with a chief complaint of low back pain. She describes the pain as gradual in onset and aching in nature. The pain started 2 days ago. She denies radiation to the abdomen or legs. She states the pain is worse with movement and is relieved by rest. She has had back pain in the past, but states that this is worse. She denies any trauma. She denies any recent physical activity to stress the back. She reports increased urinary frequency and difficulty today. She denies fever. She denies leg weakness or numbness. She denies IV drug abuse. She denies a history of diabetes or immunocompromise. She denies a history of cancer.

Her vitals are temperature 37.2, blood pressure 130/92 mm Hg, pulse 77 beats/min, respiratory rate 18 breaths/min, and oxygen saturation of 99% on room air.

On physical examination, the patient is alert and oriented. Her cardiopulmonary examination is normal. Her abdominal examination elicits mild tenderness and fullness in the suprapubic region. Her back examination shows no overlying skin changes. The pain is localized to the L5-S1 region. She does not have significant deformity or point tenderness over the spine. Her lower extremities show mildly decreased sensation in the groin region. Reflexes are normal throughout; sensation and strength are normal throughout. Her gait is normal.

1. What are the critical diagnoses for low back pain?

2. What red flags are present in this patient's history and physical examination?

3. What imaging is warranted in this patient?

Answers

1. Table 12-1 lists the critical diagnoses and red flags for a patient with a chief complaint of low back pain.

2. Ms Rivera has several concerning features to her back pain. She gives a history of "urinary frequency and difficulty." This history should be explored further to determine if she is describing the dysuria that we expect with a urinary tract infection or urolithiasis, or if she is describing the urinary retention that we may see in cauda equina syndrome. A postvoid residual may help us differentiate. On physical examination, tenderness and fullness in the suprapubic region are

Table 12-1. Critical Diagnoses and Red Flags for Low Back Pain

Critical Diagnosis	History Red Flags/ Risk Factors	Physical Red Flags
Spinal epidural abscess	Fever, chills, gradual onset, localized pain. Risk factors include immunocompromise, IV drug abuse, recent sepsis	Warmth or erythema over spine, localized tenderness over the spine. Neurological changes are a late finding
Spinal epidural hematoma	Localized pain, may not have reproducible pain. Risk factors include anticoagulant use, bleeding disorder, or recent back surgery. May be associated with trauma	Neurological changes common—may resemble radiculopathy or cauda equina syndrome
Cauda equina syndrome	History of back pain or disc disease. Development of urinary retention or overflow incontinence, bowel incontinence, saddle anesthesia, or lower extremity weakness over a period of hours	May or may not have spinal tenderness. Urinary retention evidenced by elevated postvoid residual, suprapubic tenderness or fullness. May have decreased sphincter tone or numbness in the saddle region. Hyporeflexia, lower extremity weakness
Vertebral osteomyelitis	Fever, chills, gradual onset, focal pain, stiffness. Risk factors include immunocompromise, IV drug abuse, recent sepsis	Focal tenderness, signs of sepsis, neurological changes are a late finding
Spinal fracture or subluxation	History of trauma, acute pain, acute neurological deficit	Step-offs or deformity on examination. Focal neurological findings dependent on level or injury
Spinal metastases	Mechanical pain, insidious onset, neurological symptoms may develop late. Constitutional symptoms such as weight loss and night sweats. Risk factors include known malignancy, advanced age	Focal tenderness, may have neurological deficits

(continued)

Table 12-1. Critical Diagnoses and Red Flags for Low Back Pain (*Continued*)

Critical Diagnosis	History Red Flags/ Risk Factors	Physical Red Flags
Leaking abdominal aortic aneurysm	Sudden-onset abdominal or back pain with radiation to flank or testicle. May be associated with syncope. Risk factors include known AAA, vascular disease and its associated risk factors	No spinal tenderness. Abdominal pulsatile mass. Hypotension. Bedside ultrasound with AAA or peritoneal fluid
Aortic dissection	Sudden "tearing" pain. Usually associated with chest or abdominal pain. Risk factors include hypertension, vascular disease, recent instrumentation, connective tissue disorders	Patient is likely anxious, unstable vital signs possible, unequal blood pressure in upper extremities, focal neurological changes possible. New aortic regurgitation murmur possible

concerning for urinary retention. Additionally, the patient has saddle anesthesia. Ms Rivera does not have all the history and physical examination features of cauda equina syndrome, but there are enough red flags to raise significant concern.

3. An MRI is the most sensitive test for cauda equina syndrome. MRI is also highly sensitive for epidural hematoma and abscess, and osteomyelitis. CT myelography can be used in those who cannot have an MRI. Plain or contrasted CT may identify cauda equina syndrome, but it is not sufficiently sensitive to rule it out.

CASE REVIEW

Ms Rivera has signs and symptoms concerning for cauda equina syndrome—low back pain, urinary difficulty, saddle numbness, and fullness over the bladder. A postvoid residual is elevated at 500 mL. An MRI confirms the diagnosis by demonstrating a large vertebral disc compressing the thecal sac at the level of the cauda equina. As discussed above, immediate neurosurgical decompression is required to prevent long-term sequelae such as neurogenic bladder, stool incontinence, lower extremity weakness, and impotence in men.

LOW BACK PAIN

Diagnostic Reasoning

Low back pain is a chief complaint that unfortunately carries a certain amount of negative connotation in the ED. For this reason, the EM physician needs to remain especially vigilant for the detection of critical diagnoses in the face of possible affective bias or triage cueing. Overall, however, the list of critical diagnoses for low back pain is relatively small and can many times be addressed simply by asking the correct questions and performing the correct physical examination maneuvers.

After an initial assessment for stability by reviewing the patient's vital signs and ABCs, the EM physician can begin to focus on the chief complaint. An important initial distinction in a patient who presents with low back pain is to determine if the pain is more consistent with a musculoskeletal cause or if the patient is experiencing referred visceral pain. Pain related to the spine and its associated muscles and nerves is more likely to be worse with movement, reproducible on palpation of the back, have related radicular or lower body neurological symptoms, or have a preceding traumatic event. It may also be helpful to ask the patient if she has had similar pain in the past, and, if so, how is this pain different. The critical diagnoses associated with a musculoskeletal presentation of low back pain are spinal epidural abscess, spinal epidural hematoma, cauda equina syndrome, vertebral osteomyelitis, spinal metastases, or spinal fracture and subluxation. In contrast, referred or visceral back pain is often constant, not exacerbated by movement or palpation of the back, associated with other areas of pain such as abdominal pain, and less likely to be associated with neurological changes. The critical diagnoses associated with referred or visceral back pain are leaking AAA and aortic dissection. In addition, referred back pain is associated with several emergent diagnoses such as cholecystitis, pancreatitis, PE, and retroperitoneal mass or hemorrhage. A story consistent with a musculoskeletal cause does not "rule out" a referred pain diagnosis, but it does make it less likely.

The physical examination can further narrow down the differential diagnosis. Inspection of the back should focus on evidence of trauma or infection. The EM physician should have full visualization of the back to look for bruising, abrasions, lacerations, rashes, and erythema. The entire spine should be palpated for deformity, midline tenderness, or warmth. The abdomen and chest should be examined to look for signs of a referred source of the pain. For example, an absence of back tenderness and a pulsatile mass on abdominal examination would be very concerning for a leaking AAA. The final crucial part of the examination in a patient with a chief complaint of low back pain is the neurological examination. The examination should focus on the neurological function of the lower extremities. Figure 12-1 illustrates examination techniques for nerve roots L4-S1. In addition, the patient should be assessed for urinary retention, saddle anesthesia, and decreased rectal tone. Finally, unless an unstable fracture is suspected, the patient should be examined through a standing full range of motion and assessed for gait.

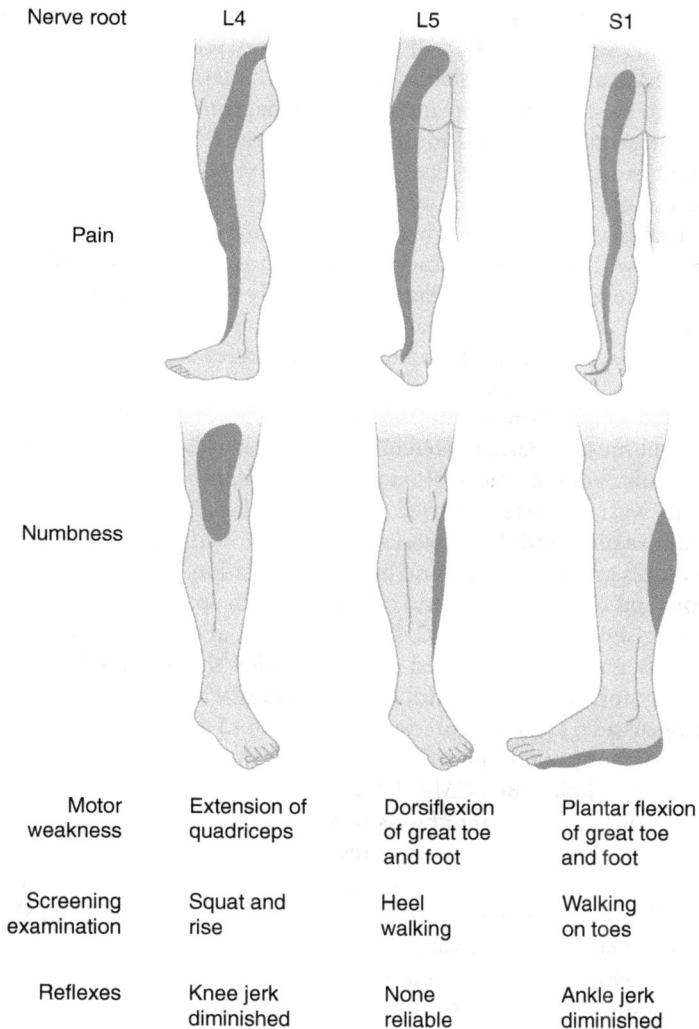

Nerve root	L4	L5	S1
Pain			
Numbness			
Motor weakness	Extension of quadriceps	Dorsiflexion of great toe and foot	Plantar flexion of great toe and foot
Screening examination	Squat and rise	Heel walking	Walking on toes
Reflexes	Knee jerk diminished	None reliable	Ankle jerk diminished

Figure 12-1. Testing for lumbar nerve root compromise. (Reproduced, with permission, from Tintinalli JE, Stapczynski JS, Ma OJ, Cline DM, Cydulka RK, Meckler GD. *Tintinalli's Emergency Medicine: A Comprehensive Guide.* 7th ed. New York: McGraw-Hill Education; 2011 [Figure 276-3] <http://www.accessmedicine.com>.

Diagnostic Workup and Management

A thorough history and physical examination will facilitate a focused diagnostic workup. The majority of patients with a chief complaint of back pain will be triaged to lower-acuity areas and in most instances this is appropriate. The first step in management is to identify any patients who may have been mistriaged by examining vital signs and ABCs. If potentially unstable patients are identified, they should have a safety net established and ABC interventions as needed. Once determined to be stable, workup and further management can begin.

A patient with a suspected musculoskeletal source of back pain and no red flags in the history or physical examination may require no additional workup. A common example of a patient who requires no additional workup is a patient with a nontraumatic, acute exacerbation of chronic pain and no red flags. In contrast, a patient with a traumatic exacerbation of chronic pain and midline tenderness, even in the absence of red flags, will typically receive an x-ray of the spine. Management of musculoskeletal back pain with no red flags and a negative x-ray (if applicable) is symptomatic. Depending on the degree of pain, IV or oral opioids may be indicated. NSAIDs such as ketorolac and ibuprofen may also be helpful. Adjuncts such as cyclobenzaprine and benzodiazepines are helpful if the patient has significant muscle spasms. Stretching routines can also play an important role in both resolution of the exacerbation and the prevention of recurrence.

Patients with suspected referred pain or red flags in the history or physical examination require additional workup. Suspected *leaking AAA* in an unstable patient requires immediate fluid and blood resuscitation, consultation of a vascular surgeon, and bedside ultrasound or CT scan if the patient is stabilized. Laboratory testing should include CBC, CMP, PT/PTT, and type and crossmatch at least 8 U. Patients with a suspected *aortic dissection* should have blood pressure control to a systolic BP <100 by titrating IV labetalol with or without the addition of IV nitroprusside; a cardiothoracic surgeon should be immediately consulted, and CT angiography of the chest/abdomen/pelvis should be obtained. Laboratory testing should include CBC, CMP, PT/PTT, and type and crossmatch. Patients with suspected *spinal epidural abscess* or *vertebral osteomyelitis* should have an MRI or CT myelogram. Laboratory testing should include CBC, CMP, blood cultures, CRP, and ESR. The most common pathogen is *Staphylococcus aureus*, but empiric antibiotics such as vancomycin and piperacillin–tazobactam should be started pending culture and possibly biopsy results. Patients with suspected *cauda equina syndrome* or *epidural hematoma* require an MRI or CT myelogram. Laboratory testing should include CBC, CMP, and PT/PTT. A patient with a suspected fracture/subluxation requires prone positioning with full spinal precautions and a CT of the spine. MRI may be indicated but should not delay surgical management in an unstable fracture/subluxation or in the presence of neurological deficits. Neurosurgical consultation is mandatory in all of the above diagnoses, but cauda equina and unstable fractures/subluxations require immediate surgery to prevent long-term sequelae. Finally, although there is variation in practice, most recommend standard- or high-dose dexamethasone or methylprednisolone in the event of a traumatic spinal cord injury with neurological symptoms and in cauda equina syndrome.

TIPS TO REMEMBER

- Do not let the negative connotations associated with low back pain inhibit a thorough history and physical examination.
- Back pain can be musculoskeletal or referred visceral pain; this differentiation will help determine the appropriate workup.
- MRI is most frequently the test of choice when considering critical diagnoses for musculoskeletal back pain.

COMPREHENSION QUESTIONS

1. Which of the following is most consistent with visceral referred back pain?
   A. The pain is worsened by flexion and extension of the back.
   B. The pain is not reproduced by palpation of the back.
   C. The pain is preceded by direct trauma to the back.
   D. Inability to ambulate.

2. What imaging should be ordered on a patient who fell off a step onto his back, has spinal and paraspinal tenderness in the L3-L4 region, and has no red flags on history or physical examination?
   A. MRI of the lumbar spine
   B. CT myelogram
   C. Noncontrasted CT of the lumbar spine
   D. Plain film x-rays of the lumbar spine

Answers

1. B. Referred pain typically is not reproducible with palpation of the back.

2. D. Musculoskeletal back pain with minor trauma and no red flags is most efficiently evaluated with plain x-rays.

SUGGESTED READINGS

Marx JA, Hockberger RS, Walls RM, eds. *Rosen's Emergency Medicine: Concepts and Clinical Practice.* 7th ed. Philadelphia: Mosby-Elsevier; 2010 [chapter 28] <http://www.mdconsult.com>.
Tintinalli JE, Kelen GD, Stapczynski JS, Ma OJ, Cline DM, eds. *Tintinalli's Emergency Medicine.* 7th ed. New York: McGraw-Hill Education; 2011 [chapters 168, 255, 276].

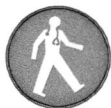

A 40-year-old Male With Low Back Pain

Charles Reeve, DO and Ted R. Clark, MD, MPP

CASE DESCRIPTION

Mr Brick is a 40-year-old male who presents to the ED with a chief complaint of worsening low back pain for 4 days. He is a manual laborer and carries heavy items daily. He reports that the pain is aching, constant, and present in the bilateral lower back. There is occasional sharp radiation of the pain down the right leg. He reports that he has had chronic pain in his lower back for the past 10 years. He has been worked up with MRI in the past and has been found to have degenerative disease and bulging discs at L4-L5. He denies any specific injury with the recent onset of worsening pain. He reports several similar flare-ups of his chronic pain in the past. He denies bowel or bladder changes. He denies fever. He denies leg weakness or numbness. He denies IV drug abuse. He denies a history of diabetes or immunocompromise. He denies a history of cancer.

His vitals are temperature 37.4, blood pressure 156/98 mm Hg, pulse 93 beats/min, respiratory rate 20 breaths/min, and oxygen saturation of 99% on room air.

On physical examination, the patient is alert and oriented. His cardiopulmonary examination is normal. His abdominal examination is normal. His back examination shows no overlying skin changes. The pain is present on palpation of L1-S1 both in the midline and in the paraspinal muscles. He does not have significant deformity or point tenderness over the spine. Sensation, strength, and reflexes are normal throughout. His gait is normal.

1. What physical examination maneuvers are required in a patient with low back pain?

2. What are the noncritical diagnoses for a chief complaint of low back pain?

3. What imaging is indicated in this patient?

Answers

1. Despite the absence of red flags in the history, it is still important to complete a thorough assessment of red flags on the physical examination. Table 12-1 describes the red flags associated with a chief complaint of low back pain. The following physical examination maneuvers are mandatory for Mr Brick:

   A. Inspection of the back for warmth, erythema, trauma, or deformity.

   B. Palpation for spinal point tenderness, deformity, or instability.

C. A complete lower extremity neurological examination, including sensation, strength, and reflexes in all dermatomes.

D. If cauda equina syndrome is suspected, the EM physician should assess for saddle anesthesia, rectal tone, and postvoid residual.

2. Although Mr Brick does not appear to have a critical diagnosis, there are several noncritical diagnoses to consider. His pain is most consistent with a mechanical cause; therefore, we will focus on mechanical causes of low back pain. Table 13-1 describes the most common causes of noncritical lower back pain.

Table 13-1. Noncritical Diagnoses for a Chief Complaint of Low Back Pain

Diagnosis	History and Risk Factors	Physical Examination
Nonspecific back pain (other names used are back strain, mechanical back pain, or lumbago)	Pain is mild-to-moderate, worse with movement, relieved with rest. Mild trauma or muscle exertion. May have had similar episodes in the past. No red flags	Tender to palpation diffusely over both the spine and the paraspinal muscles. No red flags. Imaging is basically normal
Degenerative joint disease	Gradual onset, generalized back pain. Worse with movement and lifting. Age >40. May have history of manual labor	May have spinal tenderness. No neurological changes. X-ray showing arthritis is required to make diagnosis
Sciatica	Nonspecific term for symptoms associated with back pain that radiates down the legs in a lumbosacral nerve root distribution. It is usually from disk disease, but may be from another source. The pain may be acute or chronic in nature and typically radiates unilaterally in the L4, L5, or S1 distribution	The patient may have sensory loss in the associated distribution. There may also be diminished reflexes or motor weakness in the involved area. Will likely have a positive straight leg raise test if caused by disk herniation

(continued)

Table 13-1. Noncritical Diagnoses for a Chief Complaint of Low Back Pain (*Continued*)

Diagnosis	History and Risk Factors	Physical Examination
Disk herniation with radiculopathy	May have history of back pain with an acute exacerbation. Radicular symptoms (sciatica) may be new or chronic. The severity of the neurological symptoms may worsen over time	Decreased sensation or motor deficits usually isolated to a single unilateral dermatome. More than 95% are L4, L5, or S1. Will likely have a positive straight leg raise test
Spinal stenosis	Chronic back pain with a gradual onset. Age typically >60. Pain worse with extension and exertion, relieved with flexion and rest. May have pain radiating down the legs. May have *pseudoclaudication*	May have some diffuse back tenderness. May have pain radiating down the legs and may have chronic motor deficits in the lower extremities
Ankylosing spondylitis	Back pain and stiffness that is worse at night and in the morning but improves throughout the day with mild activity. Gradual onset and chronic. No relief with conservative therapy. Usually males <40	Lumbosacral tenderness to palpation. No neurological changes

3. For an acute exacerbation of chronic low back pain, in the absence of trauma, signs of infection, suspicion for spinal metastases, or new neurological deficits, no imaging is indicated. If trauma is reported, spinal x-ray or CT is indicated. If signs of infection, cauda equina, or new neurological deficit exist, MRI is indicated.

CASE REVIEW

Mr Brick has an uncomplicated acute exacerbation of chronic back pain. Importantly, the patient reports a history of similar occurrences and has no red flags in his history or physical examination. His pain is most likely due to a strain of his paraspinal muscles and a flare-up of his degenerative disease from overuse. No further workup is indicated for Mr Brick in the ED. Management consists of rest and symptomatic relief. A comprehensive management plan includes decreased lifting, stretching exercises, and NSAIDs. Adjuncts to this therapy include muscle relaxers such as cyclobenzaprine and pain medication such as hydrocodone. Importantly, the EM physician should have a discussion regarding the expected course of the disease, the red flags to warrant immediate return to the ED, and preventive strategies for future recurrences. It is also worthwhile to discuss the need for a primary care physician to manage chronic pain.

LOW BACK PAIN WITHOUT RED FLAGS

Diagnostic Reasoning

Low back pain is a frequent chief complaint in the ED. It accounts for 2.3% of all ED visits. Although it is extremely important to maintain vigilance for the potential presence of critical diagnoses, the vast majority of patients who present with low back pain have a noncritical diagnosis. The most common diagnosis is mechanical back pain, and it is usually related to degenerative joint disease, lumbar disk disease, or muscle overuse. Despite the absence of a critical diagnosis, there are still several diagnoses that should be considered, diagnosed, and appropriately managed.

The EM physician should first attempt to determine whether back pain is musculoskeletal (mechanical) in nature, or if it is referred visceral pain. See Case 12 for an explanation of how to make this differentiation. After the EM physician has determined the cause of the back pain to be mechanical, a thorough search for red flags in the history and physical examination should be conducted. Once the back pain is determined to be mechanical and likely noncritical, the next step is determining whether the episode is an acute pain or an exacerbation of chronic pain. This can most easily be ascertained by asking the patient, "Have you ever had pain like this in the past?" If the patient has had back pain in the past, it can be helpful to ask, "In what way is this pain different from prior episodes?" Progression of the symptoms, particularly of neurological symptoms, may alert the EM physician to the need for additional testing. If the patient has stable neurological symptoms, he or she may not require additional workup.

Neurological deficits are always concerning, but if stable, they may not require additional workup. The most commonly affected nerve roots are L4, L5, and S1. See Figure 12-1 for a detailed explanation of the deficits one would expect to see for a given nerve root involvement. For example, a patient with chronic back pain and known right L4 nerve root compression may have numbness over the medial portion of the knee, a diminished patellar reflex, and weakness of knee extension on the right. If the patient is having an exacerbation of pain and the neurological findings are otherwise stable, then no additional imaging is required.

Bilateral neurological deficits, new neurological deficits, or symptoms of cauda equina syndrome will require MRI in most cases.

Diagnostic Workup and Management

A patient with a suspected musculoskeletal source of back pain and no red flags in the history or physical examination may require no additional workup. The most common clinical diagnosis given for low back pain in the ED is *nonspecific low back pain*. Management is directed at the symptoms. Depending on the degree of pain, IV or oral opioids may be indicated. NSAIDs such as ketorolac and ibuprofen may also be helpful. Adjuncts such as cyclobenzaprine and benzodiazepines are helpful if the patient has significant muscle spasms. Stretching routines can also play an important role in both resolution of the exacerbation and the prevention of recurrence. Workup and management for specific causes of noncritical mechanical low back pain are described below.

Disk herniation with radiculopathy. Although the diagnosis can be suspected clinically, a nonemergent MRI is required to confirm the diagnosis of nerve root impingement. MRI is not indicated in the emergent setting unless the neurological deficits are severe (paralysis), bilateral, involving more than 1 nerve root, or progressive in nature. Additionally, if there is reason to suspect fracture, tumor, hematoma, or infection, imaging should be obtained. Treatment is conservative and includes opioid analgesia, NSAIDs, and muscle relaxers. Stretches and mild physical activity are also important. Corticosteroids, although frequently used, have limited efficacy. Local heat and massage therapy may also provide some benefit. Regarding education, the patient should be instructed to follow up with primary care in 1 month for reevaluation. If the symptoms persist, an MRI and physical therapy may be indicated. The patient should be informed that about 80% of patients with a herniated disc recover with conservative therapy. If there is no resolution after 6 weeks, the patient will likely be referred to orthopedics for further evaluation.

Spinal stenosis can occur in multiple areas of the lumbar spine. The symptoms are dependent on the areas that are affected by the narrowing. A clinical diagnosis can be made if you have chronic pain in an elderly patient, with or without radiculopathy, that is worse with extension and relieved by flexion. CT can confirm the diagnosis, but an MRI will provide more information on the extent of the nerve compression. Management includes opioids and NSAIDs. The patient should be informed that the pain is unlikely to resolve on its own. Surgical referral may be beneficial.

Ankylosing spondylitis is an autoimmune cause of low back pain. It is unique in that it most commonly affects younger patients. Stiffness is a prominent feature. There are rarely neurological changes. Plain x-ray or CT of the lumbar spine is likely to reveal sacroiliitis and a square-like appearance to the lumbar vertebrae, referred to as "bamboo spine." This chronic condition requires pain control with opioids or NSAIDs and referral to a rheumatologist.

Degenerative joint disease is typically the result of mechanical wear and tear on the articular surfaces of the lumbar vertebrae. It is fairly nonspecific, but it may contribute to the development of lumbar disk disease, spondylolisthesis, compression fractures, and spinal stenosis. The pain is chronic, and unlikely to resolve. Plain x-rays or CT may reveal osteophytes, ragged joint surfaces, or mild spondylolisthesis. Pain control can be achieved with NSAIDs and opioids. The EM physician should provide education as to the chronic nature of the pain and the need for a primary care physician to manage chronic pain.

Compression fractures can be acute or chronic. A compression fracture in a young, healthy patient is nearly always a traumatic event. These fractures can be stable or unstable. Compression fracture in an elderly patient may occur as a result of minor or unnoticed trauma. Such fractures are usually stable. The pain is localized to the affected vertebral body and can be severe. Plain x-ray or CT confirms the diagnosis. Pain can be controlled with opioids or NSAIDs. Unstable compression fractures require urgent neurosurgical consultation and admission. Stable compression fractures can be discharged if the pain can be controlled; however, some patients require admission for pain control and due to compromised mobility.

TIPS TO REMEMBER

- Every patient with low back pain, regardless of the duration of symptoms or the number of ED visits, requires an exploration of red flags in the history and physical examination.
- A patient with back pain and stable focal neurological changes does not necessarily need imaging.
- Back stretches, exercise, heat, and muscle massage are very important adjuncts to pharmacotherapy in acute exacerbations of chronic back pain.
- Patient education on the expected course of mechanical low back pain will decrease unnecessary return visits to the ED.
- The EM physician should have a discussion about proper chronic pain management with a patient presenting with chronic pain.

COMPREHENSION QUESTIONS

1. A patient presents with low back pain radiating to the left leg. Which of the following sets of findings is consistent with an isolated L5 nerve root compression?
     A. Numbness over the left lateral calf, inability to heel walk, inability to dorsiflex the left first toe
     B. Numbness over the left medial calf, inability to heel walk, diminished left Achilles reflex
     C. Weakness to extension of the left knee, diminished left patellar reflex
     D. Saddle numbness, urinary retention

2. A 58-year-old male presents with a chief complaint of low back pain for 3 months. He reports no radiation down the legs. He has no neurological symptoms. He has no history of cancer, no trauma, and no symptoms of infection. He reports the pain to be worse with back extension and relieved with bending forward. When he walks for a long time, he develops aching in the lower extremities that is relieved with rest. His neurological examination is normal. With what diagnosis are his symptoms most consistent?

    A. Degenerative joint disease
    B. Ankylosing spondylitis
    C. Spinal stenosis
    D. Compression fracture

Answers

1. A. L5 nerve root compression is likely to cause numbness or pain over the lateral calf, diminished dorsiflexion of the foot and first toe, and difficulty with heel walking.

2. C. His history is most consistent with spinal stenosis based on the chronicity, relief with flexion, and pseudoclaudication. He is young for this disorder, but on consideration of his entire symptom complex, spinal stenosis is most likely.

SUGGESTED READINGS

Marx JA, Hockberger RS, Walls RM, eds. *Rosen's Emergency Medicine: Concepts and Clinical Practice.* 7th ed. Philadelphia: Mosby-Elsevier; 2010 [chapter 28] <http://www.mdconsult.com>.
Tintinalli JE, Kelen GD, Stapczynski JS, Ma OJ, Cline DM, eds. *Tintinalli's Emergency Medicine.* 7th ed. New York: McGraw-Hill Education; 2011 [chapters 168, 255, 276].

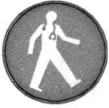

An 84-year-old Male Becomes Unresponsive

James R. Waymack, MD

CASE DESCRIPTION

Mr Brown, an 84-year-old male with a history of hypertension and coronary artery disease, is brought back immediately from the ED waiting room with a complaint of substernal chest pressure for the past 2 hours that radiates down his left arm. You proceed to the room and see that he is in moderate distress secondary to the pain, diaphoretic, and clutching his chest. While the nurse is placing the patient on the monitor and the procedural technician is placing electrodes for a 12-lead EKG, the patient suddenly becomes unresponsive.

1. Describe the initial steps in caring for an abruptly unresponsive patient?

2. Identify ventricular fibrillation (VF) and other life-threatening arrhythmias?

3. What are possible precipitants of VF?

4. What immediate interventions are required for VF?

Answers

1. It is important to assess that the patient is in fact completely unresponsive; quickly check the ABCs and consider the clinical context of the patient's presentation.

2. VF is an irregular, disorganized ventricular rhythm. It is manifested clinically by unresponsiveness and cardiovascular collapse because there is no cardiac output.

3. Possible causes or precipitants of VF include coronary artery disease, drug toxicity, hypoxemia, and electrolyte disturbances.

4. Immediate defibrillation followed by CPR should begin if the patient is unresponsive and pulseless. The "safety net" should be implemented and CPR should be continuous. Repeat cardioversion and antiarrhythmic administration per ACLS guidelines as well as addressing possible precipitants are the definitive care.

CASE REVIEW

Mr Brown's presentation as a patient with known cardiac disease, his symptom of chest pain, and signs of diaphoresis are concerning for cardiac ischemia. His deterioration to unresponsiveness with this clinical presentation suggests that he was most likely having a myocardial infarction that precipitated a cardiac dysrhythmia. The safety net should be put into place and cardiopulmonary resuscitation started once it is determined that he is pulseless. After the diagnosis of a dysrhythmia is made, appropriate treatment such as defibrillation and antiarrythmic medication administration should be completed. This patient will require consultation with an interventional cardiologist and medical intensivist for possible percutaneous intervention and further evaluation and treatment, respectively.

UNRESPONSIVE PATIENT

Diagnostic Reasoning

When a patient presents or acutely becomes unresponsive, the differential diagnosis you must consider is very broad. It is helpful to always use a systematic approach to ensure all possibilities are considered and to guide your assessment and diagnostic approach. The mnemonic AEIOU TIPS is a useful guide for the evaluation of the unresponsive patient (see Table 14-1).

The evaluation and treatment of the unresponsive patient occur simultaneously. The safety net must be enacted and the ABCs assessed immediately. While the patient is being placed on supplemental oxygen and a cardiac monitor with pulse oximetry, and intravenous access is being obtained, the physician should quickly confirm unresponsiveness, and check for respirations and a pulse. If the patient is not in cardiac arrest but has respiratory compromise, the airway and ventilation may need to be controlled with maneuvers such as jaw thrust or chin lift, an oral airway, or bag valve mask ventilation. If there is not adequate breathing or circulation, then cardiopulmonary resuscitation must be started while the etiology and treatment of the patient's unresponsiveness concurrently occurs. Dysrhythmias such as ventricular tachycardia (VT) or VF are often identified at the first pulse check. While it is often overlooked in an intense situation such as resuscitation, a full set of vital signs including temperature should be obtained so that causes of unresponsiveness such as hypothermia or hyperthermia are identified quickly.

There will be little time available for obtaining a history and performing a physical examination. If the patient has arrived via EMS, they may provide some information as far as past medical history, medications, preceding events, amount of time the patient has been down, and responses to any interventions that they have performed. Family may also be present or arrive later and could contribute to the history of the patient's situation.

Historical information may suggest the cause of the patient's unresponsiveness, such as alcohol ingestion, medication overdose, or illicit drug use. A focused physical examination may reveal an odor suggesting alcohol ingestion, cyanide toxicity (bitter almonds), or diabetic ketoacidosis (fruity). Specific toxidromes such as opioid, sympathomimetic, cholinergic, and anticholinergic can be identified on the physical examination. Focal neurologic findings such as hemiparesis or failure to withdraw extremities to pain may suggest intracranial bleeding or a space-occupying lesion.

Table 14-1. Mnemonic AEIOU TIPS Guide for Evaluation of the Unresponsive Patient

A	Alcohols (ethanol, isopropyl, methanol ethylene glycol)
E	Endocrine—myxedema coma, thyrotoxicosis
	Electrolytes—hyponatremia, hypernatremia, hypokalemia, and hyperkalemia
	Encephalopathy—hyperammonemia or carbon dioxide narcosis
I	Insulin—hypoglycemia, diabetic ketoacidosis, and nonketotic hyperosmolar state
O	Oxygen—hypoxemia or other disorders of respiration such as carbon monoxide, methemoglobinemia, or cyanide toxicity
U	Uremia
T	Toxidromes—anticholinergic, sympathomimetic, opioid, cholinergic, sedative hypnotic
	Trauma—intracranial hemorrhage or hemorrhagic shock
	Temperature—hypothermia, heat stroke, malignant hyperthermia, and neuroleptic malignant syndrome
I	Infection—sepsis and bacterial meningitis
P	Psychiatric—diagnosis of exclusion
	Porphyria
	Pharmacy—TCA, SSRI, lithium or salicylate toxicity
S	Space-occupying lesion
	Subarachnoid hemorrhage
	Stroke

Once the patient is placed on a cardiac monitor and pulse oximetry, causes of unresponsiveness such as hypoxemia or arrhythmia may be identified. Bedside glucose measurement may identify hypoglycemia or hyperglycemic causes as well and should be obtained as soon as possible on every unresponsive patient regardless of reported prehospital glucose measurements. Other point-of-care testing in the emergency department is becoming more widely available and can be invaluable in the rapid assessment of the unresponsive patient. Components of point-of-care testing can include hematocrit, lactic acid, electrolytes, creatinine, blood gas, and carbon monoxide measurement.

Further laboratory tests might include a complete blood count, complete metabolic profile, alcohol, magnesium, and cardiac markers. Urinalysis and urine toxicology may be helpful and a urine pregnancy should be obtained on all females of potential childbearing age. If there is a return of spontaneous circulation, a 12-lead EKG would be indicated to search for ischemic patterns, heart blocks, or drug toxicity. A chest radiograph would also be indicated to confirm endotracheal tube position if the patient is intubated and to assess for pneumothorax or other pulmonary processes. If there was possible head trauma or intracranial process such as intracranial hemorrhage or space-occupying lesion is suspected as the cause of unresponsiveness, computed tomography of the head should be ordered.

Diagnostic Workup and Management

VF is the totally disorganized depolarization and contraction of small areas of ventricular myocardium, and because of this there is no effective cardiac pumping activity. This erratic ventricular activity may be due to prolonged hypoxemia, myocardial ischemia, drug toxicity, electrolyte abnormality, or myocardial irritation from pacemaker leads or an intracardiac catheter. Defibrillation is performed to spontaneously depolarize the entire myocardium and allow the intrinsic pacemaker of the heart to resume in a more organized rhythm.

When a patient becomes unresponsive, it is imperative to see if arousal occurs by sternal rub or deep pressure on the fingernails. Next, assessment of airway, breathing, and circulation is necessary by looking, listening, and feeling for respiration and checking a carotid pulse. If the patient is found to be apneic and pulseless, immediate CPR must be started with high-quality chest compressions and bag valve mask ventilation. In the case presented it is very likely the patient is experiencing VF because of his history of coronary artery disease and possible acute myocardial ischemia; therefore, defibrillation is indicated as soon as possible. If the defibrillator is biphasic, the energy selected would be 200 J and if monophasic, it would be 360 J, which are the maximum settings. The quicker a patient receives defibrillation, the more likely it is to be successful. Chest compressions should be resumed immediately after the first defibrillation if there is no sign of organized cardiac activity. The antiarrhythmic medication of choice is 300 mg of amiodarone intravenously. Cardiopulmonary resuscitation can be continued and epinephrine can be given 1 mg IV push every 5 minutes. If VF persists and resuscitation continues, endotracheal intubation may be necessary.

When addressing possible precipitating events, it is important to keep a differential for VF in mind. If there is a return of spontaneous circulation, a 12-lead electrocardiogram may suggest acute myocardial ischemia and the patient may require angioplasty or thrombolytics. Routine laboratory studies would be indicated such as a complete blood count, complete metabolic profile, cardiac markers, and urine toxicology. Serum magnesium is often not part of a routine panel and may have to be specifically requested. Laboratory results will not be immediately available; so if there is clinical suspicion of an underlying cause, treatment must be started before laboratory confirmation. If point-of-care testing is available, critical values such as potassium may be available more quickly.

Other cardiac arrhythmias require rapid identification and treatment. If a rapid wide complex tachycardia suggestive of VT is identified, it must first be determined if there is a pulse present. If there is no pulse, management is similar to VF. If a pulse is palpable, you must determine if the patient is stable or unstable. A patient is considered unstable if there is altered mental status, chest pain, dyspnea, or signs of shock. If the patient is determined to be unstable, immediate intervention must be performed to terminate the arrhythmia. The safety net should be established, including IV access, and mild sedation given if the patient can tolerate it before synchronized cardioversion is performed. Energy for biphasic cardioversion may be started at 120 to 150 and 200 J for monophasic cardioversion. When a wide complex tachycardia fails to convert on the initial attempt, cardioversion can be repeated with increasing energy levels to a maximum of 200 J for biphasic or 360 J for monophasic. Consideration should also be given to starting antiarrhythmic medication such as amiodarone at 300 mg IV for the unstable patient. During the resuscitation and cardioversion of the patient with a wide complex tachycardia constant attention must be paid to the ABCs and anticipation that the rhythm may deteriorate to VF or pulseless electrical activity (PEA).

If the patient with a wide complex tachycardia is determined to be stable, the rhythm should be further analyzed to determine appropriate treatment. If the rhythm is regular, an antiarrhythmic medication such as amiodarone may be administered at a dose of 150 mg IV. If the rhythm is thought to be SVT with aberrancy (because of the patient's age being younger or subtle EKG findings such as fusion beats or escape sinus beats), a trial of adenosine may be given. If the rhythm is believed to be atrial fibrillation with aberrancy because it is irregular, rate control can be achieved with an AV nodal blocking agent such as diltiazem or beta-blockers. If there is any uncertainty, the wide complex tachycardia should be treated like VT. When torsades de pointes is encountered, the patient should be treated with IV magnesium at a dose of 1 to 2 g over 2 minutes and then an infusion begun at 1 to 2 g/h. Resistant VT may also be precipitated by cardiac ischemia and urgent percutaneous coronary intervention should be considered if this rhythm is encountered.

When the patient is found to be in a narrow complex tachycardia, it is helpful to determine if the patient is stable or unstable first, just as in the management of a patient with a wide complex tachycardia. When the rhythm is a regular narrow complex tachycardia, it is considered to be supra-VT. If the patient is stable, vagal maneuvers such as unilateral carotid massage or Valsalva may be attempted to cease the rhythm while the safety net is being established and a 12-lead EKG is being obtained. If vagal maneuvers are unsuccessful, adenosine may be given at an initial dose of 6 mg rapid IV push through a large-bore antecubital or external jugular IV. This administration is necessary due to the short half-life of adenosine. If the first dose is unsuccessful, 1 or 2 repeat doses may be given of 12 mg apiece. If AV nodal blocking with adenosine fails, the patient may be given diltiazem or a beta-blocker to slow AV node conduction. If the rhythm does convert with adenosine, underlying causes should be investigated such as cardiac ischemia, pulmonary embolus, electrolyte abnormalities, or thyroid disease. Often though, the cause of SVT is intrinsic to the conduction system of the heart and further monitoring and cardiology referral may be necessary for recurrent episodes.

If the patient has a narrow complex tachycardia and is found to be irregular once the 12-lead EKG is obtained, rhythms other than SVT should be suspected such as atrial fibrillation, atrial flutter, or multifocal atrial tachycardia. When these rhythms are suspected, the patient should be placed on a medication that slows conduction through the AV node such as diltiazem or a beta-blocker. Diltiazem is often the drug of choice for these arrhythmias and is given initially as a bolus of 10 to 20 mg IV followed by an infusion at 10 to 20 mg/h. The infusion should be titrated to a heart rate less than 100 beats/min. When these medications are started, the patient's blood pressure should be closely monitored for hypotension; IV fluid boluses may be required to prevent it. If the onset of the symptoms has occurred within the last 48 hours, consultation with a cardiologist should be obtained and the patient may be cardioverted to a sinus rhythm. If the onset cannot be determined, the patient should not be urgently cardioverted as there is concern that an atrial thrombus may have formed and could embolize to the systemic circulation if the patient were to return to a sinus rhythm. In this case the patient should be admitted to the hospital for anticoagulation and monitoring prior to cardioversion at a later time.

Another concern for the unresponsive patient is bradycardia. If the heart rate is less than 60 beats/min, the safety net should be established and assessment of perfusion should be performed. If there is adequate perfusion and the patient is comfortable, a 12-lead EKG should be obtained, the patient monitored, and further etiology of the bradycardia, if any, should be determined. Sinus bradycardia and first- or second-degree Type 1 Mobitz AV blocks often do not cause a patient to be unstable. These patients should be monitored closely and cardiology consultation obtained for further evaluation and follow-up. Patients who have a more severe AV block such as a second-degree Type 2 Mobitz or third degree should be admitted to the hospital with urgent cardiology consultation as they often require pacemaker placement.

If the patient has signs of inadequate perfusion such as altered mental status, chest pain, hypotension, or signs of shock, immediate action should be taken to improve the patient's cardiac output. While the safety net is being implemented, a 12-lead EKG should be obtained and cardiac pacing pads placed on the patient's chest. Once IV access is obtained, atropine can be given at a dose of 0.5 mg up to a total dose of 3 mg. If the response to atropine is temporary or unsuccessful, the patient should be transcutaneously paced and cardiology consultation obtained for placement of an emergent pacemaker. Epinephrine at 2 to 10 mcg/min or dopamine at 2 to 10 mcg/kg/min may also be administered to increase the heart rate. Transcutaneous pacing can be uncomfortable for the patient; therefore, light sedation with midazolam and pain control with fentanyl should be administered while monitoring the patient's ABCs. If an emergent pacemaker cannot be placed or prolonged transport times are faced, central venous access should be secured and a transvenous pacer placed.

If the unresponsive patient is found to have a rhythm on the monitor but be pulseless, the patient has PEA. If there is no electrical activity on the monitor, the rhythm is asystole. The management of PEA and asystole are similar and do not include defibrillation. In this case CPR should be started immediately while the safety net is established. Once IV access is established, epinephrine should be given at a dose of 1 mg every 3 to 5 minutes. High-quality CPR should be performed with minimal interruptions, only a pulse check every 2 minutes. Ventilation should initially be performed with a bag valve mask and an advanced airway placed if the resuscitation is prolonged. Causes of PEA should be considered and addressed while the resuscitation is continuing. Helpful reminders of the etiologies of PEA are the H's and T's (see Table 14-2). If during a pulse check, a rhythm on the monitor that can be defibrillated is identified (such as VF or VT), then defibrillation should be performed immediately and CPR resumed. CPR should only be stopped if the team has determined that their efforts have been unsuccessful, or if the patient regains consciousness or a perfusing rhythm. Determining when to discontinue the resuscitation can be difficult and multifactorial. Consideration should be made to the total down time of the patient, the patient's age and comorbidities, as well as likelihood for a meaningful recovery. Bedside ultrasound and end-tidal carbon dioxide monitoring may be helpful in determining when to stop CPR. If cardiac standstill is found on ultrasound or end-tidal carbon dioxide is less than 10 after 10 to 15 minutes of CPR, the likelihood for recovery is very low.

Table 14-2. Causes of PEA (The H's and T's)

Hypovolemia	Toxins
Hypoxia	Tamponade, cardiac
Hypokalemia/hyperkalemia	Tension pneumothorax
Hypoglycemia	Thrombosis (MI)
Hypothermia	Thrombosis (PE)
Hydrogen ion (acidosis)	Trauma

If drug toxicity is suspected, testing results would not be available immediately; therefore, intervention must be undertaken based on clinical suspicion and evidence. If there is a history of digoxin use and symptoms or EKG findings suggestive of digoxin toxicity such as a bradycardic wide-complex rhythm with scooped ST segments, digoxin immune Fab would be indicated. Correction of other electrolyte abnormalities such as hypomagnesemia with 2 g of magnesium intravenously or hyperkalemia with 10 U of regular insulin IV, 10 ml of 10% solution (0.4 meq/ml) of calcium gluconate IV, and 50 ml of 8.4% solution (1 meq/ml) of sodium bicarbonate may also be indicated.

TIPS TO REMEMBER

- A single precordial thump may be performed prior to beginning CPR if no defibrillator is at hand.
- Fine VF may be mistaken for asystole, which has a different management, that is, defibrillation is not indicated.
- If fine VF is suspected, check another cardiac monitor lead or give a trial defibrillation.
- Immediate defibrillation is key to optimizing the success of termination of the VF and having a return of spontaneous circulation.
- High-quality CPR is defined as chest compressions at a rate of 100/min with a depth of 1.5 to 2 in allowing for chest recoil after each compression and minimizing interruptions to less than 10 seconds.
- Endotracheal intubation is not immediately required.

COMPREHENSION QUESTIONS

1. A patient you are caring for suddenly becomes unresponsive and you suspect VF on the cardiac monitor. You begin CPR and call for help. You tell the ED nurse you would like to defibrillate and the ED nurse asks you what settings you would like on your biphasic defibrillator. You answer which of the following?
    A. Synchronized at 100 J
    B. Synchronized at 200 J
    C. Unsynchronized at 100 J
    D. Unsynchronized at 200 J

2. You defibrillate the patient at the correct energy level; however, VF is still present. What is your next action?
    A. Defibrillate again.
    B. Perform a pulse check.
    C. Endotracheal intubation.
    D. Continue high-quality CPR.

3. While continuing with your resuscitation, the nurse gives 1 mg of epinephrine IV per ACLS guidelines and asks you if there is any other medication you would like to give. Administration of what other drug is indicated in VF?
   A. Narcan 2 mg IV
   B. Atropine 0.5 mg IV
   C. Amiodarone 300 mg IV
   D. Metoprolol 25 mg IV

Answers

1. D. Synchronized cardioversion is not indicated when attempting to terminate the unorganized rhythm of VF. Synchronized cardioversion is usually at a lower energy level, 25 to 50 J, and is used to treat tachyarrhythmias or VT with a pulse. Unsynchronized cardioversion defibrillation with escalating energy levels is no longer indicated so the highest level should be used, 200 J with a biphasic defibrillator and 360 J with a monophasic.

2. D. If there is no immediate change in rhythm, 5 cycles of CPR should be performed. Stacked or multiple shocks are no longer recommended. If there is not an organized rhythm on the monitor, a pulse check is not indicated. Endotracheal intubation is not immediately necessary during the resuscitation; however, someone should be readying equipment if the resuscitation will be prolonged.

3. C. Besides epinephrine and defibrillation an antiarrhythmic medication is needed and amiodarone is the first choice. Lidocaine 1.5 mg/kg may also be used. Atropine is no longer recommended for the treatment of VF. Narcan and metoprolol would not be helpful in this situation.

SUGGESTED READINGS

American Heart Association. Sinz E, Navarro K, Soderberg ES, eds. *Advanced Cardiovascular Life Support: Provider Manual.* 2011.
Tintinalli JE, Kelen GD, Stapczynski JS, Ma OJ, Cline DM, eds. *Tintinalli's Emergency Medicine.* 7th ed. New York: McGraw-Hill Education; 2011 [chapter 22] <http://www.accessmedicine.com>.

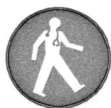

A 21-year-old Female With a Reported Overdose

Quoc V. Pham, MD and Ted R. Clark, MD, MPP

CASE DESCRIPTION

Sandy Baker is a 21-year-old previously healthy female who presents to the ED by private vehicle. The patient was brought in by friends due to a suspicion that the patient took an overdose in an attempt to kill herself. The history is difficult to obtain due to the patient being uncooperative. The history from EMS and from friends is that the patient has recently been depressed and tearful. Today she sent text messages to friends that said she was going to "end it all" about 1 hour prior to arrival. EMS states they found 2 empty 30-pill bottles of extra-strength (500 mg) acetaminophen in the room in which the patient had locked herself. The patient will not admit to an ingestion, but does report an upset stomach.

Her vitals are temperature 37.1 (98.8), blood pressure 120/70 mm Hg, pulse 80 beats/min, respiratory rate 16 breaths/min, and oxygen saturation of 98% on room air.

On physical examination, the patient is alert but tearful and with flat affect. She has a normal cardiovascular, pulmonary, abdominal, and neurological examination. She has no evidence of a toxidrome.

1. In addition to the ABCs, what are the immediate considerations in an overdose patient?

2. Does this patient need GI decontamination?

3. Does this patient need a specific antidote?

Answers

1. With regard to history, it is important to try to determine what the patient ingested. If the patient is not cooperative with history, alternate history may be available from family, friends, police, and EMS. The time of ingestion is also important, as this may affect the decision to perform GI decontamination. With regard to history, the physician should search for signs of the common toxidromes. Finally, the physician should consider the use of specific antidotes.

2. There are many forms of GI decontamination. Currently, the most commonly employed method of GI decontamination is activated charcoal. Activated charcoal is indicated if there is a patient with a significant ingestion of a substance that absorbs charcoal who presents within 1 to 2 hours. The major

contraindication to activated charcoal use is altered mental status (unless intubated and delivered by orogastric tube). According to the information we have available, Ms Baker likely took an overdose of acetaminophen approximately 1 hour prior to arrival. Since acetaminophen is readily absorbed by charcoal, its use is indicated in this patient.

3. There are several specific antidotes that are used for overdoses. In fact, "antidotes" can be thought of as an additional "A" in the ABCs for patients with toxicological exposures. The antidote for an acetaminophen overdose is N-acetylcysteine (NAC). The action and specific indications for NAC use are discussed in more detail below. Ms Baker will most likely receive NAC to prevent the toxic effects of acetaminophen overdose.

CASE REVIEW

Ms Baker most likely ingested a toxic amount of acetaminophen. Although she is currently asymptomatic, she may need NAC therapy to prevent liver failure. The safety net should be established, and a basic toxicological workup, including CBC, CMP, acetaminophen level, aspirin level, EKG, UA, UPT, and urine drug screen, should be ordered. Additional more specific tests such as toxic alcohol levels are ordered if there is suspicion of a certain toxin. Ms Baker should also receive activated charcoal because the time of ingestion appears to be about 1 hour prior to arrival. The decision to start NAC in this patient can be based on either the amount taken (if known) or the 4-hour acetaminophen level. The 4-hour level is plotted on the Rumack-Matthew nomogram (see Figure 15-1). In general, if the 4-hour level is >150 µg/mL, the patient should receive NAC. Also, because this appears to be a suicide attempt, the patient cannot leave the ED, involuntary psychiatric hold papers must be completed, and the patient should receive psychiatric screening.

ACETAMINOPHEN OVERDOSE

Diagnostic Reasoning

Collecting an accurate history is very important in the workup of a patient with a suspected overdose. The history and physical examination can be difficult at times due to the patient's mental status or willingness to cooperate. The EM physician must utilize all sources of information to get the most accurate history possible. EMS, police, and family can be very helpful resources. EMS and police can provide information such as pill bottles that were present, other information regarding the scene of the overdose, and any mental status changes that occurred during transportation. Family members can provide similar information, as well as information regarding PMH, a medication list, onset of ingestion, or history of

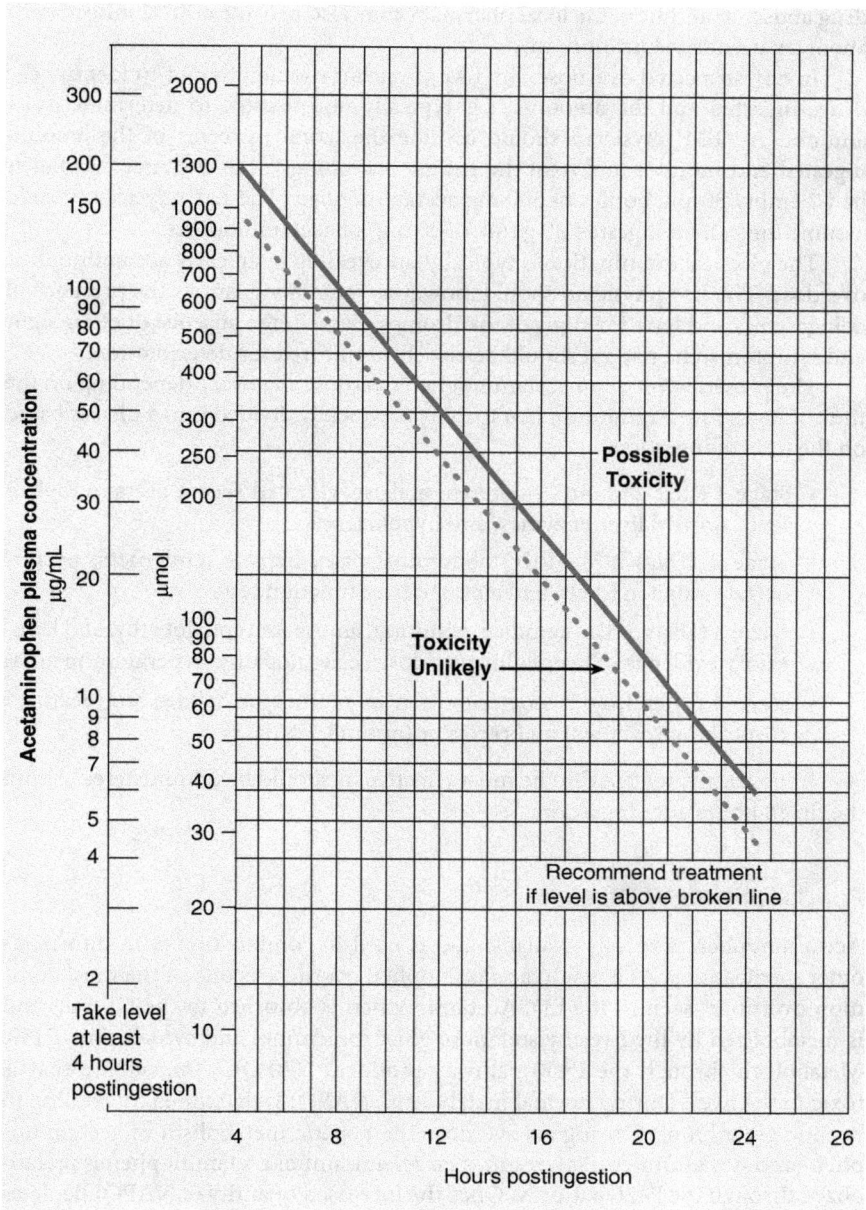

Figure 15-1. Rumack-Matthew nomogram. (From Tintinalli JE, Stapczynski JS, Ma OJ, Cline DM, Meckler GD. *Tintinalli's Emergency Medicine: A Comprehensive Study Guide.* 8th ed. New York: McGraw-Hill; 2012 [Figure 184-2] <www.accessemergencymedicine. com>. Copyright © The McGraw-Hill Companies, Inc. All rights reserved)

drug abuse. In addition, the local pharmacy may also provide crucial information about a patient's medication list.

In any suspected overdose, the EM physician should attempt to identify the drugs ingested and the amount. It is typically not possible to determine exact amount. An EM physician should assume the worst in terms of the amount ingested and monitor and treat the patient accordingly. For instance, Ms Baker had 2 empty 30-pill bottles of 500 mg acetaminophen. The EM physician should assume the patient ingested 30 g (60×500 mg) of acetaminophen.

The physical examination is typically unrevealing in an early acetaminophen overdose. The EM physician should, however, remain vigilant to the presence of coingestants and look for signs of toxidromes. Even in the absence of other signs and symptoms, the patient should be closely monitored for deterioration.

The presentation of an acetaminophen overdose may vary depending on the time of ingestion. Acetaminophen toxicity is typically divided into 4 phases based on the time of ingestion.

- Stage 1 (first 24 hours)—nausea, malaise, elevated serum acetaminophen level, normal liver enzymes, and hypokalemia
- Stage 2 (Days 2-3)—RUQ abdominal pain, hepatic tenderness, normal acetaminophen levels, and elevated liver function tests
- Stage 3 (Days 3-4)—jaundice, vomiting, anuria, encephalopathy, and laboratory evidence of liver failure (acidosis, coagulopathy, hyperammonemia)
- Stage 4 (after Day 5)—deterioration to multiorgan failure and death or clinical improvement and recovery (around 7-8 days)

Importantly, for NAC to be most effective, it should be administered within the first 8 hours after ingestion.

Fundamentals of Disease

Acetaminophen is readily available and is used in combination with numerous other medications. As a result, acetaminophen overdose is one of the most common overdoses seen in the ED. Acetaminophen is absorbed in the GI tract and is metabolized by the liver by sulfation, glucuronidation, and cytochrome P450. Metabolism through the P450 pathway produces NAPQI, a metabolite that is toxic to the liver. During normal metabolism, NAPQI is detoxified by binding to hepatic glutathione. During an overdose the hepatic metabolism of acetaminophen becomes saturated. As a result, a larger amount of acetaminophen is metabolized through the P450 pathway. Once the increased quantity of NAPQI depletes the glutathione stores, hepatic damage occurs (see Figure 15-2). NAC works by increasing the quantity of glutathione in the liver to process NAPQI to a harmless metabolite. If given within 8 hours of ingestion, NAC is nearly 100% effective in preventing liver failure.

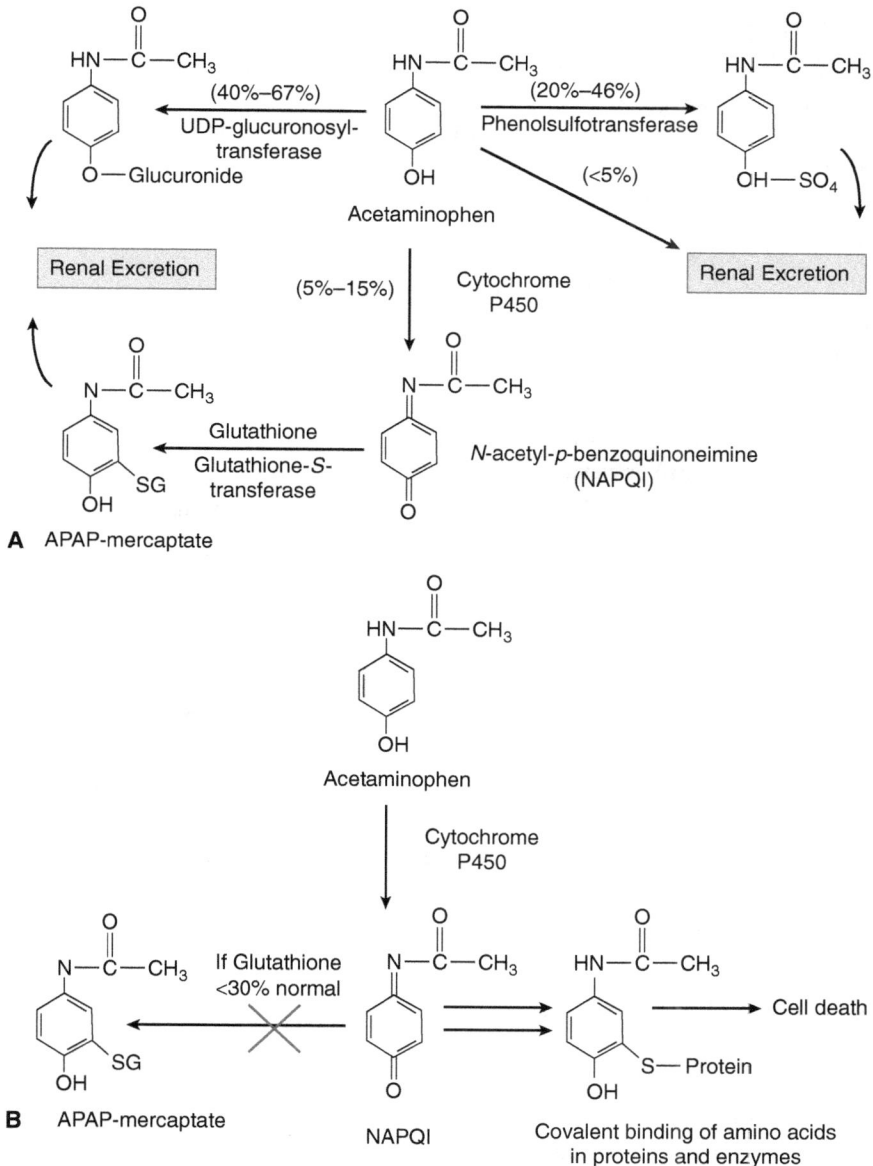

Figure 15-2. Acetaminophen metabolism. (From Tintinalli JE, Stapczynski JS, Ma OJ, Cline DM, Meckler GD. *Tintinalli's Emergency Medicine: A Comprehensive Study Guide.* 8th ed. New York: McGraw-Hill; 2012 [Figure 184-1] <www.accessemergencymedicine.com>. Copyright © The McGraw-Hill Companies, Inc. All rights reserved)

Diagnostic Workup and Management

After the safety net has been established, an acute acetaminophen overdose is fairly easy to manage. Activated charcoal should be administered if the ingestion occurred within 2 hours of arrival. NAC should be administered for acute acetaminophen overdose in the following instances:

- A 4-hour serum acetaminophen level >150 μg/mL
- A single ingestion >200 mg/kg or 10 g

Indications for NAC become more difficult in a chronic overdose or ingestion of unknown time. NAC should be administered for suspected chronic or indeterminate acetaminophen toxicity in the following instances:

- Ingestion of >150 mg/kg or 6 g on 2 consecutive days
- Suspected ingestion of unknown timing with elevated acetaminophen level (>10 μg/mL) or elevated liver enzymes
- A story/evidence of a significant ingestion of unknown timing

After the charcoal and NAC are administered, the patient should be admitted for continued NAC therapy, supportive care, and psychiatric evaluation.

TIPS TO REMEMBER

- Acetaminophen is present in many medications and is a common toxin in both intentional and unintentional overdoses.
- Activated charcoal should be used in any suspected overdose that presents to the ED within 2 hours.
- NAC should be administered for acetaminophen toxicity when the 4-hour level is >150 μg/mL.
- Patients with intentional overdose need a psychiatric consultation.

COMPREHENSION QUESTIONS

1. What is the toxic dose for a single ingestion of acetaminophen?

2. Approximately how long after a toxic ingestion of acetaminophen do you expect to see liver enzyme elevation?

3. How does NAC work?

Answers

1. >200 mg/kg or 10 g.

2. >24 hours.

3. NAC prevents liver toxicity by providing cofactors for the metabolism of NAPQI to nontoxic metabolites. In addition, it may mitigate liver cell destruction by acting as an antioxidant.

SUGGESTED READING

Tintinalli JE, Kelen GD, Stapczynski JS, Ma OJ, Cline DM, eds. *Tintinalli's Emergency Medicine*. 7th ed. New York: McGraw-Hill; 2011 [chapter 184] <http://www.accessmedicine.com>.

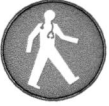

A 3-week-old Male With a Fever

Myto Duong, MB, BCh, BAO
and Erica J. Cacioppo, MD

CASE DESCRIPTION

Stevie is a 3-week-old uncircumcised Caucasian male who is brought into the emergency department by his parents at 8:00 PM. His mother states he has had a rectal temperature of 38.2°C (100.8°F) since this morning and only had 3 wet diapers after drinking 2 bottles (8 oz) of formula all day. Mom had to wake him up for his feedings overnight. The baby appears to have decreased alertness and is flushed and warm to touch. The parents deny any sick contacts or travel and state that the baby was born at 38 weeks' gestation via a normal spontaneous vaginal delivery. Mom had the normal prenatal care and labs. There were no complications, and he was discharged home with his mother after 2 days in the hospital. He has not been coughing or vomiting, nor had any change in bowel movements.

His heart rate is 164 bpm with a respiratory rate of 56 breaths/min. Temperature is 38°C. During the examination, the baby is crying and irritable but consolable. No bulging or flattening of the fontanelles is noted, nor are any rashes seen on examination. There is no erythema or bulging of the tympanic membranes; oral mucosa is mildly dry; no pharyngeal erythema or exudates are appreciated. His lungs are clear with no evidence of retractions, but he is breathing rapidly. No murmurs are heard during the cardiac examination. His crying seems to increase during palpation of the lower quadrants of the abdomen, but no masses or hernias are felt. (It is really difficult to tell if a 3-week-old crying has increased or not, and if the child has been crying a lot, the abdomen often looks distended from air in the stomach. If the child is crying during the examination, you may be easily fooled into thinking that he has guarding; 1 trick is to bend the knees and hips up to relax the rectus muscles and palpate the abdomen this way.) External genitalia are normal.

1. What is the differential diagnosis for a febrile neonate/child?

2. What are the risk factors for a pediatric UTI?

3. How do pediatric patients with a UTI usually present?

4. What findings support a diagnosis of UTI in this patient?

5. Which ancillary tests are indicated?

6. How should a urine sample be obtained?

7. What treatment should this patient receive? Does he need to be admitted?

Answers

1. The differential diagnosis for a febrile child includes meningitis, bacteremia, cellulitis, osteomyelitis, otitis media, pneumonia, urinary tract infection, gastroenteritis, viral syndrome, appendicitis, Kawasaki disease, and retained foreign body.

2. Risk factors include gender, age, circumcision status, race, sexual activity, and previous history of UTI, with 3 times higher risk for UTIs in females, an increased risk in infants and young children, 10 times higher risk in uncircumcised males, and an increased prevalence in sexually active people and those with UTIs in the past. Those at a decreased risk are African American children.

3. See Table 16-1.

4. The patient in this case displays evidence of a febrile illness without an obvious source. His risk factors include age, uncircumcised status, and race. He has not been coughing or displaying URI symptoms, and his lungs are clear on examination making pneumonia or a viral syndrome unlikely. He is irritable and fussy but consolable and interacting appropriately with family and staff despite showing increased fatigue. However, the change in mental status along with age keeps meningitis on the differential despite no evidence of rash, fontanelle bulging, or lethargy. The absence of a rash or skin changes and the ability to move all extremities make cellulitis and osteomyelitis very unlikely.

5. Given the patient's febrile neonatal status (<28 days old), he requires a sepsis workup including CBC, microscopic urinalysis (UA), urine culture, blood culture, and lumbar puncture with CSF cell count, Gram stain, and culture.

6. In a non–toilet-trained patient, a urine sample must be obtained via bladder catheterization in order to obtain a clean sample. The exception to this is if the patient has a genitourinary deformity preventing catheterization in which case suprapubic aspiration would be required. It is not uncommon for the patient

Table 16-1. Usual UTI Presentation by Age

Age	Signs and Symptoms
Infant/nonverbal	High or prolonged fever without a definitive source, prolonged hyperbilirubinemia (uncommon), vomiting, diarrhea, concurrent bronchiolitis
Toddler/verbal	Abdominal pain, back pain, dysuria, polyuria, new-onset enuresis, vomiting, associated with constipation
Adolescent	Dysuria, urinary frequency, urgency, suprapubic pain, flank pain, new-onset sexual activity, vaginal or penile discharge

to void during the preparation for urine catheterization, and a clean catch specimen obtained during this instance is acceptable.

7. This patient shows evidence of dehydration and likely pyelonephritis, with a high risk for bacteremia, meningitis, and encephalitis in this age group. He needs to be admitted for IV antibiotics and rehydration. He should be treated with a total of 2 weeks of antibiotics (IV and PO combined) tailored to his urine culture sensitivities. The patient will also require a renal/bladder ultrasound as either an inpatient or outpatient since this is his first febrile UTI.

CASE REVIEW

Stevie is a neonate with a febrile illness of 1-day duration, Tmax of 100.8°F, and no obvious source of infection. His age, uncircumcised status, and physical examination put him at risk for a UTI and most likely pyelonephritis given the fact that up to 60% of children less than 2 years of age with a UTI are found to have pyelonephritis. In children under 2 years old, pyelonephritis is usually diagnosed based on the presence of a temperature >39°C (102.2°F) and a UA or urine culture with evidence of infection. The child in this case appears ill based on the presence of tachycardia and tachypnea, anorexia, and evidence of dehydration with a history of decreased PO intake and urine output. A UA was obtained via bladder catheterization and found to have positive leukocyte esterase and nitrite with gram-negative rod bacteria seen on Gram stain and 45,000 cfu/mL on urine culture. Of note, the UA may not have nitrites in non–toilet-trained children since the urine is not in the bladder long enough for the by-products of E. coli to form. In fact, 20% of UA may be negative for nitrites but have positive urine cultures 24 to 48 hours later. Based on this information and the fact that he is 21 days old, this child requires admission for a full sepsis workup (including a lumbar puncture), fluid resuscitation, and empiric antibiotics. Prior to discharge, he will need a renal ultrasound to rule out vesicoureteral reflux and hydronephrosis.

PEDIATRIC FEVER

Diagnostic Reasoning

Fever is defined as a core body temperature greater than 38°C (100.4°F) in infants (see Table 16-2). It is responsible for 30% to 40% of pediatric emergency department visits and is the most common chief complaint seen in the pediatric population. In the community, there is a large proportion of parents with "fever phobia" due to misconceptions regarding fever. There are many causes of fever. It is not an illness but a sign or symptom. The physician needs to determine the cause and decide whether or it not it requires workup/treatment. It is a fine balance between doing unnecessary/invasive lab workup with antibiotic overuse promoting multidrug-resistant pathogens and missing life-threatening infections.

Table 16-2. Definitions of Pediatric Fever by Age

Neonate	Birth to 28 days	38°C (100.4°F)
Infant	29 days to 3 months	38°C (100.4°F)
	3 months to 1 year	39°C (102.2°F)
Toddler	1–3 years	39°C (102.2°F)
Child	>3 years	No fixed definition, based on signs and symptoms

The role of the emergency physician is to evaluate the child's severity of illness based on a thorough history and physical examination, including the patient's general appearance, age, severity and duration of the fever, immunization status, activity, and feeding patterns. It is important to clarify the parents' definition of lethargy, which is a term that is often used by parents to describe fatigue, not difficulty arousing the patient (altered mental status). Infants less than 3 months of age are at especially high risk for serious bacterial infections due to an inadequate ability to mount an IgG antibody response to encapsulated bacteria and the fact that they are nonverbal. The clinical examination of neonates (<29 days old) is the least reliable since they sleep the majority of the time. The clinically useful and reassuring social smile does not appear in infancy until 4 to 6 weeks of age. Because of these factors, the physician must maintain a high level of suspicion for a serious bacterial illness until proven otherwise and, therefore, will have to assess for the most common sources of serious febrile illness, specifically urinary tract infection, bacteremia and sepsis, pneumonia, osteomyelitis, and meningitis.

For all febrile children, it is important to determine the source of infection, the age of the child (neonate—<29 days old; young infants are 1-2 months; infants are <12 months), complications of birth (prolonged rupture of membranes) and/or pregnancy (perinatal maternal fever, GBS status, or history of herpes/STDs), and the degree of the fever in order to help determine the type of organism responsible for the infection and the severity of the infection itself. Most pediatric fevers are benign, usually with a localized source of infection, and most likely viral. Higher fevers are more likely caused by bacterial infections. The fever pattern varies with age. For example, a newborn with an infection may present with hypothermia instead of hyperpyrexia (>40°C), which is seen in slightly older children. There are also certain febrile illnesses that are characterized by specific patterns in body temperatures (periodic fever syndrome, different strains of malarial infections). A history of ill contacts may be helpful in narrowing down the differential diagnosis, as well as recent immunization, which may itself be the cause of the fever. Infants and toddlers are vaccinated at 2, 4, 6, 12, and 15 months. Patients who have been on recent antibiotic treatment are at higher risk of serious bacterial infection. In the emergency department, about 20% of pediatric patients with a fever present without a source, and the extensiveness of the workup will be dependent on the clinician's overall assessment.

As a general rule, any ill-appearing patient should undergo a complete sepsis workup composed of a CBC, blood culture, UA, urine culture, lumbar puncture with CSF analysis, plus or minus chest x-ray and stool testing, with admission to the hospital for empiric IV antibiotic treatment.

A very important component of any pediatric evaluation is the physical examination, starting with the vitals. Check pulses (brachial or femoral for neonates/infants). Check capillary refill. Blood pressures are not commonly obtained in children under the age of 2 years old, and therefore must be ordered in these patients if they are ill appearing.

The information obtained from direct observation is among the most helpful. Any time a child is inconsolable, crying but not producing tears, pale, lethargic, not moving all extremities, limp or hypotonic, or has bulging or sunken fontanelles, with poor interaction or response to the family or examiner, then that child is seriously ill and requires immediate fluid resuscitation, further workup and antibiotics, followed by admission. An otoscopic examination must be done to look for erythema, bulging tympanic membranes, or decreased light reflex to rule out otitis media, and the oral pharynx should always be visualized for signs of infection and hydration status. During the lung examination, look for signs of respiratory distress including nasal flaring and retractions, and auscultate to assess for evidence of pneumonia or bronchiolitis. The abdominal examination requires auscultation and palpation with careful attention given to increased crying or the child pushing the examiner's hand away at a certain position on the abdomen. It may be helpful to draw the legs up in an infant and palpate the abdomen to assess for guarding. If the child is old enough, it can be helpful to have him or her jump to look for signs of peritonitis. An inability to jump or increased pain after jumping may be a peritoneal sign or evidence of other severe illness. Older children and adolescents should also be assessed for costovertebral angle (CVA) tenderness. Always do a genital examination and check if the patient is circumcised or not. Being uncircumcised places a child at a higher risk of UTIs. Look for rashes, specifically viral exanthem, petechiae, or herpetic lesions.

Management of fever in infants <3 months old is guided by dividing them according to age: neonates (age 0-28 days) and young infants (29-90 days). It is recommended that *all* febrile neonates who present with a rectal temperature ≥38°C receive a full septic workup (CBC, UA, blood and urine cultures, lumbar puncture for CSF analysis and culture), and be admitted *regardless* of the neonate's clinical appearance. Chest x-rays are reserved for patients with respiratory signs or symptoms (eg, nasal flaring, grunting, increased respiratory rate, retractions, stridor). Empiric antibiotic treatment with ampicillin and gentamycin/cefotaxime should be initiated. Acyclovir should be added in suspected CNS or disseminated HSV infection in which the neonate is lethargic with vesicular skin lesions, seizures, elevated liver transaminase enzymes, a negative CSF Gram stain, and/or active maternal herpetic infection.

Table 16-3. Rochester Criteria for Low-risk Infants

Low Risk	High Risk
Well appearance	Toxic clinical appearance
Previously healthy, term infant and hospitalized no longer than the mother	Abnormal cry
Lack of obvious focal infection	Temperature ≥38.5°C
WBC 5000–15,000/mm³	Fail low-risk Rochester criteria
Band count <1500/mm³	CRP >5
Urinalysis normal (<10 WBC/high-power field and no bacteria seen)	
Stool <5 WBC/high-power field (if diarrhea present)	
CRP <5	

Data from Kourtis et al. *Clinical Pediatrics*. 2004. CRP, C-reactive protein; WBC, white blood cell.

Management of febrile young infants aged 29 to 90 days depends on whether they appear ill or not. Patients who look well are further categorized into high or low risks for serious bacterial infection based on the Rochester criteria (see Table 16-3). In this age group, high-risk infants, who appear toxic with an abnormal cry and temperatures ≥38.5°C, should be admitted for a full septic workup and antibiotics.

Infants (1-3 months) with a temperature ≥38°C, who appear well and are categorized as low risk, require a complete history and physical examination and a septic workup (without a lumbar puncture unless empiric antibiotics are given). Well-appearing infants in this group with normal lab and chest x-ray may be discharged and followed up the next day. If inadequate follow-up is likely, a more aggressive workup and admission for antibiotic therapy may be indicated.

Fever in infants aged 3 to 36 months: most children in this age category with fever have a self-limited viral or bacterial infection with a recognizable source. If the history and physical examination do not identify a source of the fever, further evaluation may be required if the fever ≥39°C, searching for an occult infection in a nontoxic child. Underlying medical conditions may place these children at higher risk of serious bacterial infection such as sickle cell disease or urinary tract reflux. Nonimmunized children are at increased risk for bacteremia compared with fully immunized children. Other risk factors for occult bacteremia include fever ≥39°C and white blood cells (WBCs) >15,000/μL.

Serious bacterial infections that occur in this age group include meningitis, pneumonia, focal skin infections, and osteomyelitis. Pneumonia and urinary tract infections are common causes of occult bacterial infections.

Children between the ages of 3 and 36 months who appear ill or have unstable vital signs should have a septic evaluation including CBC with differential, blood cultures, urine cultures, and CSF cultures if meningitis is suspected. A chest x-ray is required for children with respiratory distress, tachypnea, oxygen saturation <97%, or WBC >20,000. In these cases, empiric antibiotic treatment should be initiated.

Well-appearing children (3-36 months of age) who have no identifiable source of infection, or who are not fully immunized, are at greater risk for bacteremia, and thus need a CBC with differential and UA with urine culture. If the WBC ≥15,000/µL, a blood culture should be obtained and parenteral antibiotics strongly considered. If the WBC ≥20,000/µL, get a chest x-ray, since there is a high probability of occult pneumonia, and consider antibiotics. Children should be treated for a urinary tract infection if they have an abnormal UA.

Children >6 months who present with fever, appear well, and have received their Hib and pneumococcal vaccinations should receive urine testing. However, for girls 24 months and older, uncircumcised boys older than 12 months, and circumcised boys older than 6 months, routine UA and empiric antibiotics are not recommended.

It is very important that follow-up within 24 hours be arranged for those children aged 3 to 36 months who receive antibiotics and within 48 hours for all children with continual fever. Children should also return if their condition further deteriorates or if a positive culture is discovered.

Fundamentals of Disease

No clinical criteria are available to confirm the presence of a UTI in infants and young children. The gold standard for UTI diagnosis is urine culture with empiric antibiotic treatment to be initiated based on positive UA results. Adolescents and older children are easier to diagnose since they tend to present with more classic symptoms of UTI such as suprapubic pain, dysuria, and polyuria. However, infants and nonverbal children usually present with fever without an obvious source, as previously discussed, with 3% to 8% of these patients being diagnosed with a UTI. This age group may also present with atypical symptoms such as vomiting and abdominal pain, which may lead to the infection ascending to the upper urinary tract causing pyelonephritis before symptoms are noticed by parents and medical attention is sought.

Overall, there has been a decrease in most causes of serious bacterial illness such as meningitis and occult bacteremia in the pediatric population due to successful immunization programs, but no vaccine exists to prevent UTIs, which makes it the most common source of serious bacterial infection in the younger pediatric population. In fact, it is estimated that 3% of girls and 1% of boys will be diagnosed with a UTI before puberty. The most common organisms found to cause UTIs are bacteria, specifically *E. coli*. The majority of UTIs in all age groups occur from stool and perineal bacterial contamination of the urethra, providing an ascending route for infection of the bladder. As *E. coli* is present in large quantities in stool, it is no surprise that it is the predominant source of UTIs. Other less common pathogens include *Enterococcus faecalis* (5%) and *Staphylococcus saprophyticus* (in adolescents). Anatomic abnormalities such as vesicoureteral reflux and urinary outflow blockage, or the need for an indwelling catheter, put people at higher risk for recurrent UTIs. Children with a history of constipation are more likely to have UTIs as well.

Diagnostic Workup and Management

A UTI is diagnosed based on UA and urine culture results of a clean catch urine specimen. Urine samples are obtained in non–toilet-trained children via bladder catheterization or suprapubic aspiration if bladder catheterization is contraindicated (labial fusion, anatomic abnormality). Although suprapubic aspiration is technically the gold standard, it is invasive, painful, and infrequently performed. It is *not* acceptable to use perineal adhesive bags for urine collection since samples become contaminated with perineal flora and provide false-positive results with low specificity. Therefore, bagged urine specimens are only useful if they are negative. Toilet-trained children able to void on command may provide a urine sample that is caught midstream during urination.

Use of either a colorimetric dipstick test or microscopic UA with Gram stain may be used for relatively rapid diagnosis of a UTI. A dipstick test looks for the presence of leukocyte esterase and nitrite in urine. Leukocyte esterase is an enzyme found in WBCs and suggests the presence of pyuria. Nitrite is formed when normal urinary nitrate is reduced by coagulase-splitting bacteria, mostly gram-negative bacteria (*E. coli*), but it can also be formed by normal flora if urine is retained in the bladder. Microscopic UA is the preferred screening test for UTI since it provides more information including the number of WBCs, presence of blood (but note that you can get blood in a urine sample if it is a catheter sample), and number of squamous epithelial cells allowing the physician to ascertain whether or not the sample was contaminated. A positive test result for leukocyte esterase has a sensitivity of 67% to 85% while nitrite has a specificity of 95% to 99% for UTI. If the number of WBCs is ≥5 per high-power field and/or identification of bacteria on Gram stain is positive, then the test is positive for a UTI. Pyuria and bacteriuria are the most sensitive findings for UTI.

Once the UA returns positive or clinical suspicion of a UTI is high, a sterile urine culture must be sent for bacterial identification and antibiotic sensitivities. In children, a large percentage of negative UAs become positive on culture; therefore, catheterized urine samples should be sent for both UA and urine culture. Urine culture results are positive if there are 50,000 to 100,000 cfu/mL in a clean catch sample or 10,000 to 50,000 cfu/mL in a bladder catheterization sample, or if any single species of bacteria is grown in the presence of acute UTI symptoms in a suprapubic catheterization sample. It is very important to obtain a urine culture specimen *before* starting the patient on empiric antibiotics since initiation of antibiotics may alter bacterial growth and provide false data. For the same reason, blood cultures and CSF samples should also be obtained prior to antibiotic administration in septic children whenever possible. Afebrile patients with an isolated UTI will only need a UA and urine culture before receiving antibiotics, whereas 5% to 10% of febrile infants with UTI will have bacteremia and also need a blood culture. If the child is a febrile neonate, then a lumbar puncture and blood culture are required.

Antibiotic selection consists of gram-negative bacterial coverage for *E. coli* empirically with use of a third-generation cephalosporin and aminoglycoside or an extended-spectrum penicillin. Fluoroquinolones are to be avoided unless they are the only effective drug based on culture sensitivities. Use of trimethoprim/ sulfamethoxazole and amoxicillin should also be avoided since many local resistance patterns show high resistance to these antibiotics. All further antibiotic therapy should be adjusted based on urine culture sensitivities once available for optimal management. If a patient is to be treated as an outpatient but remains febrile after 3 days on an oral third-generation cephalosporin (or if the child is vomiting and unable to tolerate PO abx), then the patient must be admitted for antibiotic management and further assessment for pyelonephritis. See Table 16-4 for treatment considerations by age for first UTI.

Table 16-4. UTI Treatment Considerations by Age for First UTI Without an Anatomic Abnormality

Age	Comment
≤1 month	Hospital admission and IV abx for 3-5 days followed by variable course of PO abx for 10-14 days
>1 month to 2 years	If *toxic*, admit to hospital. If *nontoxic*, not vomiting, and well hydrated, give ceftriaxone 50 mg/kg in ED; follow with PO abx for 10-14 days. Follow up with pediatrician in 24 h for reevaluation and to get a renal ultrasound
>2 years	PO abx based on local resistance patterns (third-generation cephalosporin)
	If 2-13 years, treat for 7-10 days. Follow up with pediatrician in 2-3 days to assess response to therapy. Adolescent girls ≥13 years, option to treat for 3 days

Data from Magín EC, García-García JJ, Sert SZ, et al. Efficacy of short-term intravenous antibiotic in neonates with urinary tract infection. *Pediatr Emerg Care.* 2007;23(2):83–86; Hodson EM, Willis NS, Craig JC. Antibiotics for acute pyelonephritis in children. *Cochrane Database Syst Rev.* 2007;(4).

Special Considerations

The American Academy of Pediatrics 2011 guidelines continue to recommend a renal/bladder ultrasound examination after the first febrile UTI to rule out anatomic abnormalities that would warrant further evaluation. However, the new AAP guidelines no longer include a VCUG after the first febrile UTI since prophylactic use of antibiotics in children with vesicoureteral reflux has been shown to provide little, if any, benefit, in terms of renal scarring or prevention of UTIs. Due to the lack of evidence of identifying VUR, the risks, costs, and discomfort of the VCUG are hard to justify. If the child has a second or recurrent UTI, then a VCUG may be appropriate in order to assess for a rare grade V reflux.

TIPS TO REMEMBER

- Neonates (<28 days old) with a temperature ≥38°C (100.4°F) must be admitted for a sepsis workup and empiric antibiotic treatment.
- Common pediatric causes of serious bacterial illness include pneumonia, sepsis and bacteremia, meningitis, and UTI, with UTI being the most common since the successful implementation of immunization programs.
- Infants and young children have an atypical presentation of UTI including fever, vomiting, back pain, abdominal pain, and new-onset enuresis.
- Microscopic UA is the preferred screening method and urine culture is the gold standard for diagnosis of UTI.
- Urine samples should be obtained via bladder catheterization or clean catch.
- *E. coli* is the most common pathogen in UTIs and initial treatment should include a third-generation cephalosporin.
- A bladder/renal ultrasound is needed for 2- to 24-month-old children with first-time febrile UTI. VCUG is no longer required unless the presentation is that of a second febrile UTI or if hydronephrosis/renal scarring is seen on renal ultrasound.

COMPREHENSION QUESTIONS

1. Which of the following patients should be treated as an outpatient?
   - A. A 12-year-old female with right CVA tenderness, dysuria, and vomiting with Tmax 102°F
   - B. A 4-year-old girl with Tmax 101.8°F complaining of abdominal pain with a positive UA
   - C. A 26-day-old circumcised male with Tmax 100.6°F
   - D. An 8-year-old febrile girl with her third UTI this year who is oliguric

2. What is the first-line treatment for a 3-year-old girl with her first UTI? (She is afebrile and drinking juice while playing on the bed in the ED.)
    A. Amoxicillin 25 mg/kg, PO twice daily × 7 days
    B. Levofloxacin 8 mg/kg, PO twice daily × 5 days
    C. Gentamycin 1.5 mg/kg per day, IV every 8 hours × 3 days
    D. Cefdinir 7 mg/kg, PO once daily × 10 days

3. Which of the following is least likely to cause a serious bacterial illness in neonates?
    A. Pneumonia
    B. UTI
    C. Otitis media
    D. Meningitis

4. Which test result is positive for a UTI?
    A. Clean catch urine culture with 30,000 cfu/mL
    B. Bladder catheterization urine culture with 30,000 cfu/mL
    C. UA positive for leukocyte esterase, and 10 squamous epithelial cells
    D. UA with 4 WBCs and no bacteria seen on Gram stain

Answers

1. B. The patient in "B" does not have a temperature >102.2°F and has a known UTI as a source of her fever. As long as she is nontoxic, tolerating PO intake, and well hydrated, she can be treated as an outpatient with PCP follow-up in 48 hours. The patient in "A" has pyelonephritis and is not tolerating PO intake; "C" requires a neonatal sepsis workup and empiric antibiotics; "D" is febrile, has recurrent UTIs, and is not producing an adequate amount of urine that may be due to dehydration or an anatomic abnormality requiring further workup.

2. D. A third-generation cephalosporin is the first-line outpatient treatment for a child >1 month old who is nontoxic in appearance and tolerating PO intake. High resistance exists to amoxicillin, and a fluoroquinolone is only to be used in children when the bacteria are resistant to other medications based on urine culture sensitivity testing.

3. C. Causes of most serious bacterial illnesses in children include meningitis, bacteremia and sepsis, UTI, and pneumonia.

4. B. Bladder catheterization specimens are positive if they have 10,000 to 50,000 cfu/mL; clean catch specimens require 50,000 to 100,000 cfu/mL. "C" is incorrect since 10 epithelial cells are present proving the sample was contaminated.

SUGGESTED READINGS

American Academy of Pediatrics. <http://pediatrics.aappublications.org/>.

Byerley JS, Steiner MJ. Urinary tract infection in infants and children. In: Tintinalli JE, Kelen GD, Stapczynski JS, eds. *Tintinalli's Emergency Medicine: A Comprehensive Study Guide*. 7th ed. New York: McGraw-Hill; 2011 [chapter 126].

Levine BJ. *2011 EMRA Antibiotic Guide*. 14th ed. Ohio: EMRA; 2010.

Newman TB. The New American Academy of pediatrics urinary tract infection guideline. *Pediatrics* 2011;128(3):572–575. doi:10.1542/peds.2011-1818 [Epub August 28, 2011].

Shah SK, Allison ND, Tsao K. Evaluation of abdominal pain in children. Epocrates Online: BMJ Group; 2011 [updated October 19, 2010; cited March 6, 2011] <https://online.epocrates.com/noFrame/showPage.do?method=diseases&MonographId=787>.

Wang VJ. Fever and serious bacterial illness. In: Tintinalli JE, Kelen GD, Stapczynski JS, eds. *Tintinalli's Emergency Medicine: A Comprehensive Study Guide*. 7th ed. New York: McGraw-Hill; 2011 [chapter 113].

Woolridge D. *Emergency Medicine's Pediatric Top Clinical Problems*. Texas: EMRA; 2008.

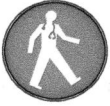

A 5-year-old Female With Fever

Myto Duong, MB, BCh, BAO and Erica J. Cacioppo, MD

CASE DESCRIPTION

Jane is a 5-year-old female who is brought to the ED by her parents for complaints of progressively worsening fever and a headache for the past few hours. She is alert with increased fatigue and keeps asking someone to please turn off the lights. Her parents state she is an otherwise healthy child, although it is not unusual for her to "pick something up" from the other children at day care. She was born full term without complications and is up to date with her vaccinations. The parents deny any recent illness, upper respiratory tract symptoms, nausea, vomiting, diarrhea, antibiotic use, a history of neurologic surgery, seizure-like activity, recent travel, or animal exposure.

On physical examination, her temperature is 39.1°C (102.4°F) with a heart rate of 160 bpm and blood pressure of 88/40. The patient is mildly drowsy but maintaining her airway and breathing appropriately though rapidly. No wheezing or abnormal breath sounds are appreciated. No murmurs or rubs are heard on the cardiac examination. She is tachycardic, with thready peripheral pulses and a delayed capillary refill of 5 seconds. There is a diffuse nonblanching petechial rash over her body, and she moans when her neck is passively flexed. There is no evidence of papilledema or focal neurologic deficits on examination. No sinus tenderness or lymphadenopathy is appreciated. Abdomen is soft and nontender.

1. What is the differential diagnosis for the patient?
2. What examination findings are the most important when considering meningitis?
3. How would a meningitis presentation differ if the patient was younger or older?
4. Which lab tests need to be performed?
5. Does anything need to be done before obtaining labs?
6. Why can this patient not be treated as an outpatient?

Answers

1. The differential diagnoses include bacterial meningitis, viral meningitis, encephalitis, brain abscess, shunt malfunction (when appropriate), sepsis, bacteremia, UTI, pneumonia, sinusitis, pharyngitis, and otitis media.

2. The most important physical examination findings for the assessment of bacterial meningitis include nuchal rigidity with passive flexion of the neck including use of Kernig and Brudzinski signs, petechial or purpural nonblanching rash (which can be evaluated by pressing glass or clear plastic against the rash), photophobia, papilledema on fundoscopic examination, and mental status changes. A thorough neurologic examination and assessment for cranial nerve palsies is critical. In any patient who is lethargic or has a decreased level of consciousness, it is vitally important to assess the airway and determine the need for intubation.

3. Infants with meningitis may present with decreased alertness or playfulness, decreased response to noxious stimuli, a bulging fontanelle, not waking up for feedings or vomiting, increased irritability when held, inconsolability, or a febrile seizure. A rash is not always present, and nuchal rigidity and Kernig or Brudzinski signs are usually absent in children less than 2 years old. Older, more verbal, patients are more likely to present with complaints of fever, headache, neck stiffness, petechial rash, vomiting, photophobia, altered mental status (AMS), positive Kernig and Brudzinski signs, lethargy, and/or hypotension. There may be a history of exposure to a sick contact.

4. CBC, CMP, UA, urine culture, blood cultures, chest x-ray, lumbar puncture with CSF analysis and cell count, differential, Gram stain, and cultures should all be obtained. Proinflammatory markers may be helpful such as CRP, ESR, or procalcitonin levels. An EEG may also be needed if seizures are present.

5. The patient must be placed in isolation with droplet precautions. Depending on the severity of the illness, patients may need immediate fluid resuscitation (20 mL/kg of normal saline which may be repeated 2-3 times) and started on empiric antibiotics within the first hour. If labs and cultures can be obtained quickly, then they may be sent before the initiation of antibiotics. However, *antibiotics should never be delayed in order to obtain labs or imaging in patients with suspected meningitis!* This patient does not have evidence of AMS, focal neurologic deficits, or seizures and has no history of malignancy or an immunocompromised state so a head CT is not required before performing her lumbar puncture.

6. This patient is sick and is in compensated shock. She has an AMS (drowsy), which suggests poor cerebral perfusion with tachycardia and delayed capillary refill. She needs emergent fluid resuscitation within the first 30 minutes of arrival and IV antibiotics. She has signs and symptoms supportive of bacterial meningitis, which is associated with high risks of morbidity and mortality, and requires droplet isolation for at least the first 48 hours of IV antibiotics. Adequate long-term follow-up must be arranged in order to prevent subsequent neurologic or learning disabilities.

CASE REVIEW

Jane has the 4 classic symptoms of meningitis including headache, fever, nuchal rigidity, and AMS. She also has had a rapid progression of symptoms and the presence of a nonblanching petechial rash, which points toward a bacterial source of infection, specifically *Neisseria meningitidis* in 64% of cases. On further evaluation, she also involuntarily lifts her legs up in response to neck flexion (Brudzinski sign) when she is lying supine and has pain and contracts her hamstrings when her knees are extended and her hips are flexed (Kernig sign). Other signs of serious infection that this patient displays are hypotension with a widened pulse pressure, thready pulse with delayed capillary refill, tachycardia, tachypnea, and fever >39°C (102.2°F). As discussed above, this patient requires a lumbar puncture, the gold standard for diagnosis of meningitis, with empiric antibiotics, steroids (if given prior to starting antibiotics), and droplet isolation to be initiated as soon as possible. A head CT is required before lumbar puncture in any patient with evidence of focal neurologic symptoms, AMS, history of malignancy, or an immunocompromised state. This patient's CSF reveals a WBC of 1250/mm^3, 87% PMN predominance, glucose 29 mg/dL, and 300 mg/dL of protein. Her opening pressure obtained in the lateral decubitus position is 415 mm and gram-negative diplococci were seen on Gram stain with identification of *N. meningitidis* on culture. (Please see Table 17-1 for typical spinal fluid results for meningeal processes.)

Table 17-1. Typical Spinal Fluid Results for Meningeal Processes

Parameter	Bacterial	Viral	Neoplastic	Fungal
Normal (<170 mm CSF)				
Opening pressure	>300 mm	<300 mm	200 mm	300 mm
WBC (<5 mononuclear)	>1000/mm^3	<1000/mm^3	<500/mm^3	<500/mm^3
PMN cells (0)	>80%	1%–50%	1%–50%	1%–50%
Glucose (>40 mg/dL)	<40 mg/dL	>40 mg/dL	<40 mg/dL	<40 mg/dL
Protein (<50 mg/dL)	>200 mg/dL	<200 mg/dL	>200 mg/dL	>200 mg/dL
Gram stain (−)	+	−	−	−
Cytology (−)	−	−	+	+

Data from Fitch MT. Emergency department management of meningitis and encephalitis. *Infect Dis Clin North Am.* 2008;22(1):33–52.

MENINGITIS

Diagnostic Reasoning

Any patient who presents with fever, AMS, headache, and nuchal rigidity has bacterial meningitis until proven otherwise. For discussion of febrile pediatric patients with a low suspicion for meningitis or fever of unknown source, please see the previous case. The main items to address in the history include onset and progression of symptoms, mental status changes, history of seizures, vaccination status, sick contacts, neurosurgical procedures, recent URI or antibiotic use, and birth history. The meningitis infection itself may be the result of an untreated otitis media or sinusitis, brain abscess, traumatic or congenital communication to the outside of the body, or a recent neurosurgical procedure. Because these are known possible sources of infection, it is important to adequately assess for them during the history and physical examination, which should include an otoscopic and pharyngeal examination and palpation of the sinuses.

Fundamentals of Disease

Bacterial meningitis is inflammation of the meninges and is diagnosed based on the presence of bacteria and demonstration of an inflammatory response of >5 WBCs in the CSF. On physical examination, 94% of patients with bacterial meningitis present with 2 of the 4 classic symptoms discussed above. A fever exists in 95% of cases and will last about 4 days. Nuchal rigidity occurs in 88% and may persist for >7 days despite other signs of clinical improvement. Mental status changes are present in 78% of patients and mostly appear as confusion or lethargy, although patients can also be comatose. Viral meningitis is less likely to present with petechiae/purpura, is usually of slower onset, and is definitively differentiated by CSF analysis (see Table 17-1). Encephalitis is a viral infection of the brain parenchyma leading to new-onset psychiatric or cognitive deficits, seizures, and/or movement disorders in addition to the classic symptoms of meningitis. Brain abscesses can also be confused with bacterial meningitis but commonly present with atypical, nonspecific symptoms most commonly including headache, focal neurologic signs (such as focal seizures), or increased intracranial pressure symptoms and fever.

The most common causes of bacterial meningitis in the United States are *Streptococcus pneumoniae* (61%), *N. meningitidis* (16%), group B *Streptococcus* (14%), *Haemophilus influenzae* (7%), and *Listeria monocytogenes* (2%), but predominance varies by age. Vaccination programs against *S. pneumoniae*, *N. meningitidis*, and *H. influenzae* have decreased the overall rate of meningitis in the population, but bacterial meningitis and septicemia remain highest in early infancy and are more common in children 2 months to 2 years old. The encapsulated bacteria mentioned above most commonly invade the body via the upper respiratory tract before being hematogenously spread and entering the subarachnoid space. Components of the bacterial capsule trigger a profound inflammatory response leading to edema of the brain and meninges, which decreases drainage of CSF and increases the intracranial pressure. The response of the body can subsequently result in ischemia and disruption of the blood–brain barrier. Major risk factors for meningitis include poor living conditions, trauma (*S. pneumoniae*), neurosurgical procedures (*S. aureus*), immunocompromised state (HIV), immunization noncompliance, antibiotic use, day care (*H. influenzae*), splenectomy, and concomitant pneumonia or endocarditis.

Diagnostic Workup and Management

Bacterial meningitis is diagnosed and differentiated from other types of meningitis based on CSF analysis as described in Table 17-1. However, CSF analysis does not always definitively point to the source of meningitis due to multiple areas of overlap in the diagnostic results. Because of this, a bacterial meningitis score consisting of 5 risk factors exists for people 2 months to 18 years of age with patients considered to be at high risk for a bacterial source if any 1 risk factor is present. The risk factors include (1) a positive CSF Gram stain, (2) CSF ANC ≥1000 cells/mL, (3) CSF protein ≥80 mg/dL, (4) peripheral blood ANC ≥10,000 cells/mL, and (5) a history of seizure before or after presentation. Any patient found to be high risk should be started on empiric antibiotics and admitted to the hospital. In addition, all children <2 months old with an elevated WBC count, any child with a toxic appearance, and even younger children with viral meningitis should be admitted to ensure adequate hydration and establishment of long-term follow-up to help avoid future sequelae. When an older child is suspected of having viral meningitis based on CSF and has a negative bacterial meningitis score, he or she should still receive ceftriaxone 100 mg/kg IV in the ED (if CSF was obtained) before discharge and then follow-up with the pediatrician within 24 hours.

Once suspicion of bacterial meningitis arises, the patient must be immediately placed in droplet isolation with steroids and empiric antibiotics (see Table 17-2) initiated as soon as possible. The use of steroids (dexamethasone 0.15 mg/kg IV) has been found to significantly decrease the morbidity and mortality in both the pediatric and adult populations with *H. influenzae B* or *S. pneumoniae* sources of bacterial meningitis. Dexamethasone should be given before (this is preferred) or at the same time as the first antibiotic administration for presumed bacterial meningitis. Labs and blood cultures ideally should be obtained at the time IV access is gained, before antibiotics are started, but antibiotics are not to be delayed due to labs or imaging. A head CT is to be done before the lumbar puncture when appropriate as described above. It is also important to perform the lumbar puncture in a timely manner since the CSF can become sterilized within 2 hours after the first IV dose of antibiotics. There will however be cases in which the patient is too ill for a lumbar puncture, and may have a coagulopathy, which would be a contraindication to a spinal tap.

Table 17-2. Bacterial Causes and Treatment of Meningitis by Age

<1 month	*E. coli*, group B *Streptococcus*, *L. monocytogenes*, *Klebsiella* spp.	Ampicillin 50 mg/kg IV Q6 h + cefotaxime 50 mg/kg IV Q8 h *or* gentamicin 2.5 mg/kg IV Q8 h
		Add vancomycin 10 mg/kg IV Q6 h if suspect MRSA *or* cephalosporin-resistant *S. pneumoniae*
1 month to 2 years	Group B *Streptococcus*, *E. coli, H. influenzae*	Vancomycin 15-20 mg/kg IV Q12 h + ceftriaxone 2 g (50 mg/kg) IV Q12 h *or* cefotaxime 2 g IV Q4 h
		Add ampicillin 2 g IV Q4 h if suspect *Listeria*
>2 years	*S. pneumoniae, N. meningitidis, S. aureus*	Same as for 1 month to 2 years

Treatment of nonbacterial sources of meningitis usually involves the use of acyclovir. Herpes (HSV-2) meningitis often presents with neurologic symptoms, which requires treatment with acyclovir (10 mg/kg IV Q8 hours). Cases of viral encephalitis are also treated with acyclovir and may require the addition of ganciclovir (5 mg/kg IV Q12 hours) if CMV is the causative agent. Bacterial sources of meningitis are to be treated by age according to Table 17-2. Penicillin is no longer a common antibiotic choice since 25% to 35% of *S. pneumoniae* strains are now resistant, but may be used once cultures and sensitivity results are available if appropriate.

Special Considerations

Prophylaxis: People who have had high-risk contact with patients documented to have *N. meningitidis* or *H. influenzae B* meningitis should be prophylactically treated with rifampin 10 mg/kg (maximum dose 600 mg/dose) every 12 hours for 2 days, ceftriaxone 250 mg IM once (125 mg if ≤15 years old), *or* ciprofloxacin 500 mg PO once. High-risk contact includes people not vaccinated with the Hib or meningococcal vaccines, household contacts, school or day care contacts within 7 days of diagnosis, direct exposure to the patient's secretions through kissing, shared utensils or toothbrushes, mouth-to-mouth CPR, or anyone who intubated the patient while not wearing a face mask. Patients are considered no longer contagious after they have received 48 hours of IV antibiotics.

TIPS TO REMEMBER

- The classic symptoms of bacterial meningitis include fever, headache, AMS, and nuchal rigidity. Other common symptoms are photophobia, nausea, and a petechial or purpuric rash.
- Diagnosis is based on CSF analysis.
- The ideal diagnostic and therapeutic sequence of events in a patient suspected of having bacterial meningitis is isolation, fluid resuscitation if septic (within 30 minutes), labs/cultures, steroids, empiric antibiotics (within the first hour), head CT, and lumbar puncture.
- Antibiotic selection is age dependent.
- Exposed contacts must be prophylactically treated with rifampin, ceftriaxone, or ciprofloxacin.

COMPREHENSION QUESTIONS

1. Which of the following is the least sensitive for bacterial meningitis?
    A. Fever
    B. Headache
    C. Kernig and Brudzinski signs
    D. AMS

2. A patient presents with lethargy, headache, fever, and neck stiffness. What is the proper sequence of treatment that should occur immediately?
    A. Isolation, steroids, antibiotics, CT, lumbar puncture
    B. CT, lumbar puncture, steroids, antibiotics, isolation
    C. Antibiotics, steroids, CT, lumbar puncture, isolation
    D. Isolation, steroids, CT, lumbar puncture, antibiotics

3. A 6-year-old boy is brought to the ED by his parents with a temperature of 39.4°C (103°F) and a complaint of a headache. His parents also state he has been talking to the wall and having conversations with people who are not present. During his stay, the patient has a generalized tonic–clonic seizure. What is the most likely diagnosis?
    A. Bacterial meningitis
    B. Viral meningitis
    C. Viral encephalitis
    D. Brain abscess

4. What antibiotics should a neonate with suspicion of bacterial meningitis receive if she was born prematurely and discharged from the hospital 2 weeks ago?
   A. Ampicillin, gentamicin, and cefotaxime
   B. Vancomycin, ampicillin, and cefotaxime
   C. Vancomycin and ceftriaxone
   D. Ampicillin, gentamicin, ceftriaxone, and vancomycin

Answers

1. **C.** Combined, the presence of the Kernig and Brudzinski signs is only 5% sensitive but 95% specific for bacterial meningitis when present.

2. **A.** Droplet isolation precautions must be instituted immediately on suspicion of bacterial meningitis, followed by administration of dexamethasone before IV antibiotics. A head CT is needed before lumbar puncture any time the patient has AMS, focal neurologic deficits, seizures, or a history of malignancy or an immunocompromised state.

3. **C.** Encephalitis presents with new-onset psychiatric or cognitive deficits, seizures, or movement disorders in addition to fever, headache, nuchal rigidity, or AMS. Viral meningitis has a slower onset than bacterial meningitis and is diagnosed on CSF analysis. Brain abscesses may present with focal neurologic symptoms (focal seizures), fever, or elevated ICP.

4. **B.** The patient is less than 1 month old so requires treatment with ampicillin plus either gentamicin or cefotaxime. However, she is at high risk for a MRSA infection given her recent prolonged hospitalization so she should also receive vancomycin.

SUGGESTED READINGS

American Academy of Pediatrics. <http://pediatrics.aappublications.org/>.
Levine BJ. *2011 EMRA Antibiotic Guide*. 14th ed. Ohio: EMRA; 2010.
Loring KE, Tintinalli JE. Central nervous system and spinal infections. In: Tintinalli JE, Kelen GD, Stapczynski JS, eds. *Tintinalli's Emergency Medicine: A Comprehensive Study Guide*. 7th ed. New York: McGraw-Hill; 2011 [chapter 168].
Wang VJ. Fever and serious bacterial illness. In: Tintinalli JE, Kelen GD, Stapczynski JS, eds. *Tintinalli's Emergency Medicine: A Comprehensive Study Guide*. 7th ed. New York: McGraw-Hill; 2011 [chapter 113].

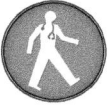

A 5-year-old Male With Abdominal Pain

Myto Duong, MB, BCh, BAO and Julie Fultz, MD, MDiv

CASE DESCRIPTION

J.R. is a 5-year-old boy with a history of constipation who presents to the ED with the chief complaint of abdominal pain. He has had intermittent diffuse abdominal pain for the past 1.5 weeks. He is unable to describe the pain. Mom reports an increase in frequency and intensity of the abdominal pain for the past 2 days. The pain is so severe that it makes him double over sometimes. The pain does not wake him up at night. There are no relieving or exacerbating factors. On review of systems, mom reports that his last bowel movement was 2 weeks ago. She states that he strains a lot when he is on the toilet. Patient reports pain with passing of stool. No bloody stool. No fever or vomiting, but mom notes her son has had a decreased appetite and decreased oral intake. No diarrhea. Normal urination. No weight loss.

His vitals are temperature 37.2, blood pressure 90/65 mm Hg, pulse 80 beats/min, respiratory rate 15 breaths/min, and oxygen saturation of 100% on room air.

On physical examination, the patient is alert and in no apparent distress. His cardiopulmonary examination was normal. His abdomen was soft but diffusely tender. There was no guarding or rebound. No palpable masses. The back examination was normal with no overlying skin changes. He had normal genitalia with bilateral cremasteric reflexes present. No hernias were appreciated. Rectal examination demonstrated normal tone with a hard fecal mass in the rectal vault. Stool hemoccult test was negative.

1. What are the critical diagnoses for pediatric abdominal pain? What are the red flags for pediatric abdominal pain?

2. How is constipation defined in the pediatric population?

3. What workup is warranted in this patient?

4. What is the treatment of constipation in infants and children?

Answers

1. In a child presenting with abdominal pain, it is important to be aware of the critical diagnoses and be able to recognize red flags in the history and physical examination. Importantly, the most likely critical diagnoses can vary by age. Table 18-1

159

Table 18-1. Important Differential Diagnoses for Abdominal Pain Based on Age of Presentation

Diagnosis	Key Features
Newborn	
Volvulus with malrotation	90% <3 months old; abdominal distension with bilious emesis, no bowel movement and septic appearance; requires high index of suspicion, potentially fatal
Hirschsprung disease	No passing of meconium within 24 hours; vomiting, abdominal distension, enterocolitis, primarily in **first year of life**
Necrotizing enterocolitis	Feeding intolerance, apnea, lethargy, bloody stools, abdominal distension and tenderness, abdominal erythema, hematochezia, bradycardiac, primarily in **premature infants but also in full-term babies in first month of life**
Pyloric stenosis	Nonbilious projectile emesis with hypochloremic metabolic alkalosis in <3 months old; may find palpable olive in RUQ during feeding; ensure the patient is NPO 2-3 h prior to abdominal ultrasound
Trauma (ie, during birth)	
Hernia	Seen on physical examination; usually in premature babies
Gastroesophageal reflux	Crying and vomiting after feedings associated with arching of the back
Infant (<2 years)	
Constipation	Hard pellet-like stool
Acute gastroenteritis	History of vomiting and diarrhea with ill contacts; diffuse abdominal pain without guarding or rebound
Intussusception	Similar presentation to volvulus but intussusception tends to occur >3 months old; colicky pain, flexing of legs, fever, lethargy, vomiting, peak incidence in children at **6 months of age**; jelly current stool is a late finding; ultrasound diagnosis; air enema reduction or surgery is the treatment

(continued)

Table 18-1. Important Differential Diagnoses for Abdominal Pain Based on Age of Presentation (*Continued*)

Diagnosis	Key Features
Trauma	Look for stigmata of child abuse
Toxin ingestion	Anticholinergics such as Benadryl; botulism (nonpasteurized honey) resulting in constipation and abdominal pain
Colic	Diagnosis of exclusion
Infantile dyschezia/ pseudoconstipation	Cries with passing of flatus or stool with parental concern of straining around 4–6 weeks of age
Respiratory illness	Lower lobe pneumonia may present as abdominal pain, tachypnea, cough, diminished breath sounds or crackles on auscultation
Children (2–18 years)	
Acute gastroenteritis	History of vomiting and diarrhea with ill contacts; diffuse abdominal pain without guarding or rebound
Constipation	Infrequent bowel evacuations, difficult or painful defecation, can see blood in stool from anal fissures, low-fiber diet, high milk consumption (>2-3 cups per day)
Urinary tract infection/ pyelonephritis	Urinary frequency, dysuria, fever, and/or vomiting, flank/suprapubic/CVA tenderness
Peptic ulcer disease	Epigastric tenderness, pain related to eating a meal, ulcer can **perforate**
Intestinal obstruction	
Testicular torsion	Must do GU examination, absent cremasteric reflex, high riding testes on affected side
Pneumonia	History of coughing and fever
Mesenteric adenitis	History of recurrent respiratory tract/intercurrent infection
Trauma	External evidence of trauma such as bruising, abrasions, or lacerations
Henoch-Schonlein purpura	Palpable purpuric rash in lower extremities, buttock, and extensor surfaces of upper extremities. Abdominal pain may be due to intussusception

(*continued*)

Table 18-1. Important Differential Diagnoses for Abdominal Pain Based on Age of Presentation (*Continued*)

Diagnosis	Key Features
Appendicitis	Initial periumbilical pain migrating to RLQ with low-grade fever, anorexia, nausea, and vomiting. Patient avoids movement, rebound tenderness, McBurney sign (pain at 2/3 between umbilicus and right ASIS), Rovsing sign (pain in RLQ on left-sided palpation), psoas sign (pain in RLQ with left and right hip hyperextension), obturator sign (pain in RLQ on internal rotation of flexed right thigh). Can rupture and cause sepsis
Pancreatitis	Steady and sudden-onset pain radiating to the back, nausea, vomiting, history of cholelithiasis
Cholecystitis	Abdominal pain worse after food, especially spicy or fatty foods
Adolescents (12-18 years)	
Trauma	Bruise
Dysmenorrhea	
Pelvic inflammatory disease	Sexual history, history of STIs
Ovarian torsion/cysts	Acute pain with vomiting
Pregnancy (ie, ectopic)	Nausea and vomiting, review sexual history and consider **ectopic pregnancy and associated ruptures**
Testicular torsion	Acute pain with vomiting, must do GU examination
Cholecystitis	
Nephrolithiasis	Acute renal colic, flank pain radiating to groin; check UA
Toxin ingestion, food poisoning	
Gastroenteritis	
Constipation	
Irritable bowel syndrome	Change in stool frequency, bloating, abdominal distension, may be associated with **certain foods**; periumbilical tenderness. No guarding or rebound

(continued)

Table 18-1. Important Differential Diagnoses for Abdominal Pain Based on Age of Presentation (*Continued*)

Diagnosis	Key Features
Ulcerative colitis	Bloody and/or chronic diarrhea, crampy lower abdominal pain, anorexia, weight loss, fever, fecal urgency, can develop to **toxic megacolon**
Crohn disease	Intermittent diarrhea, weight loss, crampy right lower quadrant pain, anorexia, weight loss, fatigue

lists the most important critical diagnoses and red flags by age. Red flag symptoms at any age include:

- Bilious vomiting
- Bloody stool or emesis
- Nighttime waking with abdominal pain
- Hemodynamic instability
- Weight loss

2. Constipation is defined as a delay or difficulty in defecation present for 2 or more weeks, and sufficient to cause significant distress to the patient. Normal number of bowel movements per day depends on the age of the patient (see Table 18-2). It may be normal for a breastfed baby to not have stools for up to 7 to 10 days if the stools that are passed are soft and not pellet-like. Once defined, it is important to determine if the cause of the constipation is functional (exists in isolation) or organic (due to some underlying physiological problem). Table 18-3 describes the typical history, physical examination findings, and differential diagnosis for a pediatric patient with constipation.

A history of stool-withholding behavior (dance-like behavior in which children rise on their toes and rock back and forth while stiffening their buttocks and legs, or wriggle, fidget, or assume unusual postures; often misconstrued as straining) reduces the likelihood that there is an organic disorder for the abdominal pain.

Other features that are helpful in distinguishing functional from organic constipation include weight loss or failure to thrive (therefore, the weight and growth curves are useful), abdominal distension, spinal dimple/hair tuft, explosion of liquid stool and air from rectum on withdrawal of finger during a digital examination (suggestive of Hirschsprung disease), occult blood in stool, absent anal wink, absent cremasteric reflex, decreased lower extremity tone and/or strength, and absence or delay in relaxation phase of lower extremity deep tendon reflexes (concerning for hypothyroidism).

Table 18-2. Normal Number of Bowel Movements Per Day

Age	Mean Number of Bowel Movements Per Day
0-3 months	
Breast milk	2.9
Formula	2
6-12 months	1.8
1-3 years old	1.4
>3 years old	1.0

Data from Fontana M, Bianchi C, Cataldo F, et al. Bowel frequency in healthy children. *Acta Paediatr Scand*. 1989;78(5):682–684.

Table 18-3. History, Physical Examination, and Differential Diagnosis for Constipation

History	Physical Examination	Differential Diagnosis
Constipation history	General appearance	Developmental/ cognitive handicaps
Frequency and consistency of stools	Vital signs: temperature, pulse, respiratory rate, blood pressure	Attention deficit disorders
Pain or bleeding with passing stools	Growth parameters: failure to thrive	Situational
Abdominal pain • Waxing and waning of symptoms	Head, ears, eyes, nose, throat	Coercive toilet training
Age of onset	Neck: goiter	Toilet phobia
Toilet training	Cardiovascular	School bathroom avoidance
Fecal soiling	Lungs and chest	Excessive parental interventions

(continued)

Table 18-3. History, Physical Examination, and Differential Diagnosis for Constipation (*Continued*)

History	Physical Examination	Differential Diagnosis
Withholding behavior	**Abdominal examination:** • Distension • Palpable liver/spleen or fecal mass • Guarding • Rebound tenderness • Bowel sounds	Colonic inertia
Change in appetite	**Rectal examination:** • Anal wink/tone • Fecal mass • Stool presence and consistency • Other masses • Explosive stool on withdrawal of finger (seen with Hirschsprung disease) • Occult blood in stool	Genetic predisposition
Nausea or vomiting	**Back and spine examination:** • Dimple • Tuft of hair	Reduced stool volume and dryness
Weight loss		Low fiber in diet, dehydration
Perianal fissures, dermatitis, abscess, or fistula	**Neurological examination:** • Tone • Strength • Cremasteric reflex • Deep tendon reflexes	Underfeeding or malnutrition

(continued)

Table 18-3. History, Physical Examination, and Differential Diagnosis for Constipation (*Continued*)

History	Physical Examination	Differential Diagnosis
Current Treatment		
Current diet (24-h recall): high fiber and <2-3 cups of milk		Anatomic malformations: • Imperforate anus • Anal stenosis • Anterior displaced anus • Pelvic mass (sacral teratoma)
Current medications (for all medical problems): oral, enema, suppository, herbal		Metabolic and gastrointestinal: • Hypothyroidism • Hypercalcemia • Hypokalemia • Cystic fibrosis • Diabetes mellitus • Multiple endocrine neoplasia type 2B • Gluten enteropathy
Results of Prior Tests		
Previous treatment or prior successful treatments: • Diet • Behavioral treatment		
Estimate of parent/patient adherence		Neuropathic conditions: • Spinal cord abnormalities • Spinal cord trauma • Neurofibromatosis • Static encephalopathy • Tethered cord

(continued)

Table 18-3. History, Physical Examination, and Differential Diagnosis for Constipation (*Continued*)

History	Physical Examination	Differential Diagnosis
Family history: • Constipation • Hirschsprung disease • Thyroid • Parathyroid • Cystic fibrosis • Celiac disease		Intestinal nerve or muscle disorders: • Hirschsprung disease • Intestinal neuronal dysplasia • Visceral myopathies/ neuropathies
Medial history: • Gestational age • Time of passage of meconium • Condition at birth • Acute injury or disease • Hospital admissions • Immunizations • Allergies • Surgeries • Delayed growth and development		Abnormal abdominal musculature: • Prune belly • Gastroschisis • Down syndrome
Review of system: • Sensitivity to cold • Coarse hair • Dry skin • Recurrent urinary tract infections • Daytime urinary incontinence		Connective tissue disorders: • Scleroderma • Systemic lupus erythematosus • Ehlers-Danlos syndrome

(continued)

Table 18-3. History, Physical Examination, and Differential Diagnosis for Constipation (*Continued*)

History	Physical Examination	Differential Diagnosis
Social history:		Medications:
• School performance		• Opiates
• Psychosocial disruption of child or family		• Phenobarbital
		• Sucralfate
• Interaction with peers		• Antacids
• Temperament		• Antihypertensives
• Toilet habits at school		• Anticholinergics
		• Antidepressants
		• Sympathomimetics
		Other:
		• Heavy-metal ingestion (lead)
		• Vitamin D intoxication
		• Botulism
		• Cow's milk protein intolerance

3. Constipation is primarily a clinical diagnosis, and, therefore, should not require significant workup. However, some basic workup may need to be done to exclude organic causes. A stool test for occult blood is recommended in all constipated infants and in those children who also have abdominal pain, failure to thrive, diarrhea, or a family history of colon cancer or polyps. In selected patients, an abdominal radiograph, when interpreted correctly, can be useful to diagnose fecal impaction or megacolon, especially if a digital rectal examination was not performed. Rectal biopsy with histopathological examination and rectal manometry are the only tests that can reliably exclude Hirschsprung disease, and thus the patient may be referred to pediatric surgery. Routine labs are not generally required (including TSH level) in the ED setting.

4. In infants, rectal dismpaction can be achieved with glycerin suppositories. Enemas are to be avoided. In infants, juices that contain sorbitol, such as prune, pear, and apple juices, can decrease constipation. Barley malt extract, corn syrup, lactulose, or sorbitol (osmotic laxatives) can be used as stool softeners. Mineral oil and stimulant laxatives are not recommended for infants.

In children, disimpaction can be achieved with either oral or rectal medication, including enemas. In children, a balanced diet, containing whole grains, fruits, and vegetables, is recommended as part of the treatment for constipation. The use of medications with behavioral modification (ie, scheduled toilet time, blowing out candle, etc) can decrease the time to remission in children with functional constipation. Mineral oil (a lubricant) and magnesium hydroxide, lactulose, and sorbitol (osmotic laxatives) are safe and effective medications. Rescue therapy with short-term use of stimulant laxatives, such as senna and bisacodyl, can be useful in selected patients who are more difficult to treat. Polyethylene glycol electrolyte solution, given in low dosage, may be an effective long-term treatment for constipation that is difficult to manage. Biofeedback therapy can be an effective short-term treatment of intractable constipation. Difficult cases may be referred to pediatric gastroenterologists.

CASE REVIEW

J.R. has constipation with fecal impaction on examination. Since his physical examination was not concerning for an acute abdomen, he was discharged home with a short-term use of high-dose MiraLAX for disimpaction, followed by a lower, daily dose, for maintenance to ensure soft bowel movements. He has scheduled toilet time (3 times a day, for 10 minutes), at home and school, and he practices the Valsalva maneuver by pretending to blow out candles while on the toilet.

PEDIATRIC ABDOMINAL PAIN

Diagnostic Reasoning

Pediatric abdominal pain is an extremely common chief complaint in the ED. It is the most common presentation with both trivial and life-threatening etiologies, ranging from functional pain to acute appendicitis. Fortunately, the majority of pediatric abdominal complaints are relatively benign (eg, constipation), but it is extremely important to look for and detect red flags suggestive of more serious underlying disease.

In addition, diagnosing abdominal pain in the pediatric patient can be a challenging task. Stranger anxiety may contribute to the challenge with the patient not being forthcoming with information. Children may not be able to describe the pain or localize it. Fear of painful procedures such as blood draw may also result in half-truths. Try to engage the patient but include him or her in the conversation. The physical examination will start from the doorway and distraction techniques may be employed to get a more accurate examination of an anxious/fearful patient.

The first thing to consider for the patient presenting with abdominal pain is whether or not this is an acute or chronic condition. Acute pain lasts several hours to days while chronic pain can last from days to weeks to months. The abdominal pain may be an acute exacerbation of a chronic issue, such as constipation.

The differential diagnoses for some common and serious causes of pediatric abdominal pain vary with age (see Table 18-1). When taking a history and examining a child with abdominal pain, also consider the organs surrounding the abdomen as a source of the abdominal pain, such as pneumonia and testicular/ovarian torsion.

If available, the characterization of the abdominal pain can be helpful in narrowing down the differential diagnosis. Have the child identify a specific location by asking him or her to use 1 finger to point to the area of greatest pain. The quality of the pain can be sharp and stabbing (ie, trauma) or achy/crampy (ie, mittelschmerz). The patient may be able to report radiation down the groin (ie, nephrolithiasis) or to the right lower quadrant (acute appendicitis). The severity of the pain is helpful in documenting improvement and may require the use of face or number scales (from 1 to 10 out of 10). The most important information to solicit is if the pain was severe enough to wake the child up from sleep. Is the pain constant or intermittent? The duration and course of the pain during the day is helpful. Alleviating and exacerbating factors may also be informative (ie, worsens with food). Associated symptoms may be extremely useful in narrowing the differential diagnosis. Associated symptoms can include hematemesis (suggestive of peptic ulcer disease or gastritis), vomiting, nausea, hematochezia (seen with GI bleed, IBD, NEC, dysentery, or constipation), melena (consistent with upper GI bleed), diarrhea (gastroenteritis or protein-losing enteropathy), fever, and weight loss. Ask about bowel movement patterns and stool quality (size, hard/soft, odor). Joint swelling/pain with various skin lesions is associated with HSP (palpable purpura) and IBD (erythema nodosum). Abdominal pain associated with vaginal or penile discharge is suggestive of STI. If dysuria or urinary frequency is present, think urinary tract infection.

The past medical history can provide important clues. For example, cystic fibrosis predisposes to gallstones and intussusception, sickle cell disease predisposes to splenic autoinfarction, recurrent respiratory tract infections suggest mesenteric adenitis, and spina bifida/cerebral palsy/developmental delay predisposes to constipation. A sexual history should be obtained with screening for STI in adolescents, including LMP if applicable.

Past abdominal surgeries increase the patient's risk for adhesions and obstructions. Acute appendicitis can be ruled out if an appendectomy has been performed in the past. There are some diseases that are inherited and thus a family history would be helpful (ie, IBD). Obtain travel, social, and psychiatric (potential stressors) history. Explore risks for nonaccidental trauma. For patients with constipation, get a detailed dietary history. In young children, too much milk (>2-3 cups per day) can lead to constipation.

The physical examination starts with the vitals and growth parameters, especially if there are reports of weight loss or failure to thrive. The abdominal examination starts with a general inspection, looking for contour, symmetry, hernias (wall protrusion), signs of trauma (bruises or swelling), and abdominal distension. Auscultate the abdomen before palpation, and listen for bowel sounds, or abdominal bruits. The stethoscope pressure on the abdomen may provide a more accurate assessment of tenderness in children. The liver and splenic tip may be percussed. Ascites may be detected by change in tone of the percussion. Light and deep palpation can be used to assess guarding and rebound tenderness. Digital rectal examination should be considered, unless the child has a history of sexual abuse/molestation.

Diagnostic Workup and Management

A thorough history and physical examination will facilitate a focused diagnostic workup. The urgency of the workup and management is dependent on whether or not the abdominal pain is an acute or chronic issue.

Abnormal vital signs should alert the providers to more concerning conditions. The general appearance of the patient will quickly identify sick and not sick patients. If potentially unstable patients are identified, they should have a safety net established and ABC interventions as needed. Once they are stable, workup and further management can begin.

A patient with a suspected benign cause of the abdominal pain (no red flags) in the history or physical examination may require no additional workup, such as the case with constipation. In contrast, a patient with an acute abdomen will need screening blood work (CBC, BMP, hepatic panel, and lipase) and KUB. An upper GI study is required to diagnose malrotation with volvulus. Ultrasound is recommended for the diagnosis of pyloric stenosis and intussusception. To reduce radiation exposure in the pediatric patient, abdominal ultrasound is recommended as the initial imaging study in the workup of acute appendicitis, which may also detect mesenteric adenitis. Inability to visualize the appendix on ultrasound may require a CT scan of the abdomen/pelvis to rule out appendicitis. The other option is to admit and observe the patient, depending on the clinical examination. Ultrasound with Doppler is also invaluable in the evaluation of testicular and ovarian torsion. See Table 18-4 for other laboratory investigations specific for the differential diagnosis.

Depending on the degree of pain, IV or oral opioids may be indicated. NSAIDs such as ketorolac and ibuprofen may also be helpful. Fluids should be started if the patient is made NPO. In persistent vomiting, an NGT should be placed. Intravenous antibiotics may be required prophylactically for an acute abdomen presentation.

Table 18-4. Laboratory Investigations for Common Differential Diagnoses of Abdominal Pain

Medical Condition	Relevant Diagnostic Tests
Gastrointestinal	
Constipation	None if history does not suggest an alternative diagnosis
Acute appendicitis	CBC (WBC normal or elevated), urinalysis, urine pregnancy
Gastroenteritis	BMP, stool culture, stool for virology
Irritable bowel syndrome	None, based on history and clinical findings
Trauma	CBC for blood loss, UA, FAST, abdominal/pelvic CT with IV contrast
Celiac disease	Anti-TTG, IgA
Inflammatory bowel disease	CBC, ESR/CRP, electrolytes, albumin, LFTs, bilirubin, stool culture, AXR (megacolon)
Genitourinary	
Urinary tract infection	Urine dipstick (for leukocyte esterase and nitrite), urine microscopy, urine culture (cath)
Primary dysmenorrhea	None, based on history and clinical findings
Pulmonary	
Pneumonia and empyema	Chest x-ray, sputum culture

TIPS TO REMEMBER

- The differential diagnosis for abdominal pain is extensive. A complete history and physical examination will provide the majority of diagnosis for pediatric abdominal pain complaints. Is this acute or chronic? Are there red flags?
- A high index of suspicion is often required to diagnose emergent causes of abdominal pain, especially in the nonverbal patient, and age of presentation may help narrow the differential.

COMPREHENSION QUESTIONS

1. Constipation can be quantified in a number of bowel movements per week? True or False.

2. Which of the following is *false* concerning constipation in the pediatric population?

  A. It is usually a surgical emergency.
  B. It can and should be treated medically.
  C. Age is critical in the differential diagnosis.
  D. Lab work and imaging are often unnecessary.

3. Which of the following is contraindicated in the evaluation and treatment of constipation?

  A. Attempting to discern inciting event/recent change
  B. Long-term stimulant laxatives
  C. Long-term lactulose use
  D. Establishing regular times for defecation

Answers

1. **False.** Constipation does have to do with decreased frequency of bowel movements, but it also is characterized by pain with defecation and hard stool. No specific numbers can be used to characterize constipation.

2. **A.** There are many causes for abdominal pain in children and adolescents, and while some of them do require emergency surgery, that number is not the majority.

3. **B.** The long-term use of stimulant laxatives can cause electrolyte abnormalities and is thus contraindicated.

SUGGESTED READINGS

Marx JA, Hockberger RS, Walls RM, eds. *Rosen's Emergency Medicine: Concepts and Clinical Practice.* 7th ed. Philadelphia: Mosby-Elsevier; 2010 <http://www.mdconsult.com>.

Misra S. Approach to Acute Abdominal Pain in Children. Pediatric Oncall. 2005 [updated May 1, 2005; cited March 6, 2010] <http://www.pediatriconcall.com/fordoctor/diseasesandcondition/gastrointestinal_disorders/acute_abdominalpain_children.asp>.

Neuman MI, Ruddy RM. Emergent evaluation of the child with acute abdominal pain. *UptoDate.* 2010 [updated August 2, 2010; cited March 6, 2011].

Shah SK, Allison ND, Tsao K. Evaluation of abdominal pain in children. Epocrates Online: BMJ Group; 2011 [updated October 19, 2010; cited March 6, 2011] <https://online.epocrates.com/noFrame/showPage.do?method=diseases&MonographId=787>.

Tintinalli JE, Kelen GD, Stapczynski JS, Ma OJ, Cline DM, eds. *Tintinalli's Emergency Medicine.* 7th ed. New York: McGraw-Hill; 2011 <http://www.accessmedicine.com>.

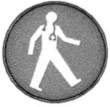

A 9-month-old Female With Abdominal Pain, Vomiting, and Diarrhea

Myto Duong, MB, BCh, BAO and Julie Fultz, MD, MDiv

CASE DESCRIPTION

Sally is a 9-month-old girl with a 4-day history of vomiting and diarrhea who presents to the ED with intermittent episodes of lethargy and drawing up of her legs as if she is in pain. Initially, she had 4 to 5 episodes of loose watery stool for 2 days. In the last 2 days she has not had any bowel movements but started vomiting, 3 to 5 episodes per day of greenish substance. Her last bowel movement was bloody with some mucous. Mom was worried about her color and lack of activity. The patient has not had anything to eat or drink for the past 36 hours. No urine output today. Her vitals are HR 190 bpm, BP 70/45, RR 40, and SaO_2 100% on RA. On examination, she is afebrile, pale with a capillary refill of 5 seconds. She is awake but minimally responsive. Lungs are clear to auscultation bilaterally. No retractions. She is tachycardic with no murmur. She squirms with palpation of her slightly distended abdomen. Diminished bowel sounds. Her genital examination was normal.

1. What are the 2 most pertinent/useful components of the history in narrowing your differential diagnosis?

2. What is the next appropriate step in the management of this patient?

3. What is on your list of differential diagnoses?

4. What imaging studies are indicated?

Answers

1. Vomiting characteristics and age of presentation. Patients with bilious emesis are worrisome for an obstructive process, and for her age of presentation, intussusception would be highest on the list of differential diagnoses. If she was presenting with the same complaint at the age of 3 weeks old, malrotation with volvulus would be more concerning. A 4-week-old baby with nonbilious projectile emesis would be more consistent with a diagnosis of pyloric stenosis.

2. Currently her airway and breathing appear to be intact. The patient needs immediate fluid resuscitation with 20 mL/kg bolus of normal saline or lactated Ringer's, followed by reassessment of her mental status, HR, and capillary refill. The fluid bolus may be repeated 2 to 3 more times. Infants, especially newborns, who have had poor feeding, are at high risk of hypoglycemia. It is pertinent to

obtain a bedside glucose in this baby. If she is persistently vomiting, a nasogastric tube would need to be placed to prevent aspiration. Antibiotics should be started and appropriate imaging obtained.

3. Intussusception, gastroenteritis with hypoglycemia and dehydration, appendicitis, incarcerated hernia, pyelonephritis, and sepsis. Malrotation with midgut volvulus is less likely at her age but should also be considered.

4. KUB with left lateral decubitus film can be obtained immediately to confirm an obstructive condition, while the patient is getting her fluid resuscitation. An ultrasound should be ordered to look for intussusception. If the patient was younger and the concern for malrotation with a volvulus was higher, an upper GI study would be required to make the diagnosis.

CASE REVIEW

Sally is presenting in compensated hypovolemic shock with a history of poor feeding, vomiting, diarrhea, and decreased urine output. She is tachycardic with delayed capillary refill and has a decreased interaction with her environment. The history of bilious emesis suggests a gastrointestinal obstruction. KUB demonstrated air-fluid levels with dilated loops of small bowel. Ultrasound demonstrated an ileocolic intussusception. With multiple fluid boluses, the patient's heart rate decreased to 150 bpm and her capillary refill improved to 2 to 3 seconds. Patient was more alert and interactive with her parents. Her abdomen was soft and nontender. She was taken to the operating room since she had arrived to the ER with signs of sepsis and peritonitis, putting her at increased risk for perforation with air enema reduction under fluoroscopy.

INTUSSUSCEPTION

Diagnostic Reasoning

Most infants with intussusception have a history of intermittent severe abdominal pain in which they scream and draw their legs up to their abdomens. They may also look pale. These episodes last only a few seconds but occur every 5 to 30 minutes. In between episodes, they may appear calm with normal appearance and activity, but some infants may become quite lethargic and somnolent between attacks. Parents will report having difficulty arousing the baby, and thus raise concerns for complex partial seizure activity with postical periods.

Initially, the infant may vomit undigested food, but with time, it will become bilious. Stool will eventually become dark red and mucoid (resembling currant jelly), a sign of intestinal ischemia and mucosal sloughing, which is a very late finding.

In terms of the physical examination, between attacks, the infant may appear somnolent or normal with an unremarkable abdominal examination. During an attack, the infant suddenly appears startled or anxious and begins to scream. Initially, the abdomen may appear scaphoid, but during the spasms, it may be rigid, with distension and signs of peritonitis as late findings. In ileocolic intussusceptions, a sausage-shaped mass may be palpable in the RUQ with an empty RLQ (known as the Dance sign) if the baby is not crying with a rigid abdomen from muscle straining.

The rectal examination should commence with inspection of fecal material in the diaper. Normal-appearing stool should be tested for occult blood. The presence of mucoid or frankly bloody stool supports the diagnosis. Rarely, inspection of the anus reveals the prolapsed tip of the intussusception. A digital rectal examination should be performed routinely, looking for blood or a mass higher in the anal canal.

Lab studies include a CBC and BMP, to assess for leukocytosis, anemia, and hydration status.

Imaging should start with KUB with a left-side-down decubitus view to improve diagnostic accuracy since it is the fastest and most readily available study in the ED. Early in the course of the illness, abdominal plain films may be unremarkable. Findings suggestive of intussusception include dilated loops of small bowel with or without air-fluid levels, an airless or opacified right lower quadrant, or both. Occasionally, the intussusceptum is apparent on plain abdominal radiography.

Ultrasound is the imaging study of choice, but is operator dependent. Findings consistent with intussusception include target (transverse section) and pseudokidney signs (longitudinal section). Ultrasound measurements may be useful in determining the type of intussusception (AP diameter measures 1.5 cm for transient small bowel in the RLQ and periumbilical region vs 3.5 cm for large bowel) and identifying those requiring surgery (based on lengths of the intussusception that are >3.5 cm).

Fundamentals of Disease

Intussusception, which is defined as the telescoping or invagination of a proximal portion of intestine (intussusceptum) into a more distal portion (intussuscipiens), is one of the most common causes of bowel obstruction in infants and toddlers (3 months to 2 years of age) with a male predominance of 3:2. The different types of intussusception are ileoileal, colocolic, ileoileocolic, or ileocolic, which is the most common (80%). The incidence is 2 to 4 cases per 1000 live births with seasonal peaks correlating with gastroenteritis and upper respiratory tract infections periods when there is Peyer's patch lymph node hypertrophy from rotavirus or adenovirus infections. Most intussusception (95%) is idiopathic in patients <2 years of age. A pathological lead point is often found in older patients, such as malignancy, Meckel diverticulum, or polyps. Children with cystic fibrosis may develop intussusception from inspissated meconium in the terminal ileum, including neonates with meconium plug syndrome. When intussusception occurs, the mesentery comes with it, causing obstruction of venous return and engorgement. Vascular compromise with subsequent bowel necrosis, perforation, and sepsis may occur.

Diagnostic Workup and Management

Intussusception results in bowel obstruction; thus, complications such as dehydration and aspiration from emesis can occur. Management starts with rapid fluid resuscitation (20-60 mL/kg). Some patients may present with hypovolemic and/or septic shock. An NG tube should be placed to intermittent suction for stomach decompression, especially if the child is actively vomiting. Ischemia and bowel necrosis can cause bowel perforation and sepsis; therefore, antibiotics should be started in a timely manner. Adequate pain medication should be provided prior to reduction with air enema via a lubricated straight catheter that is placed in the rectum and taped to the buttock. A manometer and blood pressure cuff are connected to the straight catheter and air is insufflated slowly to a pressure of 70 to 80 mm Hg (maximum 120 mm Hg) and followed fluoroscopically. The radiologist will often request that a pediatric surgeon be present or be on standby while the enema reduction is being performed. Patients should be admitted following the procedure to monitor for recurrences.

Special Considerations

Contraindications to reduction via enema include signs of peritonitis, sepsis, and shock. Factors significantly predictive of bowel perforation during enema reduction are younger age and a longer duration of symptoms (>24 hours).

Recurrence rates following nonoperative reduction and surgical reduction are approximately 5% and 1% to 4%, respectively. They tend to occur within the first 24 to 48 hours. Mortality rate is <1%. Other long-term complications include short bowel syndrome if a large length of bowel was necrotic with delayed presentation, diagnosis, or management. Whether treated by operative or radiographic reduction, late stricture (4-8 weeks) may occur within the length of intestine involved.

TIPS TO REMEMBER

- Profound lethargy without preceding history of abdominal pain may be the only presenting sign of intussusceptions and can be misdiagnosed as sepsis or a postictal state, resulting in a delay in diagnosis and management.
- Bilious emesis and the age of presentation are extremely helpful in narrowing down your list of differential diagnoses.

- Always start with the ABCs since infants with intussusception may present in extremis, and thus will require aggressive fluid resuscitation.
- The classic triad of intussusceptions is intermittent colicky abdominal pain associated with bilious emesis and bloody stool, but this triad is not always present.
- Bilious emesis in an infant is due to lower GI obstruction, and should be taken seriously, until proven otherwise.
- Intussusception may present with intermittent episodes of lethargy, especially in infants.
- Currant jelly stool is a late presentation.

COMPREHENSION QUESTIONS

1. Which of the following is not seen in intussusceptions?
   - A. Episodic abdominal pain
   - B. Bilious emesis
   - C. Painless bloody stool
   - D. Lethargy

2. The gold standard for imaging to make the diagnosis of intussusception is which of the following?
   - A. Plain film
   - B. Ultrasound
   - C. CT scan
   - D. MRI

3. After making the diagnosis of intussusceptions, all of the following are appropriate except which of the following?
   - A. PO pain medication
   - B. IV antibiotics
   - C. NG tube placement
   - D. Notification of the radiologist and surgeons

Answers

1. C. Painful bloody stool is seen in intussusceptions. Painless bloody stool is consistent with Meckel diverticulum.

2. B. The diagnostic study of choice is an ultrasound. Plain film findings may be nonspecific. Too much radiation with CT scans. MRI is too expensive.

3. A. IV pain medication should be given not PO.

SUGGESTED READINGS

Caterino J, Kahan S. *In a Page Emergency Medicine*. Baltimore: Lippincott Williams & Wilkins; 2003:236.
Tintinalli JE, Kelen GD, Stapczynski JS, Ma OJ, Cline DM, eds. *Tintinalli's Emergency Medicine*. 7th ed. New York: McGraw-Hill; 2011 [chapters 123–124] <http://www.accessmedicine.com>.

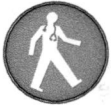

A 32-year-old Female With Headache

Christopher M. McDowell, MD, MEd

CASE DESCRIPTION

Sheila Hopkins is a 32-year-old female who presents to the emergency department with a severe headache. She describes it as very intense and rapid in onset. She is accompanied by her husband and presents in the late evening. On further questioning, she describes a sudden-onset postcoital headache. The intensity was immediately 10/10 and has not remitted. She has some associated nausea and has vomited twice, and complains of dizziness. She was able to walk into the emergency department under her own power. Her past medical history is significant for depression for which she takes sertraline (Zoloft) and 2 caesarean sections with childbirth. She does not usually get headaches and describes this as "the worst headache of her life." Her sister had "some type of brain bleed" at age 35 as well.

Her vitals are temperature 37.1°C (98.9°F), blood pressure 180/100 mm Hg, pulse 110 beats/min, respiratory rate 22 breaths/min, and oxygen saturation of 98% on room air.

On examination you note that Mrs Hopkins is in distress. She is holding her head and moaning in pain. She is mildly diaphoretic and vomits during the examination. She is tachycardic with a benign abdominal examination. Her pupils are reactive, her cranial nerves are intact, and her strength is equal bilaterally. She has no pronator drift and no past pointing. The remaining neurologic examination is unremarkable.

1. What is your differential diagnosis?

2. What are the red flags in Mrs Hopkins' history and physical examination?

3. What test must be ordered immediately?

Answers

1. The differential for headaches is vast, but must be prioritized as critical, emergent, and nonemergent causes. This patient is sick and needs immediate intervention and diagnosis. Table 20-1 contains the critical, emergent, and nonemergent causes of headache.

2. Mrs Hopkins' history and physical examination contain several concerning features. Table 20-2 contains the important red flags for headache with Mrs Hopkins' features in bold.

3. Mrs Hopkins needs an immediate CT scan of her head. A picture of her head CT is listed in Figure 20-1.

Table 20-1. Emergency Physician Differential Diagnosis for Headache

Critical Diagnoses	Emergent Diagnoses	Nonemergent Diagnoses
Intracranial hemorrhage	Intracranial mass	Tension headache
• Subacrachnoid	Benign intracranial hypertension (pseudotumor cerebri)	Migraine headache
• Epidural		Cluster headache
• Subdural		Sinusitis
• Intraparenchymal	Carbon monoxide toxicity	Eye strain
Meningitis	Concussion	Dehydration
Temporal arteritis	Cervical artery dissection	
Acute angle-closure glaucoma		

Table 20-2. Critical Diagnoses and Red Flags for Headache

Critical Diagnosis	History Red Flags	Physical Red Flags
Subarachnoid hemorrhage	**"Worst headache of life"**	Altered mental status, **diaphoresis**
Epidural hematoma	A lucid interval following an initial loss of consciousness	Rapid progression to coma
Subdural hematoma	New-onset seizure with history of trauma in the last month; alcoholics, elderly	Postictal confusion
Intraparenchymal hemorrhage (stroke)	Sudden-onset mental status change	Focal neurologic deficits
Meningitis	Fever with neck stiffness (meningismus)	Meningismus with Brudzinski or Kernig sign
Temporal arteritis (giant cell arteritis)	Temporal headache, polymyalgia rheumatic history, or vision changes	Tenderness to palpation over temporal artery
Carbon monoxide poisoning	Sick household contacts or pets, worsening symptoms while at home	Nausea, fatigue
Acute angle-closure glaucoma	New-onset blurred vision, "seeing halos around objects"	Mid-dilated pupil with increased intraocular pressure

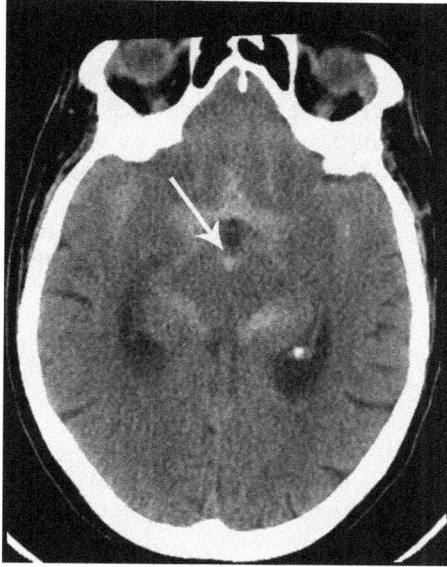

Figure 20-1. The appearance of a subarachnoid hemorrhage on CT scan. (Reproduced, with permission, from Henry GL, Little N, Jagoda A, Pellegrino TR. *Neurologic Emergencies.* 3rd ed. New York: McGraw-Hill Education, 2010 [Figure 2-5A] <http://www.accessemergencymedicine.com>. Copyright © The McGraw-Hill Companies, Inc. All rights reserved)

CASE REVIEW

Mrs Hopkins is having a subarachnoid hemorrhage (SAH). The general principles of SAH management include establishing the safety net, emergent airway management in those patients unable to protect their airways, emergent noncontrast head CT, and neurosurgical consultation. Management of hypertension can reduce risk of rebleed with care taken not to induce hypotension. Vasospasm is common and may be treated with nimodipine. SAH patients require very specialized treatment and are best managed at centers with neurosurgical and/or radiologic interventionalists, as well as neurologic intensive care units.

HEADACHE

Diagnostic Reasoning

Headache is a very common chief complaint and is responsible for 3% to 5% of visits to the emergency department. Emergency physicians must quickly decipher which patients are at risk for critical or emergent diagnoses and provide stabilization as well as a diagnosis. Even in patients with suspected noncritical diagnoses, it can be difficult to determine who needs imaging and what type of analgesia patients require. The emergent diagnoses for headache can be found in Table 20-1.

A focused history opens the differential diagnosis for headaches. Identifying the onset as acute or gradual and whether the patient has experienced a headache like this before helps to focus the differential. Other characteristics including location, severity, constitutional symptoms, vision changes, and new neurologic symptoms are important as well. The physical examination will depend somewhat on the historical information, but all headache patients need vital signs and a complete neurologic assessment.

Diagnostic Workup and Management

All patients who appear ill or have characteristics of emergent diagnoses need the "safety net" or "IV-O$_2$-pulse-ox-monitor" established. This should be done while simultaneously gathering historical and physical examination data.

Adjunctive testing is often necessary and sometimes emergently needed in the workup of headache patients. Perhaps the most important of these is the noncontrast head CT. It allows for quick diagnosis of potentially life-threatening hemorrhages, many mass lesions, and cerebral edema. The bigger question is which patients require emergent imaging? Most authorities would agree that all those with new-onset focal deficits require an emergent head CT. The American College of Emergency Physicians' (ACEP) clinical policy on acute headache suggests imaging 2 additional groups of patients: HIV patients with new-onset headache and those over 50 with new headache even with no focal neurologic deficits.

The lumbar puncture (LP) is another key adjunctive test. The LP allows for definitive diagnosis of infectious causes of headache such as meningitis and/or encephalitis. It is also employed in the diagnostic algorithm for SAH and is diagnostic or therapeutic for idiopathic intracranial hypertension (IIH) (formerly known as pseudotumor cerebri). Controversy exists regarding the use of CT prior to LP. Due to the risk of herniation, most sources suggest noncontrast head CT in those patients with abnormal neurologic examinations, papilledema, or abnormal mental status prior to LP.

SAH is one of the most critical diagnoses for the emergency physician to make. Students are taught to consider this in all "worst headache of my life" patients. Another important factor to consider is the immediate or "thunderclap" onset. One might expect debilitating neurologic deficits to accompany this etiology. Yet nearly half of all SAH patients have normal neurologic examinations. Asking about family medical history is crucial, as those with first- or second-degree relatives with a SAH are at much higher risk for SAH as well. The workup starts with a noncontrast head CT. Despite the advances in technology, patients with negative head CT studies still require LP for further evaluation. The presence of red blood cells and/or the presence of the breakdown product of xanthochromia is diagnostic for SAH. There is much debate about the role of CT angiogram in the workup of SAH. New algorithms are being tested, but no clear evidence exists for CT angiogram to supplant LP at this time.

Epidural hematoma results from sudden traumatic disruption of the middle meningeal artery. Classic teaching describes an acute loss of consciousness or altered sensorium, followed by a lucid interval, and then rapid deterioration. However, this pattern varies greatly across epidural hematoma patients. Regardless of clinical presentation, concern for rapid deterioration necessitates emergent neurosurgical consultation for surgical drainage.

Subdural hematoma represents another life-threatening intracranial hemorrhage. These patients develop slowly expanding hematomas after sudden acceleration–deceleration trauma. The time course of subdural hematoma is much slower than that of epidural hematoma, due to venous bleeding of disrupted bridging veins. It should be noted that the elderly and alcoholics are at higher risk due to cerebral atrophy. These patients often have a remote history of trauma extending back as far as 1 to 2 weeks.

Intraparenchymal hemorrhage, also known as intracerebral hemorrhage, can be the result of trauma or secondary to long-standing hypertension. Neurologic deficits depend on the area of brain involved and may include extension into the ventricles as well. Treatment depends on the involved area and extent of neurologic dysfunction.

Meningitis is an infectious and potentially life-threatening etiology of headache. Although we often think of meningitis in the face of fever and neck stiffness, not all patients will have these findings. Immunocompromised patients or those already being treated for head and neck infections must also be considered at higher risk. These patients require LP. Remember, patients with bacterial meningitis are at very high risk for long-term morbidity and mortality. Antibiotics are the lifesaving intervention. Therefore, do not delay antibiotics for anticipated LP.

Temporal arteritis is a critical diagnosis of headache most often seen in patients over 50 years of age. Temporal headache associated with a history of jaw claudication or polymyalgia rheumatica is highly suggestive of the diagnosis. The biggest complication is vision loss secondary to ischemic optic neuritis. Diagnostic criteria include age over 50, new-onset localized headache, temporal artery tenderness or decreased pulse, erythrocyte sedimentation rate >50 mm/h, and abnormal arterial biopsy. Three of the 5 criteria are required for diagnosis. Emergent treatment for suspected cases includes oral prednisone, follow-up with ophthalmology, and referral for temporal artery biopsy.

Acute angle-closure glaucoma is a critical diagnosis of headache that must be made in order to prevent blindness. Glaucoma causes vision loss secondary to increased intraocular pressure and optic neuropathy. Obstruction to aqueous humor outflow results in acute angle-closure glaucoma. Symptoms are usually precipitated by pupillary dilation and include abrupt onset pain, headache, and even nausea or vomiting. Examination reveals the classical description of the mid-position pupil, hazy cornea, and hard globe. Diagnosis is confirmed by measuring intraocular pressure that exceeds the normal 10 to 20 mm Hg. In many cases, this elevation can be severe and greater than 50 mm Hg. Treatment is based on 3 strategies and should be completed simultaneously with ophthalmology consultation. Aqueous humor production is decreased by administration of beta-blockers (timolol), alpha-adrenergic agonists, and carbonic anhydrase inhibitors (acetazolamide). Mannitol reduces the amount of vitreous humor and is rapidly effective in lowering intraocular pressure. Finally, definitive care requires iridectomy by ophthalmology.

TIPS TO REMEMBER

- Noncontrast head CT is the imaging test of choice for workup of severe headache.
- Delayed presentations of subdural hematomas are common. Ask about remote history of trauma.
- Ask about both the onset of symptoms and whether this headache is similar to previous ones in your history.
- Do not forget cerebellar testing as part of the neurologic examination.
- Do not delay antibiotics for LP.
- Remember to consider acute glaucoma in your differential for headache.

COMPREHENSION QUESTIONS

1. In patients with sudden-onset severe headaches and a negative emergent head CT, what test should be ordered or performed next?
    A. MRI
    B. CTA
    C. LP
    D. ICP monitor
    E. Endotracheal intubation

2. In patients with severe headache, fever, and new rash, antibiotic/antiviral therapy should be started:
    A. Once the urine and CXR are completed
    B. Once the LP is completed
    C. Once the cerebrospinal fluid results are back
    D. Immediately in those whom you have a high suspicion
    E. Once an emergent head CT is completed

3. An elderly man presents to the emergency department after a new-onset seizure. He had a fall approximately 2 weeks ago and takes clopidogrel. Which of the following is most likely seen on his head CT?

      A. Epidural hematoma

      B. Intracranial hematoma

      C. Subdural hematoma

      D. Hydrocephalus

      E. CNS abscess

4. EMS brings in a patient with difficulty speaking and right-sided weakness. What is the most important question to address regarding potential treatment?

      A. Is the patient taking aspirin?

      B. When was the patient last seen at his or her baseline?

      C. Is the patient left or right hand dominant?

      D. Has the patient had a stroke previously?

      E. What risk factors does the patient have for stroke?

Answers

1. **C.** In a patient with red flags for SAH and negative head CT, LP is the most appropriate next step in the workup.

2. **D.** In patients with a high-risk presentation for meningitis, antibiotics should be started emergently. Antibiotics may be lifesaving and should not be delayed for head CT, LP performance, or CSF results.

3. **C.** This patient exhibits a classic story for the delayed development of a subdural hematoma.

4. **B.** In patients who present with symptoms of acute stroke, it is imperative to determine the time of onset or last known well time. Thrombolytic therapy may be considered out to 6 hours after onset and/or interventional therapy may be considered even longer.

SUGGESTED READINGS

Marx JA, Hockberger RS, Walls RM, eds. *Rosen's Emergency Medicine: Concepts and Clinical Practice.* 7th ed. Philadelphia: Mosby-Elsevier; 2010 [chapter 16] <http://www.mdconsult.com>.

Tintinalli JE, Kelen GD, Stapczynski JS, Ma OJ, Cline DM, eds. *Tintinalli's Emergency Medicine.* 7th ed. New York: McGraw-Hill; 2011 [chapters 159–161, 217, 236] <http://www.accessmedicine.com>.

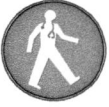

A 47-year-old Male With Headache

Christopher M. McDowell, MD, MEd and Ted R. Clark, MD, MPP

CASE DESCRIPTION

Stephen Andrews is a 47-year-old male who presents to the emergency department with a chief complaint of headache. He has had many similar headaches in the past and they usually occur weekly. Today's headache started gradually along his forehead but has steadily increased. He complains of mild photophobia but denies nausea, vision changes, dizziness, fever, or neck stiffness. He presents to the ED today because his usual Motrin and sleep combination did not alleviate the headache. He denies trauma or loss of consciousness. Mr Andrews' past medical history is significant for hypertension. He denies history of migraines, SAH, or family medical history of cerebral aneurysms. His social history is negative for tobacco usage or recreational drug usage. He drinks approximately 2 beers per week. He is employed as a stock analyst with a major financial firm and is under a significant amount of stress.

His vitals are temperature 37.1 (98.9), blood pressure 132/82 mm Hg, pulse 74 beats/min, respiratory rate 16 breaths/min, and oxygen saturation of 99% on room air.

On physical examination, Mr Andrews appears in no acute distress. He is interactive and has a normal cranial nerve examination, no temple tenderness to palpation, and the rest of his neurologic examination is unremarkable.

1. Review the critical diagnoses and red flags for a chief complaint of "headache." What red flags does this patient have?

2. What emergent and nonemergent diagnoses should be considered?

3. Does this patient require emergent imaging?

Answers

1. Mr Andrews has a headache but has a long-standing history of same. This headache started gradually and his neurologic examination is normal. His headache is similar to those in the past; he is afebrile and not immunocompromised. Therefore, Mr Andrews has no red flags to suggest emergent or critical diagnoses.

2. All patients presenting with headache must have emergent and critical diagnoses considered. However, Mr Andrews' history and physical examination lack red flags to suggest any critical diagnoses. The gradual onset and lack of trauma are inconsistent with subarachnoid hemorrhage, epidural hematoma,

and subdural hematoma. He is afebrile and not immunocompromised making infection unlikely. He has no temporal pain or vision changes to suggest temporal arteritis or acute angle-closure glaucoma. His headache is similar to previous episodes. This presentation fits well for tension headache, migraine headache, or cluster headache.

3. Mr Andrews is under 50 years of age, has a nonfocal neurologic examination, is not immunocompromised, and has a headache that is similar to those in the past. Therefore, Mr Andrews does not require emergent imaging (noncontrast head CT).

CASE REVIEW

Mr Andrews does not appear to have a critical or emergent diagnosis. He is most likely suffering from a tension headache. He is afebrile, normotensive, and in no distress with a nonfocal neurologic examination. He does not need emergent imaging. Treatment options vary, but it would be reasonable to start with IV prochlorperazine. Diphenhydramine is often added to prevent the side effect of akathisia. His discharge instructions should emphasize red flag symptoms mandating return to the ER and follow-up with his primary care provider.

HEADACHE

Diagnostic Reasoning

Although Mr Andrews has the same chief complaint as Mrs Hopkins, he is a very different patient. His history and physical examination reveals no red flags or focal neurologic deficits. His history of previous headaches similar to this one, the gradual onset, and normal mental status are reassuring. A focused history and physical examination quickly rules out the emergent and critical diagnoses discussed in our previous case and listed in Table 21-1.

Diagnostic Workup and Management

After considering Mr Andrews' history and physical information, there is very little concern about critical diagnoses. Mr Andrews' presentation is stable and his neurologic examination is nonfocal. This makes it unlikely that he will need the "safety net" established. His presentation does not require emergent head imaging or lumbar puncture.

Intracranial mass is certainly a consideration in the patient with headache. Mr Andrews is middle-aged but has a nonfocal neurologic examination. His history of chronic headaches, no previous malignancy, no trauma, and a normal physical examination do not suggest the need for emergent imaging. This patient

Table 21-1. Emergency Physician Differential Diagnosis for Headache

Critical Diagnoses	Emergent Diagnoses	Nonemergent Diagnoses
Intracranial hemorrhage	Intracranial mass	Tension headache
• Subacrachnoid	Benign intracranial hypertension (pseudotumor cerebri)	Migraine headache
• Epidural		Cluster headache
• Subdural		Sinusitis
• Intraparenchymal	Carbon monoxide toxicity	Eye strain
Meningitis	Concussion	Dehydration
Temporal arteritis	Cervical artery dissection	
Acute angle-closure glaucoma		

can easily be referred to his primary care office for consideration of neuroimaging if symptoms persist or change.

Benign intracranial hypertension (formerly known as pseudotumor cerebri) is a cause of chronic headache. Although the etiology is unclear, it results in elevated intracranial pressure. This pressure elevation can lead to vision loss if untreated. Patients may present with nausea, vomiting, decreased visual acuity, or visual deficits. Diagnosis is made by measurement of opening pressure on lumbar puncture. Treatment includes acetazolamide or serial lumbar punctures to remove cerebrospinal fluid. In severe cases, shunts may be placed for long-term treatment.

Carbon monoxide poisoning is an insidious cause of life-threatening headache. Exposure can occur in numerous settings including vehicle exhaust, gas heaters, space heaters, wood-burning stoves, charcoal fires, and many others. Generally these poisonings occur more commonly during fall and winter months due to gas heating. However, as noted above, the etiologies for carbon monoxide can be found anytime during the year. Symptoms include headache, nausea, and altered mental status extending even to coma. The variable nature of disease presentation makes diagnosis difficult. Sick contacts or ill pets living in the same environment may be key to diagnosis. Diagnosis is made by blood testing for carboxyhemoglobin (COHb) levels. Hemoglobin has a much greater affinity for carbon monoxide than oxygen. The resultant COHb leads to uncoupling of oxidative phosphorylation and tissue hypoxia or death. COHb levels greater than 10% suggest toxicity. Treatment is rapid administration of 100% oxygen to displace the COHb. Hyperbaric treatment has been employed but is not considered first-line treatment. Young children and pregnant females are at especially high risk for carbon monoxide poisoning.

Concussion is a form of mild traumatic brain injury (TBI). Usually mild TBI is defined as a Glasgow coma scale (GCS) of 14 to 15 following an acceleration–deceleration injury. Associated symptoms may include loss of consciousness, headache, nausea, vomiting, memory changes, and other neurologic symptoms. Treatment is usually supportive and focused on prevention of a second injury. Second-impact syndrome represents a poorly understood but severe complication of repeated concussions. This is the basis for not allowing patients with a concussion to participate in high-risk activities until all symptoms have resolved. Therefore, the decision to return to competition or high-risk activities must be addressed in the treatment or discharge process.

Tension headache was originally thought to be related to extracranial muscle tension. Tension headaches are typically defined as bilateral and nonpulsating headaches that are not associated with nausea or vomiting. However, more recent information suggests that tension headache and migraine headache may actually represent different ends of the same disease spectrum. Treatment is often focused around the use of oral agents such as acetaminophen and nonsteroidal anti-inflammatory agents (NSAIDs). More severe cases may benefit from treatment similar to migraine headaches as listed below.

Migraine headache is a very commonly seen condition in the emergency department. The mechanism behind migraines has been evolving over many years, but is now regarded as a result of vasoactive peptide release that results in arterial dilation. Thus, it is no surprise that many treatment options mitigate this vasodilation. Migraines are more common in females and may even start in childhood. They are typically slow in onset and described as unilateral with pulsation or throbbing. Nausea, vomiting, photophobia, and phonophobia frequently accompany these headaches. They may present with auras such as the classic scintillating scotoma, but may also start with other neurologic symptoms. There are many options for treatment with most sources calling for nonnarcotic approaches first-line. 5-HT serotonin receptor agonists (triptans), metoclopramide, prochlorperazine, droperidol, ketorolac, and dexamethasone are all reasonable options in the emergency department. Imaging is usually not indicated unless new focal neurologic signs are present or the headache syndrome itself is different from the patient's usual migraine.

TIPS TO REMEMBER

- Carbon monoxide poisoning can occur any time of year.
- Ask about the onset of the headache: gradual versus thunderclap.
- Ask if this headache is similar to previous headaches.
- Don't forget to check intraocular pressure.
- The EM physician should explore red flags and risk factors for all presentations of headache.

COMPREHENSION QUESTIONS

1. A 27-year-old male presents with a gradually worsening headache. He has had similar headaches before. He denies weakness, numbness, or vision changes. He has some associated nausea and has vomited twice. He has been diagnosed with migraine headaches in the past. Which of the following is *not* appropriate first-line treatment?

      A. Metoclopramide
      B. Morphine
      C. Ketorolac
      D. Sumatriptan

2. A 67-year-old female presents with a new-onset headache. She is holding her head and complains of pain in her left eye. She just left an orchestra concert and notes some vision changes as well. Which of the following diagnostic tests is most important?

      A. Emergent head CT
      B. Lumbar puncture
      C. Erythrocyte sedimentation rate (ESR)
      D. Intraocular pressure (tonometry)

Answers

1. B. Although morphine may help his pain, narcotics are generally regarded as secondary agents for the treatment of acute headaches. Each of the other choices would be appropriate first-line treatment.

2. D. This patient describes symptoms that are concerning for acute glaucoma. She needs to have her intraocular pressure assessed rapidly to confirm the diagnosis. If elevated, emergent contact with ophthalmology and treatment should be initiated.

SUGGESTED READINGS

Marx JA, Hockberger RS, Walls RM, eds. *Rosen's Emergency Medicine: Concepts and Clinical Practice.* 7th ed. Philadelphia: Mosby-Elsevier; 2010 [chapter 18] <http://www.mdconsult.com>.
Tintinalli JE, Kelen GD, Stapczynski JS, Ma OJ, Cline DM, eds. *Tintinalli's Emergency Medicine.* 7th ed. New York: McGraw-Hill; 2011 [chapters 159, 254] <http://www.accessmedicine.com>.

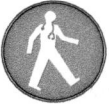

A 32-year-old Female With Vaginal Bleeding

Christi M. Lindorfer, MD and Christopher M. McDowell, MD, MEd

CASE DESCRIPTION

Mrs Bradley is a 32-year-old female G1P0 at 7 weeks gestation by date of last menstrual period presenting with a 1-day history of vaginal bleeding. She states that she has used 4 sanitary pads during this time. She reports suprapubic abdominal pain that radiates to her lower back. The pain is cramping, constant, and currently 4/10 in intensity. There are no aggravating or relieving factors for her pain. She denies any fever, chills, nausea, vomiting, constipation, diarrhea, melena, hematochezia, hematuria, or dysuria. She has no known medical problems. Her current medications include prenatal vitamins. She has no known drug allergies and has never had surgery. She denies any tobacco, alcohol, or illicit drug use. Family medical history is noncontributory.

Her vital signs are temperature 37.1 (98.8), heart rate 82 beats/min, blood pressure 115/60 mm Hg, respiratory rate 20 breaths/min, and oxygen saturation of 99% on room air.

Physical examination reveals an anxious female who appears her stated age in no acute distress. Cardiac examination is significant for normal rate and rhythm without any murmurs, rubs, or gallops heard on auscultation. Respiratory examination is unremarkable. Abdominal examination reveals normal bowel sounds. Abdomen is soft and nondistended with no tenderness on palpation. Pelvic examination is significant for moderate amount of blood in the vaginal vault without any purulent discharge, adnexal tenderness, or cervical motion tenderness. The cervical os is closed.

1. What is your differential diagnosis?

2. What are the red flags in Mrs Bradley's history and physical examination?

3. What tests and treatments should be completed?

Answers

1. While ectopic pregnancy is one of the most concerning diagnoses to consider, there are other important causes warranting investigation and management during early pregnancy including abortion (threatened, inevitable, missed, or incomplete), implantation bleeding, cervicitis, cervical cancer, and other cervical conditions (see Table 22-1). The most important diagnoses to consider in late-term vaginal bleeding are placental abruption and placenta previa. Other

Table 22-1. Emergency Physician Differential Diagnosis for Vaginal Bleeding in Pregnancy

Critical Diagnoses	Emergent diagnoses	Nonemergent Diagnoses
Ectopic pregnancy	Septic abortion	Cervical lesion
Placental abruption	Complete abortion	Vaginitis/cervicitis
Placenta previa	Incomplete abortion	
Vasa previa	Threatened abortion	
Uterine rupture	Inevitable abortion	
	Missed abortion	
	Molar pregnancy	

causes of vaginal bleeding in late pregnancy include vasa previa, uterine rupture, preterm labor, infections, and genital tract lesions. In all cases of vaginal bleeding throughout pregnancy, be sure to consider bleeding from other sources such as the urinary or gastrointestinal tracts.

2. The red flags in Mrs Bradley's history include her pregnancy and her vaginal bleeding with use of 4 sanitary pads. All pregnancies should be considered at risk for ectopic until confirmed as intrauterine by ultrasound. Her physical examination red flag is a moderate amount of blood in the vaginal vault (see Table 22-2).

3. Pertinent laboratory tests in this clinical situation include a urine pregnancy test, urinalysis, hemoglobin, quantitative beta-hCG, blood type, screen, and antibodies. If an infectious cause of bleeding is suspected, cervical cultures and tests are important to order. Bedside or formal ultrasound is crucial for diagnosis. Treatment must include initial fluid resuscitation with stabilization, transfusion of blood products if appropriate, RhoGAM administration for rhesus (Rh) negative patients, treatment of infectious causes of bleeding, and counseling.

CASE REVIEW

Vaginal bleeding in pregnancy is a concerning presentation that warrants immediate evaluation and care. During the initial management of a pregnant patient with vaginal bleeding, it is important to establish a "safety net" (include fetal monitoring in those over 20 weeks) while assessing the patient and to start resuscitation if necessary. Diagnostic workup must contain a minimum of hemoglobin,

Table 22-2. Critical Diagnoses and Red Flags for Vaginal Bleeding in Pregnancy

Critical Diagnosis	History Red Flags	Physical Red Flags
Ectopic pregnancy	History of maternal smoking, advanced age, pelvic inflammatory disorder, prior spontaneous abortion, medical abortion, infertility, fallopian tube abnormalities, abnormal endometrium, presence of an intrauterine device, or prior ectopic pregnancy. History of present illness including vaginal bleeding or abdominal pain	Tachycardia, hypotension, vaginal bleeding, abdominal tenderness, cervical motion tenderness, adnexal tenderness, adnexal mass, peritoneal signs
Placental abruption	History of increased maternal age, toxins, number of previous pregnancies resulting in live births, hypertension, preeclampsia, thrombophilia, prior placental abruption, blunt abdominal trauma, and history of physical violence during pregnancy. History of present illness including vaginal bleeding, abdominal pain, contractions	Tachycardia, hypotension, uterine tenderness, uterine irritability or contractions, vaginal bleeding, fetal distress
Placenta previa	History of increased maternal age, multiple pregnancies, smoking, and prior cesarean section. History of present illness including vaginal bleeding and sometimes abdominal pain	Tachycardia, hypotension, vaginal bleeding, uterine irritability
Vasa previa	History of artificial reproductive techniques, accessory lobes of the placenta, placenta previa, some fetal anomalies, and abnormalities of the placental insertion of the umbilical cord. History of present illness including painless vaginal bleeding in late pregnancy following rupture of membranes	Tachycardia, hypotension, vaginal bleeding
Uterine rupture	History of prior uterine surgery. History of present illness including active labor in late pregnancy, abdominal pain, or vaginal bleeding	Tachycardia, hypotension, vaginal bleeding, fetal distress, loss of fetal station, palpable uterine defect, abdominal tenderness

quantitative beta-hCG, type and screen, and ultrasound. Mrs Bradley's bed-side transvaginal ultrasound shows an empty uterus. Her quantitative hCG is 2000 mIU/mL that, in conjunction with her ultrasound, suggests an ectopic pregnancy. Since she is hemodynamically stable, it is reasonable to contact the Obstetrics/Gynecology service for management decisions including possible medical management. If hemodynamically unstable, emergent consultation is required with expectant operative management.

FIRST TRIMESTER VAGINAL BLEEDING

Diagnostic Reasoning

Vaginal bleeding in pregnancy may best be considered in the context of early (before 14 weeks gestation) versus late (14-24 weeks gestation and above) pregnancy, as gestational age and viability have a large effect on differential diagnosis and clinical management. Approximately one fourth of clinically detectable pregnancies are complicated by vaginal bleeding, making this a common clinical presentation.

It is important to have a high clinical suspicion for ectopic pregnancy in patients with bleeding or abdominal pain in early pregnancy. If ectopic pregnancy is suspected, consult Obstetrics/Gynecology immediately.

While ectopic pregnancy is one of the most concerning diagnoses to consider, there are other important causes of early vaginal bleeding that warrant investigation and management including abortion (threatened, inevitable, missed, or incomplete), implantation bleeding, cervicitis, other cervical conditions, and cervical carcinoma. In late-term pregnancies, vaginal bleeding may be caused by placental abruption, placenta previa, vasa previa, and uterine rupture.

Diagnostic Workup and Management

As mentioned earlier, the diagnosis and management of vaginal bleeding in pregnancy is different for patients during early versus late pregnancy (previable vs postviable). Regardless of gestational age, patients who appear sick or have concerning vital signs should have a "safety net" in place on arrival to the emergency department.

Mrs Bradley's symptoms and physical examination do not provide sufficient information to differentiate between ectopic pregnancy and spontaneous abortion. Workup for vaginal bleeding in early pregnancy should include a urine pregnancy test, urinalysis, hemoglobin, quantitative beta-hCG, and blood type, screen, and antibodies. A formal or bedside ultrasound must also be performed. Patients should receive supportive care including fluids and blood products if necessary. RhoGAM should be administered to any Rh negative woman who suffers vaginal bleeding or pregnancy loss.

If Mrs Bradley presented with these symptoms in late pregnancy, the first step in her care would be to establish a "safety net," assess her for signs of hemodynamic instability, resuscitate with fluids, provide continuous fetal monitoring, and obtain an obstetric consultation with transfer to an obstetric unit. Appropriate laboratory tests would include a baseline hemoglobin level, platelet count, type and crossmatch, PT, PTT, fibrinogen level, and testing for the presence of fibrin split products. A transabdominal ultrasound would be obtained in order to assess for possible placenta previa and placental abruption.

In this late-term clinical scenario, no bimanual examination, speculum examination, or transvaginal ultrasound is appropriate until placenta previa is ruled out. A patient with significant bleeding or signs of shock requires emergent obstetric consultation prior to diagnostic results. Vaginal delivery is appropriate management of third trimester bleeding unless the patient has placenta previa. If there is placenta previa, fetal distress, severe placental abruption, or severe hemorrhage, or a trial of labor has failed, then cesarean section is indicated. Other treatments include blood products and RhoGAM administration in Rh negative patients.

Ectopic pregnancy results when a fertilized ovum implants in a location other than the endometrium and must be considered during the assessment of female patients with vaginal bleeding or abdominal pain. It occurs in 2% of pregnancies and causes 6% of mortality in pregnancy. Ectopic pregnancy occurs in approximately 10% of pregnant women presenting to the ED with vaginal bleeding or pain in the first trimester. It is important to have a high suspicion for ectopic pregnancy as half of patients presenting with ectopic pregnancy have no risk factors and symptoms are often intermittent. Ectopic pregnancy can result in abortion, involution, or rupture. Risk factors for ectopic pregnancy include pelvic inflammatory disorder, smoking, advanced age, prior spontaneous abortion, medical abortion, infertility, fallopian tube abnormalities, abnormal endometrium, and the presence of an intrauterine device.

Examination findings may include vaginal bleeding, abdominal tenderness, cervical motion tenderness, adnexal tenderness, or peritoneal signs. Ten percent to 20% of patients will have an adnexal mass found on examination. In cases of suspected ectopic pregnancy, a pelvic ultrasound and quantitative beta-hCG must be performed. A pelvic ultrasound can show a normal intrauterine pregnancy, be indeterminate, or sometimes is diagnostic for ectopic pregnancy. When an hCG is less than 1000 mIU/mL given an indeterminate pelvic ultrasound, the risk of ectopic pregnancy is increased by 4 times. A normal intrauterine pregnancy may be visible on transvaginal ultrasound with a beta-hCG as low as 1500 mIU/mL (6500 mIU/mL on transabdominal ultrasound). Beta-hCG levels can be monitored in the outpatient setting and used for diagnostic information. In a normal pregnancy, beta-hCG levels double every 1.8 to 3 days for the first 6 or 7 weeks and a slow rise or decrease in beta-hCG levels can be associated with ectopic pregnancy (see Table 22-3).

Table 22-3. Association of Ultrasound Findings With Gestational Age and Beta-Human Chorionic Gonadotropin Level

Weeks Since Last Menstrual Period	Quantitative Beta-hCG Level (mIU/mL)	Ultrasound Findings
5	1,000	Gestational sac
5-6	1,500-2,000	"Discriminatory zone" at which a normal intrauterine pregnancy can usually be seen on transvaginal ultrasound
6	2,500	Yolk sac
6-7	3,000	Upper "discriminatory zone" at which a normal intrauterine pregnancy should be seen on transvaginal ultrasound
7	5,000	Fetal pole
8	17,000	Fetal heart motion

Other diagnostic tests include serum progesterone levels, culdocentesis, and laparoscopy. Laparoscopy is accurate as well as therapeutic and is appropriate in stable patients in the first trimester of pregnancy with peritoneal signs or a large amount of peritoneal fluid. As in all patients with vaginal bleeding in pregnancy, patients suspected to have an ectopic pregnancy should have a blood type and crossmatch as well as a baseline hemoglobin level. Patients should also receive fluids and blood products as appropriate. Medical treatment is most suitable for patients with a tubal mass less than 4 cm, no fetal heart activity, and no evidence of rupture on ultrasound. Methotrexate is the most common medication given. Medical therapy is successful 85% to 93% of the time. Those patients who are unstable or do not meet criteria for medical treatment should be taken for laparoscopy or laparotomy.

Spontaneous abortion is the most common complication in pregnancy. It most often occurs in the first trimester (approximately 80%) and occurs in almost one half of patients who experience vaginal bleeding in early pregnancy. Patients with spontaneous abortion most often present during weeks 8 to 12. Fetal death usually occurs several weeks prior and ultrasound studies in most cases indicate fetal death before 8 weeks gestation. It is important to correlate examination, laboratory, and pelvic ultrasound findings in order to differentiate between a threatened, complete, missed, and septic abortion. Threatened abortion is present when vaginal bleeding occurs with a closed cervical os. Complete abortion is the expulsion of all of the products of conception. On pelvic examination, the patient will have a closed cervical os and a firm uterus. An incomplete abortion results in expulsion of a portion of the products of conception, but some products of conception are retained. On examination, the cervical os is open. Inevitable abortion refers to uterine bleeding before 20 weeks gestation with an open cervix, but no expulsion of the products of conception. In missed abortion, the embryo or fetus dies, but the products of conception are not expelled. Septic abortion involves intrauterine infection that occurs due to retained product after fetal demise. Treatment of patients with spontaneous abortion must include initial fluid resuscitation, RhoGAM administration for Rh negative patients, treatment of infectious causes of bleeding, and transfusion of blood products if appropriate. It is important to counsel and reassure patients as they may have feelings of guilt as well as uncertainty regarding their prognosis.

Placental abruption causes approximately 30% of vaginal bleeding during the second half of pregnancy. It can occur as spontaneous hemorrhage or following trauma that results in shearing of the placenta from the uterine wall. Approximately 70% of patients with placental abruption have vaginal bleeding. About two thirds of patients have uterine pain or tenderness and one third have uterine irritability or contractions. However, up to 20% of women with placental abruption will have no pain or bleeding. Placental abruption can lead to fetal distress, hypotension, and disseminated intravascular coagulation. Ultrasound is the test used to diagnose placental abruption, but it is not a very sensitive test. As with all patients with vaginal bleeding in late pregnancy, workup should include a baseline hemoglobin level, platelet count, type and crossmatch, PT, PTT, fibrinogen level, and testing for the presence of fibrin split products. Bimanual or speculum examination should be avoided until placenta previa is ruled out. Continuous fetal monitoring must be provided. Treatment should include obstetric consultation and transfer, fluid resuscitation, blood products when needed, and RhoGAM for Rh negative patients.

Placenta previa occurs when the placenta implants over the cervical os. It is more likely to occur in patients of advanced age, who are multiparous, with a history of smoking and prior cesarean section. Bleeding occurs when placental blood vessels in the lower uterus are torn by uterine wall stretching during growth or by cervical dilation. Patients present most commonly with painless vaginal bleeding, but can also experience uterine irritability. Bimanual examination and speculum examination should be avoided so as not to cause further bleeding or complications. In most patients, placenta previa resolves by the time of delivery due to lengthening of the lower uterine wall. Twenty percent of patients with placenta previa have complete previa, which can cause significant hemorrhage. Ultrasound is very accurate in diagnosing placenta previa. Other testing and treatment is similar to that previously discussed in this case.

Vasa previa classically presents as painless vaginal bleeding in late pregnancy following rupture of membranes. It requires emergent cesarean section as well as the workup and treatments mentioned previously for all patients with vaginal bleeding late in pregnancy.

Risk factors for vasa previa include placenta previa, presence of accessory lobes of the placenta, abnormalities of the placental insertion of the umbilical cord, and some associated fetal anomalies.

Uterine rupture is a full-thickness perforation of the uterine wall that occurs during late pregnancy and often during labor. It can present with vaginal bleeding, abdominal pain, loss of fetal station, and uterine defect on examination. The severity of rupture and fetal extrusion correlates with the fetal mortality rate, which can range from 1% to 20%. Uterine rupture can occur without pain or bleeding. Prolonged fetal heart rate decelerations can signal fetal extrusion. Treatment includes emergent cesarean section. Prior uterine surgery is the risk factor most often associated with uterine rupture.

TIPS TO REMEMBER

- Obtain urine pregnancy test in all female patients of childbearing age.
- Every pregnant patient with vaginal bleeding must have a hemoglobin, type and screen, and a quantitative beta-hCG checked.
- Every pregnant patient with vaginal bleeding who is Rh negative must be given RhoGAM.
- In cases of suspected ectopic pregnancy obtain Obstetrics/Gynecology consults sooner than later.
- Vaginal bleeding in late pregnancy always necessitates fetal monitoring, obstetric consultation, appropriate workup, and supportive treatment with RhoGAM if appropriate.

COMPREHENSION QUESTIONS

1. A 27-year-old G2P0 female at 34 weeks gestation presents with a 3-hour history of vaginal bleeding, but vital signs are stable. She has some mild abdominal pain but denies contractions. Which of the following should be avoided in this patient's diagnostic workup?

    A. Transabdominal ultrasound
    B. CBC with type and crossmatch
    C. Obstetrics/Gynecology consultation
    D. Pelvic examination

2. A 20-year-old female presents with a 1-hour history of suprapubic abdominal pain. Her pain is sharp, constant, and 9/10 in intensity. She is unsure when her last menstrual period was. Vital signs are heart rate 110 beats/min, blood pressure 75/45 mm Hg, respiratory rate 22 breaths/min, oxygen saturation 97% on room air, and temperature 37.5. She is in moderate distress. Examination shows suprapubic tenderness on abdominal examination. Pelvic examination is significant for left adnexal tenderness. Urine pregnancy test is positive. What is the most important next step in caring for this patient?

    A. Culture specimens from pelvic examination
    B. Pelvic ultrasound
    C. Quantitative beta-hCG
    D. Immediate Obstetrics/Gynecology consultation
    E. Discharge home with close follow-up

Answers

1. **D.** This patient is presenting in late pregnancy with new vaginal bleeding. She needs to be placed on the fetal monitor, have the safety net established, and have a consultation from Ob/gyn. Her presentation puts her at risk for placenta previa, vasa previa, placental abruption, or uterine rupture. She should have an urgent bedside transabdominal ultrasound. However, pelvic examination and transvaginal ultrasound should be avoided until placenta previa has been ruled out.

2. **D.** This patient is pregnant with abdominal pain and unstable vital signs. She has an ectopic pregnancy until proven otherwise. She requires emergent fluid resuscitation, blood typing, and emergent Obstetrics/Gynecology consultation. Pelvic ultrasound and laboratory tests such as quantitative beta-hCG levels may be obtained if they do not involve transferring an unstable patient or delay necessary interventions. Pelvic cultures are unlikely to change short-term management of this patient. It would be inappropriate to discharge this patient home given the patient's unstable vital signs and likelihood of ectopic pregnancy.

SUGGESTED READINGS

Bope ET, Kellerman RD, eds. *Bope & Kellerman: Conn's Current Therapy 2013.* 1st ed. Philadelphia: Saunders-Elsevier; 2013 [chapter 19] <http://www.mdconsult.com>.
Marx JA, Hockberger RS, Walls RM, eds. *Rosen's Emergency Medicine: Concepts and Clinical Practice.* 7th ed. Philadelphia: Mosby-Elsevier; 2010 [chapters 21, 26, 27, 98, 175, 176, 179] <http://www.mdconsult.com>.

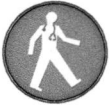

A 19-year-old Female With Vaginal Bleeding

Christopher M. McDowell, MD, MEd and Ted R. Clark, MD, MPP

CASE DESCRIPTION

Tonya Adams is a 19-year-old female who presents to the emergency department with vaginal bleeding. She describes a several-year history of irregular periods that seem to be worsening. She is presenting today because this period has been especially heavy. She is changing pads every 2 hours and is feeling very fatigued. Ms Adams is sexually active with 1 partner. She denies abdominal pain. Her past medical history is significant for obesity and severe acne. She takes no medications.

Her vitals are temperature 37.1 (98.8), blood pressure 132/84 mm Hg, pulse 70 beats/min, respiratory rate 16 breaths/min, and oxygen saturation 99% on room air.

On examination you note an overweight 19-year-old female in no distress. Her heart is regular without murmur and lungs are clear. Abdominal examination reveals an obese abdomen without distention or tenderness. Pelvic examination reveals blood from the os, no cervical motion tenderness, and normal bilaterally palpable adnexa.

1. What is the most likely cause of Ms Adams' vaginal bleeding?

2. What test must be ordered immediately?

3. What are the red flags in Ms Adams' history and physical examination?

Answers

1. The most likely cause of Ms Adams' vaginal bleeding is anovulation.

2. In all females of childbearing age who present with vaginal bleeding, pregnancy must be ruled out. The priority should be stabilization of unstable patients and the quick use of a urine pregnancy test to rule out pregnancy.

3. The differential in vaginal bleeding can be separated into 2 categories: pregnant and not pregnant. If the patient is not pregnant and stable, there is more time to diagnose, treat, and develop a follow-up plan as an outpatient. Table 23-1 includes the differential for vaginal bleeding.

Table 23-1. Emergency Physician Differential Diagnosis for Vaginal Bleeding

Critical Diagnoses	Pregnant Diagnoses	Other Diagnoses
Ectopic pregnancy	Ectopic pregnancy	Dysfunctional uterine bleeding
Coagulopathy-induced	Pregnancy-related	
	Implantation bleeding	Trauma/laceration
	Threatened abortion	Ovarian hyperstimulation syndrome
	Placenta previa	
	Placental abruption	Coagulopathy
		Uterine/cervical neoplasm
		Leiomyomas (fibroids)
		Systemic disease (Cushing syndrome, polycystic ovary syndrome, thyroid disease)

CASE REVIEW

Ms Adams is most likely experiencing dysfunctional uterine bleeding. She presents in stable condition and needs a workup. Her pregnancy test is negative, hemoglobin is 12 g/dL, and her platelet count is normal at 175,000/mm^3. She has no contraindications to estrogen therapy and can be placed on oral contraceptives if desiring contraception. NSAIDs may also alleviate any associated pain. This patient should be given a follow-up appointment with her primary care doctor or gynecologist.

VAGINAL BLEEDING (NONPREGNANT)

Diagnostic Reasoning

Vaginal bleeding is a frequently encountered chief complaint in the ED. The first priority as always is stabilizing unstable patients. In the case of vaginal bleeding, pregnancy must be ruled out urgently. Once pregnancy is excluded, the provider can proceed through the differential of nonpregnant diagnoses. A discussion of vaginal bleeding should begin with some definitions:

- Menorrhagia—menses lasting over 7 days or recurring in less than 21 days
- Metrorrhagia—irregular vagina bleeding outside the normal menstrual cycle
- Menometrorrhagia—excessive irregular vaginal bleeding
- Dysfunctional uterine bleeding—abnormal vaginal bleeding usually due to anovulation

The first priority in all patients who present with vaginal bleeding is to establish the "safety net." All patients of childbearing age must quickly have pregnancy ruled out. If the patient is hemodynamically stable and pregnancy excluded, the provider has more time to make the diagnosis. Historical red flags for vaginal bleeding include pregnancy, history of ectopic pregnancy, postcoital bleeding, postmenopausal bleeding, and history of severe anemia requiring blood transfusions. The physical examination must include a pelvic examination with both speculum and bimanual examination. Additional laboratory studies may be necessary. Imaging is best accomplished with pelvic ultrasound, but not all vaginal bleeding patients will require urgent imaging.

Diagnostic Workup and Management

The workup for a nonpregnant patient with vaginal bleeding is relatively straightforward. Once pregnancy has been excluded, attention can be turned to the other etiologies of vaginal bleeding. A pelvic examination with speculum and bimanual assessment is critical to directing the workup. Laboratory studies are useful in certain instances. All patients require a quick urine pregnancy test. Those with symptoms suggestive of severe anemia, such as fatigue or near syncope, may need a hemoglobin and hematocrit and consideration of a type and screen as well. Coagulation testing should be considered in those with historical features suggesting coagulopathy.

In addition to laboratory testing, significant information can be obtained from ultrasonography. If pregnancy has been ruled out and ectopic pregnancy is no longer a concern, many of these patients can wait for their imaging as part of the follow-up period. Patients with postmenopausal bleeding need gynecologic referral for endometrial biopsy as well.

Management depends on the patient's hemodynamics and overall condition. If the patient is hemodynamically unstable, she requires intravenous fluid resuscitation with type and screen for possible blood transfusion. If the bleeding is significant, it may require vaginal packing or Foley insertion into the cervix. These patients require emergent gynecologic consultation and may need an examination under anesthesia to rule out laceration or an urgent dilation and curettage (D&C). Intravenous estrogen may be started at 25 mg every 6 hours until bleeding stops. In those patients who are hemodynamically stable, oral contraceptives can be initiated. Recommended regimens for mild bleeding include combination pills with 20 to 35 µg of ethinyl estradiol twice a day for 5 to 7 days. For those with suspected anovulatory bleeding, progesterone withdrawal therapy of medroxyprogesterone acetate 10 mg for 10 days may stabilize immature endometrium and lessen future bleeding.

Dysfunctional uterine bleeding is the most common cause of vaginal bleeding in the nonpregnant patient. The great majority of these cases are the result of anovulatory bleeding. There are many causes of anovulation including endocrine disease, polycystic ovary syndrome, exogenous hormone use, and liver disease.

Cervical neoplasms include cervical dysplasia and cervical cancer. They should be suspected in all females with postcoital vaginal bleeding and/or a history of abnormal Pap smears. Pelvic examination may reveal cervical abnormalities, but these women should be referred for further gynecologic evaluation including Pap smear.

Uterine neoplasms are most commonly found in 2 forms: leiomyomas and endometrial cancer. Approximately 25% of white females and 50% of black females will develop leiomyomas or fibroid tumors. These benign tumors are usually diagnosed on ultrasound and can lead to bleeding and significant pain. They are treated with NSAIDs, progesterone agents, or surgical therapy. The more concerning uterine neoplasm is endometrial cancer. All women >35 years old with abnormal vaginal bleeding are at risk for endometrial hyperplasia or cancer. Postmenopausal vaginal bleeding is especially concerning for endometrial cancer. Thus, women >35 years old with abnormal vaginal bleeding must be referred for endometrial biopsy and ultrasound.

TIPS TO REMEMBER

- Pregnancy must be ruled out in all vaginal bleeding in women of childbearing age.
- Vaginal bleeding can lead to significant drops in hemoglobin.
- Both male and female providers should be accompanied by a chaperone.
- Postmenopausal bleeding is abnormal. These women need referral for ultrasound and endometrial biopsy.
- Ultrasound is an important adjunct, but not all patients with vaginal bleeding need emergent imaging.

COMPREHENSION QUESTIONS

1. A postmenopausal female presents with vaginal bleeding for 1 week. In addition to a pelvic examination, which diagnostic tests are indicated?
    A. Hemoglobin and hematocrit
    B. Pelvic ultrasound
    C. Endometrial biopsy
    D. All of the above

2. All of the following are causes of dysfunctional uterine bleeding *except* which one?
    A. Anovulation
    B. Polycystic ovary syndrome
    C. Hypothyroidism
    D. Leiomyoma

Answers

1. D. Each of the above is indicated in the workup of a postmenopausal patient with vaginal bleeding. Both the ultrasound and the endometrial biopsy can be deferred if prompt gynecologic follow-up can be arranged.

2. D. Each of the above are causes of dysfunctional uterine bleeding except for leiomyomas. These fibroid tumors are common causes of vaginal bleeding in later childbearing years. Surgical treatment is sometimes necessary if the bleeding becomes excessive.

SUGGESTED READINGS

Marx JA, Hockberger RS, Walls RM, eds. *Rosen's Emergency Medicine: Concepts and Clinical Practice.* 7th ed. Philadelphia: Mosby-Elsevier; 2010 [chapters 27, 98] <http://www.mdconsult.com>.
Tintinalli JE, Kelen GD, Stapczynski JS, Ma OJ, Cline DM, eds. *Tintinalli's Emergency Medicine.* 7th ed. New York: McGraw-Hill; 2011 [chapter 99] <http://www.accessmedicine.com>.

Section III.
The Trauma Service

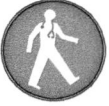

A New Emergency Medicine Resident Joins the Trauma Team

James R. Waymack, MD
and Ted R. Clark, MD, MPP

CASE DESCRIPTION

During your ED months, you have become more comfortable with patient care, but now you have a new challenge—you must join the ranks of the surgical trauma service. You have likely worked on a trauma service in medical school and have certainly seen trauma in the ED, but the trauma service has new challenges and new expectations.

1. Why is a trauma rotation important?
2. How is the trauma service different from ED months?

Answers

1. The trauma service and the ED and ICU rotations make up the 3 pillars of emergency residency. The trauma service provides a focused experience in the management of high-level trauma. On completion of residency, most EM physicians will be managing high-level trauma without a dedicated trauma team; thus, the development of trauma management skills is vital.

2. During the EM rotations, the EM resident will participate in trauma resuscitations that occur in the ED during regular ED shifts. The trauma service, in contrast, responds to all high-level traumas and provides care during the initial resuscitation, the hospital stay, and subsequent clinic follow-up. The longitudinal view of trauma provides important perspective for the EM physician. Simply, the EM physician needs to understand not only the acute management of trauma but also the projected course and the needs of the trauma service.

INTRODUCTION TO THE TRAUMA SERVICE

The trauma rotation is an integral component of EM education. A large portion of patient presentations to the ED will be traumatic injuries. Many may be less than life-threatening but will require knowledge and specific management; others may require urgent identification and intervention to prevent further morbidity and mortality.

How trauma patients are managed is variable from 1 institution to another. After arrival to the hospital patients may be managed solely by the trauma service or they may encounter EM physicians first who may direct management until the trauma service can arrive or until major injuries are identified. At other institutions EM physicians may focus on airway management while the trauma team is concerned with the remainder of the resuscitation.

Traditionally, the ED is notified of an incoming trauma patient by the prehospital providers en route to the hospital. Depending on the relationship of the ED and the trauma service the patient may initially be managed in the ED or may be sent to the trauma bay if severe injuries are involved. If the trauma team is needed, members will often be notified on the "trauma pager." Information conveyed in the page will typically include the age of the patient, the mechanism of injury, possible injuries, unstable vital signs, level of consciousness, and estimated time of arrival. Depending on the severity of the mechanism of injury and the condition of the patient the trauma will be classified as either a Level II (which is less severe) or a Level I (suggesting a high-energy injury or unstable patient). On receiving the page all members of the trauma service will assemble in the bay and await the arrival of the patient.

The trauma service consists of a multidisciplinary team. It will often be led by a Chief or senior resident who has had 3 to 4 years of experience and practices under the supervision of the attending trauma surgeon. The team will also include other junior or intern level surgery residents and residents from various other specialties, including EM and surgical subspecialties. Other participants in the trauma resuscitation may be nurses, ED technicians, prehospital providers, radiographers, pharmacists, and spiritual staff. Effective leadership and teamwork are critical to performing a satisfactory trauma resuscitation.

When you begin rotating on the trauma service, you can expect to be an active member of the team. Once the patient is brought into the trauma bay, there will be many things happening simultaneously. The team leader will obtain a report from the prehospital providers while nurses begin attaching monitor leads and starting intravenous lines. As a medical student or intern your role may include removing the patient's clothes as soon as the transfer to the trauma bay stretcher occurs. The team leader may delegate responsibilities to other team members such as initial evaluation of airway, breathing, and circulation. As the resuscitation continues there may be an opportunity for you to evaluate the patient, identify injuries, and perform procedures under the direction of the resident and attending physicians.

Another aspect of being a member of the trauma service is following patients on the floors who have been admitted for further evaluation and treatment. Depending on your institution you may have the opportunity to round on patients in the intensive care unit. You should also take this opportunity to see patients on the general floor as well. One of the objectives of your rotation is to become familiar with the management of both critical and minor traumatic injuries, not just acutely but also during recovery from injuries. This includes management in the first 24 hours of hospitalization and also in the long term through following a patient's recovery in the trauma clinic.

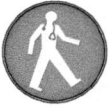

A 23-year-old Female Status Post High-speed Motor Vehicle Accident

James R. Waymack, MD
and Ted R. Clark, MD, MPP

CASE DESCRIPTION

You are beginning your rotation on the trauma service when your team receives a trauma page for a 23-year-old female who was involved in a high-speed motor vehicle rollover. The only other information you are given is that the patient may have had a loss of consciousness and is hypotensive while en route to the hospital. You proceed to the trauma bay, don appropriate personal protective equipment, and await the arrival of your patient.

On arrival the patient is somewhat drowsy but appears to be speaking clearly. You observe that the patient is tachypneic and appears to have an unequal rise and fall of her chest. You auscultate the patient's chest and do not hear breath sounds on the right side.

1. What are the components of the primary survey?

2. How are the patient's airway and breathing assessed?

3. What interventions may need to be performed during the initial assessment of the trauma patient's airway and breathing?

Answers

1. The components of the primary survey include assessment of the airway, breathing, circulation, and disability (neurologic function) and exposure of the patient so that examination for injuries may be fully performed.

2. Airway and breathing can be quickly assessed on physical examination by asking the patient to speak, observing respiration, and auscultating the lungs for breath sounds bilaterally.

3. The purpose of the initial assessment of the trauma patient's airway and breathing is to determine if endotracheal intubation or needle decompression must be performed immediately on patient arrival.

THE APPROACH TO TRAUMA

The Primary Survey—Airway and Breathing Assessment

Once the prehospital report has been obtained, the primary survey should be performed as rapidly as possible to exclude any life-threatening injuries. While

215

the trauma team is performing the primary and secondary surveys, assistants should be placing the patient on a cardiac monitor, obtaining a blood pressure, attaching a pulse oximeter, placing 2 large-bore intravenous lines, and supplying supplemental oxygen as required.

The patient's airway can be assessed by listening to hear if the speech is clear and noting whether there is any gurgling or difficulty in protecting the airway. Facial fractures or foreign bodies may cause airway obstruction and can be observed quickly while the patient is coming into the trauma bay. If there is any concern that a trauma patient's airway is compromised, or there is an expectation that the patient's clinical course will require airway protection, then endotracheal intubation should be performed.

The purpose of the primary survey is to identify life-threatening injuries as soon as the patient arrives (see Table 25-1 for a list of primary survey goals). Physical examination is the key component of the primary survey. There are no laboratory or diagnostic tests needed. If a patient has clear speech and is protecting his or her airway, as in this patient's case, then the trauma leader can move on to assess breathing. If the airway is not secure, then it must be addressed before moving on to the next step of the assessment.

The assessment of breathing includes the initial observation of the patient's respirations as described in the patient case. Further useful observations that may be included in the breathing assessment are observation of the neck veins for jugular venous distension and the trachea for deviation. The chest wall can be observed for open chest wounds and palpation for crepitus at the neck or chest can be performed to assess for subcutaneous emphysema.

Early in your trauma experience learning to follow a stepwise approach to the primary and secondary surveys should be emphasized to avoid error. When a trauma patient arrives, the members of the team often function autonomously at previously determined tasks. Therefore, multiple members of the team may simultaneously evaluate components of the primary survey or secondary survey. For example, the emergency physician may be assessing the airway while the trauma team leader is auscultating the chest for bilateral breath sounds.

Diagnostic Workup and Management

If the patient is alert and maintaining a patent airway by demonstrating clear speech, then no airway intervention is required and you may move on to the assessment of breathing. If there is question of an inadequate airway, the first intervention should be to attempt a jaw-thrust maneuver to improve the alignment of the airway and relieve anatomic obstruction. While this is being performed, an oropharyngeal airway can be placed as well. If a patient requires an oral airway, endotracheal intubation will eventually be needed. This is a more definitive airway, which provides not only patency because it is placed in the

Table 25-1. Primary Survey Goals

Identify	Intervene
Airway	
Inadequate airway	Securing and protection of airway
Cervical spine injury	Stabilization of cervical spine
Breathing	
Apnea	Positive pressure ventilation
Hypoxia	Supplemental oxygen administration
Tension pneumothorax	Needle decompression, tube thoracostomy
Massive hemothorax	Tube thoracostomy
Open pneumothorax	Occlusive dressing, tube thoracostomy
Circulation	
Hypovolemic shock	Fluid bolus, blood products
Pericardial tamponade	Fluid bolus, pericardiocentesis, thoracotomy
Cardiac arrest	Chest compressions (CPR)
	ED thoracotomy if penetrating trauma
Disability	
Spinal cord injury	Immobilization, steroids
Cerebral herniation	Mild hyperventilation, mannitol
Exposure	
Hypothermia	Warmed fluids, external warming
Exsanguinating hemorrhage	Direct pressure, air splints

Reproduced, with permission, from Tintinalli JE, Stapczynski JS, Cline DM, et al. *Tintinalli's Emergency Medicine: A Comprehensive Study Guide*. 7th ed. New York: McGraw-Hill Education; 2011 [Table 251-1].

trachea but also airway protection from aspiration because of the air-filled cuff that surrounds the tube.

Of note, it is important to remember to maintain cervical spine in-line stabilization while performing all aspects of your assessment, especially the airway. Most frequently the trauma patient will arrive with a cervical collar in place when coming to the hospital via EMS. However, there may be exceptions or the patient may arrive via private vehicle. Cervical spine protection, while often placed further down in the primary assessment, should be performed in conjunction with the assessment of the airway. If endotracheal intubation is deemed necessary, using a video-assisted laryngoscope as compared with direct laryngoscopy may allow easier visualization of the vocal cords while maintaining in-line stabilization.

Once the airway is completely addressed, the trauma leader can proceed to assess the patient's breathing. If the patient is breathing spontaneously, supplemental oxygen should be placed to improve tissue oxygenation. Supplemental oxygen will prevent hypoxia and improve tissue oxygenation if the patient is in a shock state. If the patient is unresponsive or a definitive airway has been placed, the patient will need to be ventilated with a bag-valve mask attached to 100% oxygen.

The main concern during the breathing assessment is to determine if there is a tension pneumothorax present. A pneumothorax is caused by a defect in the pleural lining of the lung, often by direct injury from fracture, but also from increased airway pressure from a high-energy impact to the body, rupturing the pleura. As air accumulates in the chest wall the mediastinal structures, including the airway and great vessels of the heart, are displaced to the opposite side of the thorax by increasing pressure. This deviation causes an obstruction to cardiac filling and eventual hypotension. Simultaneously, there is decreased pulmonary function due to the collapsed lung. A patient with a tension pneumothorax will present with not only respiratory distress but potential cardiovascular collapse as well; therefore, prompt identification and intervention is essential.

If a tension pneumothorax is suspected, the first action is to needle decompress the chest. This is performed by first identifying the appropriate side of the chest that contains the pneumothorax. The site of needle decompression is the second intercostal space in the midclavicular line (see Figure 25-1). A large-bore (usually 18-gauge), and as long as possible, intravenous catheter is placed into this space and advanced into the pleural cavity. If performed correctly, there will be a rush of air and the patient's hemodynamic status should improve. The needle is subsequently withdrawn and the plastic catheter is left in place inside the pleural cavity. A chest tube thoracostomy must now be performed because you have essentially converted the tension pneumothorax into an open pneumothorax. The remainder of the primary survey can be rapidly completed while an assistant to the trauma team sets up that equipment.

Chest tube thoracostomy is first performed by identifying the proper site and prepping it with a sterilizing solution. There are multiple sizes of chest tubes available; however, when drainage of blood from a hemothorax is needed, a large-caliber tube such as 36 or 40 French is preferable. After identifying the proper side, the appropriate site is the fourth intercostal space, approximately at the nipple line or inframammary fold, at the midaxillary line. Local infiltration of anesthetic can be performed if time permits, as this is a very painful procedure. A curved Kelly clamp is placed on the proximal end of the tube to aid insertion and a towel clamp can be placed at the distal end to prevent expulsion of fluid after insertion. An incision is made at the site of insertion with a scalpel and then blunt dissection is performed with a Kelly clamp in a superior fashion over the rib to avoid damage

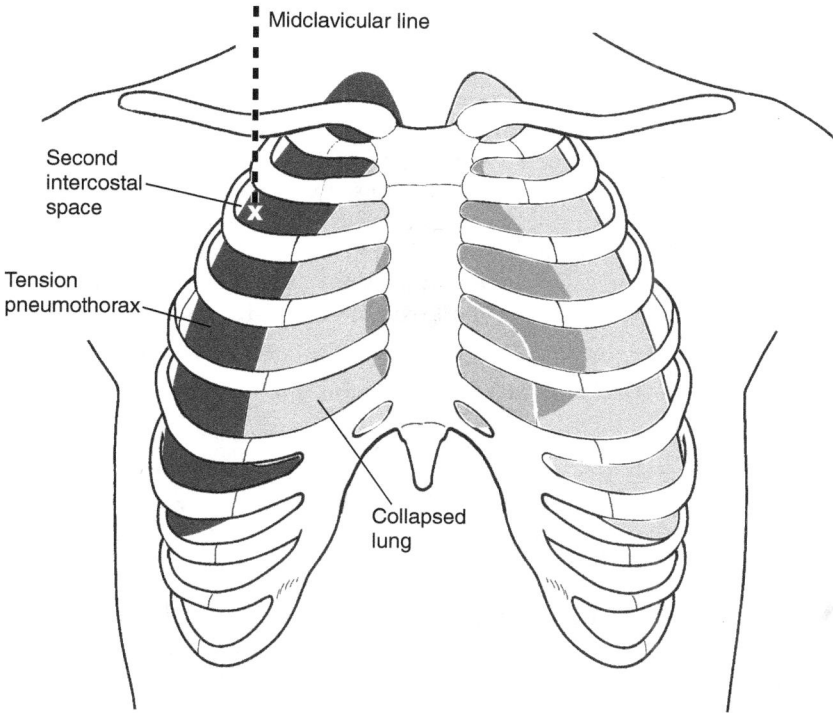

Figure 25-1. Position of the needle for tension pneumothorax decompression. (Reproduced, with permission, from Reichman EF, Simon RR. *Emergency Medicine Procedures*. New York: McGraw-Hill Education; 2004 [Figure 27-1]. <http://www.accessemergencymedicine.com>. Copyright © 2004 Eric F. Reichman, PhD, MD, and Robert R. Simon, MD. All rights reserved.)

to intercostal vessels and nerves. After dissecting through soft tissues the pleura will be met and can then be punctured with the blunt end of the Kelly, taking care to prevent deep penetration and injury to lung parenchyma. There should be a rush of air and possibly expulsion of blood if a hemothorax is present. With the Kelly still in place the opposite hand index finger should be placed into the incision to maintain identification of your tract. The Kelly clamp is withdrawn and the pleural cavity should be swept with the index finger of the dominant hand to identify any pleural adhesions. The tube is then inserted into the chest cavity, making sure to include all suction ports of the tube into the chest cavity. The distal clamp is removed and the tube is attached to wall suction to monitor output. The chest tube is then secured in place with suture. An air-occlusive dressing covers the incision and is secured in place with multiple bandages. A chest radiograph is required following insertion to demonstrate appropriate placement and improvement of the pneumothorax or hemothorax.

PATIENT CASE CONTINUED

The patient in this case demonstrates a patent airway at this time. She is speaking clearly and appears to be protecting her airway. However, there was an EMS report of hypotension in the field and on her arrival you note unequal breath sounds and some respiratory distress. These findings suggest a possible tension pneumothorax and immediate intervention is required. You successfully needle decompress the right side of her chest and place a chest tube with return of 50 mL of blood.

The patient's respirations improve. The ED tech now obtains a blood pressure of 90/60, the cardiac monitor shows a sinus tachycardia of 120 beats/min, and pulse oximetry reads 96% on 100% oxygen via non-rebreather mask.

1. What are the components of the traumatic circulatory assessment?

2. What are the physical examination findings suggestive of hemorrhagic shock?

3. What immediate interventions are required if hemorrhage is suspected?

4. What are the common locations of hemorrhage in the trauma patient?

5. What definitive treatments are available for traumatic hemorrhage?

Answers

1. During the assessment of the trauma patient's circulatory status one would observe overall peripheral perfusion and vital signs. Other causes of hypotension besides hemorrhage should also be suspected such as cardiac tamponade.

2. Patients in a shock state may have a decreased level of consciousness, cool, diaphoretic skin, and diminished peripheral pulses. These findings can often be assessed even before a blood pressure is obtained in the trauma bay.

3. All trauma patients should receive 2 large-bore intravenous lines, warm crystalloid solution, and blood typing and antibody screening. If massive hemorrhage is suspected early, identification of the need for red blood cell and other blood product transfusion is beneficial to the critically ill trauma patient.

4. Abdominal organ injury often causes traumatic hemorrhage. Other areas include external sites such as scalp lacerations, the chest cavity due to hemothorax, and pelvic or long bone fracture.

5. Management of shock due to bleeding may include direct pressure or wound closure for external sites, splinting of long bone fractures, pelvic stabilization, surgical intervention, or angiographic embolization.

The Primary Survey—Circulatory Assessment

After airway and breathing have been assessed and any necessary interventions performed, attention should be turned to assessing the trauma patient's circulatory status with a focus on identifying and treating hemorrhagic shock. There is often a focus on the blood pressure; however, this may take a few moments to obtain and physical examination can provide valuable clues to the patient's circulatory volume status even before these numbers are available. By definition, shock is hypoperfusion that leads to tissue hypoxia and eventually end-organ dysfunction. In the trauma patient the first organ to be affected is the brain and decreased mental status, lethargy, or drowsiness may be signs of shock. The finding of cool, clammy skin may signal hypoperfusion, as will decreased capillary refill or diminished peripheral pulses.

There are also vital sign abnormalities that may suggest hemorrhagic shock before the patient demonstrates hypotension. There are 4 classes of shock based on physical examination and vital signs (see Table 25-2). The first signs of hemorrhagic shock may simply be anxiousness with a mild tachycardia or tachypnea. As the patient's volume status decreases there will be a resultant decrease in blood pressure followed by mental status deterioration. As hypoperfusion increases the patient will have decreased renal blood flow and oliguria.

While hemorrhagic shock is being recognized, a causative source must be identified concurrently so that control may be achieved swiftly. The average adult has a circulating blood volume of 5 L, so prompt identification and control of bleeding is imperative. The most common sites of bleeding in the trauma patient include intra-abdominal organs such as the spleen, liver, kidneys, and small bowel. Patients may also have retroperitoneal hemorrhage; however, this is much more difficult to identify on the initial trauma examination without further imaging studies. The patient may have bleeding in the chest cavity causing a massive hemothorax. Pelvic fractures are notorious for causing severe hemorrhage due to the shearing of the venous plexus surrounding this bony structure. Long bone fractures such as the femur can contain multiple liters of blood. Sites of external bleeding such as scalp lacerations are often the most obvious.

Table 25-2. Classification of Hemorrhage Based on Estimated Blood Loss at Initial Presentation

	Class I	Class II	Class III	Class IV
Blood loss (mL)[a]	Up to 750	750-1500	1500-2000	>2000
Blood loss (% blood volume)	Up to 15	15-30	30-40	40
Pulse rate (beats/min)	<100	100-120	120-140	>140
Blood pressure	Normal	Normal	Decreased	Decreased
Pulse pressure	Normal or increased	Decreased	Decreased	Decreased

[a]Assume a 70-kg patient with a preinjury circulating blood volume of 5 L.

Reproduced, with permission, from Tintinalli JE, Stapczynski JS, Cline DM, et al. *Tintinalli's Emergency Medicine: A Comprehensive Study Guide.* 7th ed. New York: McGraw-Hill Education; 2011 [Table 250-6].

A nonhemorrhagic source of hypotension or cardiac arrest in the setting of acute trauma is most likely a pericardial effusion. This injury may be suggested by hypotension, distended neck veins, and muffled heart sounds. The increasing use of ultrasound during the trauma assessment has made the rapid identification of pericardial effusion much easier.

As with the other components of the primary survey, laboratory and radiographic imaging is not necessary to initially identify and treat injuries that are contributing to circulatory problems in the trauma patient. Hemoglobin concentrations are often normal in the setting of acute hemorrhage and are unreliable to exclude life-threatening hemorrhage. The only laboratory tests that should be obtained in regard to the evaluation and management of the trauma patient's circulatory status are a blood type and antibody screen. While a patient can be transfused with only type-specific blood, being mindful of this laboratory test can expedite the patient receiving cross-matched red blood cells.

An anterior–posterior chest radiograph is often quickly obtainable during the initial evaluation of the trauma patient. While not essential, the chest radiograph may be helpful in identifying massive hemothorax. Fractures of the long bones and pelvis will often be obvious on examination of the patient and treatment should not be delayed for radiographic studies. Another useful diagnostic modality for the assessment of the trauma patient is bedside ultrasound. Please see Chapter 38 for further detail on the focused assessment of shock.

Diagnostic Workup and Management

Once the patient arrives into the trauma bay, intravenous access should be obtained to enable the start of resuscitation. Customarily this is done with 2 L of warm crystalloid solution. If intravenous access is difficult to obtain, an intraosseous line can be placed until venous access is possible. Common sites for intraosseous line placement include the proximal tibia and proximal humerus. Central venous access is also an option, but it should only be performed if large-bore intravenous lines cannot be obtained, since the flow rate through an 18-gauge intravenous catheter is much greater than through the narrow lumens of a triple lumen central line. If central venous access is to be obtained, an introducer should be placed because it has much higher flow rates than a triple lumen catheter. If massive transfusion is anticipated, the blood bank should be alerted and resuscitation with blood products begun quickly. Infusion can also be done through a level 1 rapid transfuser, which is capable of moving 1 L/min into the patient's circulatory system. Of note, gravid patients should be immediately placed in the left lateral decubitus position to prevent compression of the inferior vena cava, which prevents adequate preload to the heart.

Once resuscitation is begun, the primary survey is continued and sites of hemorrhage may be identified on further examination or radiographic study. However, if life-threatening exsanguination is a concern, bleeding should be controlled immediately before proceeding. If external sources are seen, the easiest intervention is direct pressure. Scalp wounds can be quickly sutured closed with a running large silk suture or Raney clips may be applied. If the patient is bleeding extensively from an extremity, a manual blood pressure cuff can be placed proximal to the bleeding and inflated to 250 mm Hg.

PATIENT CASE CONTINUED

You continue to resuscitate your patient in the trauma bay. Intravenous crystalloid is infusing rapidly and you begin to assess for disability. She opens her eyes to voice. The patient cannot recall the events of the accident. Her words are clear but seem inappropriate. She continually asks what happened and where she is. She does not spontaneously move her extremities or follow commands but withdraws appropriately to pain in all 4 extremities. You observe pupils that are 4 mm, symmetrical bilaterally, and reactive to light.

You continue your primary survey and completely expose the patient. You note abrasions to both arms with no active bleeding and find no other obvious external injuries at this time. You apply warm blankets to the patient and ensure that the intravenous fluids are warm while they infuse.

1. What are the components of the Glasgow Coma Scale (GCS)?

2. How do you perform a rapid trauma assessment of neurologic function?

3. What are the key components of exposure during the trauma resuscitation?

4. Why is there concern for hypothermia in the trauma patient and what interventions can be undertaken to prevent it?

Answers

1. The GCS includes eye, verbal, and motor responses (see Table 25-3).

2. Neurologic function can be quickly assessed on the trauma patient by asking the patient to move each extremity. If the patient cannot follow commands, motor function can be assessed by applying a painful stimulus to each extremity.

3. Complete exposure is essential during the rapid trauma evaluation to avoid missing injuries. The patient should be completely disrobed. The back, axilla, rectal, and perineal areas should be inspected to avoid missing occult injuries. After the patient is exposed, care should be taken to avoid hypothermia.

4. Hypothermia may contribute to coagulopathy and continued hemorrhage in the trauma patient. Increasing the room temperature, covering the patient with warm blankets following exposure, and infusing warmed intravenous fluids may all help prevent hypothermia.

Table 25-3. Glasgow Coma Scale

Component	Score	Adult	Child <5 Years	Child >5 Years
Motor	6	Follows commands	Normal spontaneous movements	Follows commands
	5	Localizes pain	Localizes to supraocular pain (>9 months)	
	4	Withdraws to pain	Withdraws from nail bed pressure	
	3	Flexion	Flexion to supraocular pain	
	2	Extension	Extension to supraocular pain	
	1	None	None	
Verbal	5	Oriented	Age-appropriate speech/ vocalizations	Oriented
	4	Confused speech	Less than usual ability; irritable cry	Confused
	3	Inappropriate words	Cries to pain	Inappropriate words
	2	Incomprehensible	Moans to pain	Incomprehensible
	1	None	No response to pain	
Eye opening	4	Spontaneous	Spontaneous	
	3	To command	To voice	
	2	To pain	To pain	
	1	None	None	

Modified from Teasdale G, Jennett B. Assessment of coma and impaired consciousness. A practical scale. *Lancet.* 1974;2(7872):81–84.

The Primary Survey—Disability and Exposure

During the disability assessment of the trauma patient, the goal is to quickly identify mental status and assess for massive intracranial hemorrhage and spinal cord injury. It is very important during the entire trauma evaluation to maintain cervical spine precautions with a cervical collar and in-line stabilization. Every time a patient is moved or rolled, the neurologic status should be reassessed.

The GCS is a simple and rapid method to evaluate a patient's mental status. It should be performed once the patient arrives and can be repeated to monitor for deterioration. When performing this examination, remember the exact responses the patient gives because a neurosurgeon may request more information than simply the GCS number. In the setting of trauma any patient with a GCS less than 8 will require endotracheal intubation to protect the airway. If a trauma patient is going to be intubated and paralyzed, a quick assessment of motor function prior to sedation is helpful.

After determining the GCS of the patient an evaluation of the central and peripheral nervous system follows. Pupils should be examined for size and reactivity. They should also be compared with one another to assess for asymmetry, which may be a sign of increased intracranial pressure (ICP) due to intracranial hemorrhage and brain herniation. A rapid motor examination with assessment of each extremity for movement and strength is adequate during the primary survey when looking for spinal cord injury. More extensive neurologic examination can be performed during the secondary survey.

Adequate exposure is essential during the rapid trauma assessment in order to avoid missing occult injuries. All of the patient's clothes should be removed quickly by cutting them away to avoid moving the patient any more than necessary. Once the patient is completely exposed, he or she should be protected from hypothermia by covering with warm blankets and infusing warm intravenous fluids. Trauma resuscitation bays are often kept very warm as well to prevent hypothermia, because lowering body temperature can cause coagulopathy and difficulty controlling bleeding. If cutaneous wounds are identified, consideration should be given to boosting the patient's tetanus prophylaxis if it has not been received in the last 5 years or if the patient is uncertain as to when the last tetanus prophylaxis occurred.

There are no laboratory or radiographic tests indicated during the initial assessment of disability. After the initial assessment is complete, further testing may be warranted such as a CT of the head to evaluate for intracranial bleeding or skull fractures. Computed tomography of the thoracic and lumbar spine may also be helpful to evaluate for spinal fracture, dislocation, or intrusion into the spinal canal that may be causing neurologic disability.

Diagnostic Workup and Management

If a closed head injury is expected, maintaining cerebral perfusion and preventing further brain injury is the primary concern. This is achieved by continuing measures already implemented during the resuscitation, preventing hypoxia by administering supplemental oxygen, and preventing hypoperfusion by providing volume resuscitation. If there is concern that the patient's mental status is decreasing, it must be continually reassessed. If the mental status decreases below a GCS of 8, the patient must be intubated to protect the airway.

If there is concern for intracranial bleeding and increased ICP because of either the presence of pupil asymmetry or the results of a CT scan of the head, interventions should be performed to decrease ICP as soon as possible. These interventions include elevating the head of the bed, hyperventilating the patient to a goal partial pressure of a carbon dioxide of 35 mm Hg, and administering intravenous mannitol. Care must be given to maintaining blood pressure so that there is adequate cerebral perfusion pressure while administering this potent diuretic. Prompt consultation with a neurosurgeon is necessary if there is concern for increased ICP.

Management of suspected spinal cord injury includes maintaining spine precautions until the patient can have temporary fixation placed. It is important to have adequate blood flow to the spinal cord, which reemphasizes the importance of resuscitation. If a central or peripheral neurologic injury is suspected, prompt consultation with a neurosurgeon or orthopedic spine specialist is imperative.

Of note, while exposing the patient, it is important to avoid damaging possible articles of evidence. If the patient is a victim of violence or has been attacked with a weapon, it is preferred by law enforcement that clothing be left intact where bullet or stab holes are present. Clothing and other personal articles should be handled with care, placed in appropriate evidence containers, and immediately transferred to law enforcement to maintain a chain of custody.

PATIENT CASE CONTINUED

You suspect a closed head injury in your patient and believe there is no spinal cord injury based on your findings. You continue the resuscitation and begin your secondary survey. You recall that taking a stepwise head-to-toe approach is helpful to ensure that all injuries are identified. The patient continues to be drowsy, but she is able to answer some of your questions. She states that she has pain located mostly in her head, neck, abdomen, and hips.

You begin by examining her head looking for any obvious external trauma such as a scalp laceration. Examination of the ears shows no Battle's sign, no gross blood in the ear canals, and no hemotympanum. The patient is somewhat cooperative and demonstrates intact extraocular movements. No subconjunctival hematoma or proptosis is seen. The nose appears midline. There is a small amount of blood in the nares bilaterally, but there is no septal hematoma present. Dentition is intact and alignment appears maintained. You palpate the frontal, zygomatic, maxillary, and mandibular areas of the face and do not appreciate any facial instability.

You begin to examine the chest by looking for any external or penetrating wounds and palpating for clavicular or chest wall tenderness or deformity, but do not appreciate any. While you continue to examine the patient, you note a seat belt sign across her chest and abdomen, but do not identify any external signs of bleeding or extremity deformity. There does not appear to be any penetrating trauma to the abdomen. It is mildly distended and diffusely tender to percussion and palpation. You are unable to appreciate bowel sounds. When you apply posterior pressure to the iliac crests, the patient reacts in pain. At this time you are concerned about a possible pelvic injury, which may be causing the patient's hypotension. The chief resident asks you how you would like to treat this injury.

1. What are the components of the secondary survey?

2. What are the immediate interventions for a possible pelvic injury?

Answers

1. The secondary survey is a thorough but rapid head-to-toe examination of the trauma patient with the intention of identifying all possible injuries.

2. Pelvic fractures can be bound with a sheet or a commercial pelvic binder. External fixation may be performed later by orthopedics. Pelvic bleeding can be controlled by angiographic embolization.

The Secondary Survey—Anterior

When performing the secondary survey, it is important to do so in a stepwise fashion. By proceeding head-to-toe injuries are less likely to be missed. Performing the examination the same way every time will provide a source of repetition and thus aid proficiency.

Beginning by examining the head, one should look for external signs of trauma. Are there open or depressed skull fractures? If a scalp laceration is identified, it is most likely bleeding profusely and hemostatic control should be obtained quickly. You should inspect for signs of basilar skull fracture such as Battle's sign (mastoid ecchymoses), raccoon eyes (orbital ecchymoses), hemotympanum, and cerebrospinal fluid rhinorrhea. Examination should continue by inspecting for nasal bone deformity or fracture, epistaxis, or septal hematoma. Pain, instability, or crepitus on palpation of the facial bones may suggest facial bone fractures. Inspect the mouth for blood, dental trauma, and malalignment of the dentition, which may suggest a mandibular fracture.

The chest should be inspected for external signs of injury and penetrating trauma. If the patient is stable and by mechanism of injury or inspection it is not obvious that the penetrating wound is deep, it may be probed by the trauma surgeon to determine if the patient should proceed to the operating room for thoracotomy or laparotomy. Beginning at the clavicles, apply pressure to assess for clavicular pain or instability, which may suggest fracture. The chest wall is palpated to assess for rib fracture. Respirations should be observed to note if there is paradoxical motion of the chest, which may suggest a flail segment of ribs.

The abdomen should be observed for signs of external trauma and penetrating injuries. If there are contusions on the abdominal wall, they may suggest areas that received trauma with energy transferred internally causing injury to underlying abdominal organs. Tenderness on percussion and palpation may also prompt one to be concerned about certain organs depending on location of the pain. If the abdomen is distended or tense, or demonstrates rebound or guarding, one should be concerned about intra-abdominal injury or hemorrhage.

After performing the abdominal examination focus can be directed toward the pelvis. Pelvic rocking is no longer recommended because it can cause further shearing to the pelvic venous plexus and worsen hemorrhage. Pressure should be applied to the iliac crests bilaterally and in an anterior to posterior fashion. If this does not produce instability or pain, then pressure can be applied toward the midline. If there is any suggestion of pelvic injury on examination, further manipulation should not be performed to limit injury. Immediate stabilization should be applied.

After the primary survey has been performed and life-threatening injuries addressed, further injuries may be found on the secondary survey. At this point in the resuscitation blood may have been drawn and laboratory studies can be ordered. Often a complete blood cell count, complete metabolic profile (which will include transaminases), and a blood type and antibody screen will be sent. Some centers will have different laboratory panels stratified by the severity of the patient. Other studies that may be requested include coagulation studies, serum alcohol level, and toxicology screens. A urinalysis is routinely sent to evaluate for hematuria. One should not forget to obtain a rapid pregnancy test on all female patients of possible childbearing age who present to the trauma bay.

Radiographic imaging is invaluable for evaluating trauma patients for injuries once they are stabilized and urgent operative management is deemed unnecessary. In smaller hospitals, or if the patient is too unstable to go to the CT scanner, plain radiographs of the chest and pelvis can be useful in identifying injuries to the chest and pelvis (see Figure 25-2). One would look for a widened mediastinum in a chest radiograph suggesting injury to the aorta. Other findings on the chest radiograph could include pneumothorax, hemothorax, pulmonary contusion, and rib fractures.

CT has become a valuable adjunct to the evaluation of the trauma patient. CT scanning of the head can identify skull fractures and intracranial hemorrhages. If there is a suspicion of facial or orbital injuries, dedicated CT scans of the facial bones can be done to look for facial and orbital fractures, retro-orbital hematoma, and maxilla or mandible injuries. A CT scan of the chest with contrast can be

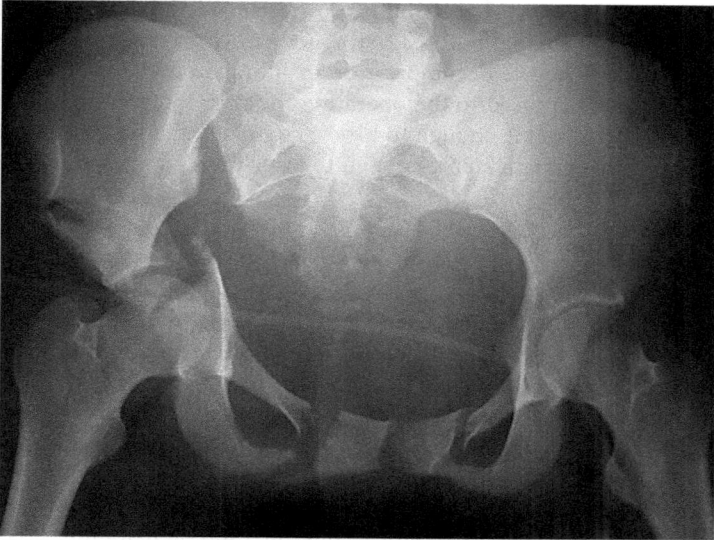

Figure 25-2. Pelvic fractures as seen on radiograph. (Reproduced from Schwartz DT. *Emergency Radiology: Case Studies.* New York: McGraw-Hill Medical; 2008. <http://www. accessemergencymedicine.com>.)

performed to look for injuries to the lungs, great vessels, and ribs. Occasionally a smaller pneumothorax or hemothorax that was not appreciated on a plain chest radiograph may be discovered.

CT scan of the abdomen with contrast will provide great detail of the solid organs of the abdomen. These are often injured from blunt trauma. Injuries may include liver or spleen lacerations or renal hematomas. Hollow organ injury to the small and large bowel and the pancreas is more difficult to identify on the CT scan. An abdominal scan is almost always accompanied by a pelvic CT, which can identify injury to the bladder, distal ureter, and the pelvic bones.

If a CT scanner is not available, the patient is too unstable, or you would prefer to limit radiation, a FAST examination may be done. Using the ultrasound you can rapidly identify free fluid in the abdomen or pelvis. If free fluid is found in the hypotensive trauma patient, it can be presumed to be intra-abdominal hemorrhage and the patient should be dispositioned to the operating room or interventional radiology suite for control of the hemorrhage.

If extremity injuries are suspected on examination by deformity or point tenderness, plain radiographs with a sufficient number of views should be obtained to assess for fracture or dislocation. Some injuries, such as tibial plateau or acetabular fractures, are more difficult to identify on plain radiographs and proceeding to CT imaging may be more beneficial.

Beyond the surveys what should also be considered is "How critical is this patient?" Does the patient need an emergent lifesaving procedure in the trauma bay such as needle decompression or thoracotomy? Should the patient be immediately transported to the operating room or interventional radiology suite? Is this patient stable enough to have a complete trauma evaluation in the trauma bay? Is this patient stable enough to leave the trauma bay and go to the CT scanner?

Diagnostic Workup and Management

The diagnostic workup and management of the injuries found on the secondary survey are often done simultaneously. As injuries are identified they may be initially managed while radiology results are returning.

If a depressed or basilar skull fracture is present or there is concern for increased ICP from an intracranial hemorrhage, a neurosurgeon should be consulted immediately. Temporizing measures that may help alleviate elevated ICP include elevating the head of the bed 30°, hyperventilating the patient to produce cerebral vasoconstriction, and administrating the diuretic mannitol. It is important to remember to continue to adequately perfuse and oxygenate the brain during episodes of ICP, so attention must be paid to adequate resuscitation.

If a scalp laceration is identified, bleeding should immediately be controlled with Raney clips or a running suture because patients, especially pediatric, can lose a significant portion of their circulating blood volume from these wounds. If the patient has a proptotic eye, decreased extraocular movements, and facial trauma, a retrobulbar hematoma must be suspected and emergent lateral canthotomy may be necessary to relieve elevated intraocular pressure and preserve future vision. If other injuries are found to the head and face, appropriate specialist intervention may be needed including plastic and reconstructive surgery, otolaryngology, and ophthalmology.

In the case of thoracic trauma one is most concerned about injury to the great vessels such as aortic disruption and pericardial effusion. These injuries may often be fatal prior to arrival in the trauma bay, but should be considered in any patient who presents in cardiac arrest. Injuries can be identified with radiography but may be even more apparent with ultrasound looking for free fluid around the heart. If a patient goes into cardiac arrest shortly before arrival to or in the trauma bay, thoracotomy may be an option if there is proper surgical backup to care for the patient resuscitation. Thoracotomy can provide access to the chest cavity to relieve a pericardial effusion, identify and repair defects in the myocardium or aorta, and allow the surgeon to cross-clamp the aorta to control distal bleeding. Internal cardiac massage can be performed through the thoracotomy. If the patient is more stable, a pericardiocentesis can be performed to relieve effusion. However, in the setting of acute trauma, the patient will likely require the care of a cardiothoracic surgeon to identify its source.

If massive hemothorax is identified, the patient should have a large-caliber chest tube placed. If initial output is greater than 1500 mL of blood, the patient should proceed to angiography or the operating room for identification of the bleeding and its control. If the initial output is substantial but less than 1500 mL, the output can be followed and if it does not decrease over a short interval of time intervention may be warranted.

Evaluation of the abdomen and pelvis may suggest intra-abdominal injury on CT scanning, but significant trauma can also be identified on physical examination. If the patient is unstable and has penetrating trauma to the abdomen or obvious free fluid on a FAST examination, he or she should proceed immediately to the operating suite for exploratory laparotomy to identify the source of the bleed and gain control. In the more stable trauma patient CT scanning may reveal injuries that are not as apparent on examination but may still be just as life-threatening such as a splenic laceration with active extravasation of contrast material suggesting ongoing hemorrhage. Patients who have ongoing bleeding from the liver or spleen may benefit from exploration in the operating room. Another treatment option is angiographic embolization by interventional radiology. In the even more stable patient who has a small hematoma or laceration of an intra-abdominal organ, bed rest and serial hemoglobin concentrations may be adequate.

Pelvic fractures are notorious for producing large hemorrhage volumes. Once a pelvic fracture is suspected, the pelvis should not be examined again and should be bound tightly with a sheet or commercial pelvic binder to increase the likelihood of internal tamponade. If a fracture is then identified on pelvic radiography or CT scanning, more definitive treatment, such as external fixation, may be necessary. If the patient is already destined for the operating room to address intra-abdominal injuries, the pelvis can be packed until control is achieved. If the patient remains unstable and ongoing hemorrhage is a concern, the pelvic vessels can be embolized by interventional radiology.

If extremity fractures are suspected from physical examination or radiographic findings, they should be splinted once other life-threatening injuries have been addressed. If there are open wounds near the fracture, the patient will likely need antibiotics and possibly debridement in addition to copious irrigation. Any fracture or dislocation that does not have adequate distal perfusion should be emergently reduced and splinted. Once fractures and dislocations are reduced and splinted, neurovascular status should be reassessed frequently.

PATIENT CASE CONTINUED

You bind the patient's pelvis with a bed sheet and continue your secondary survey for other traumatic injuries. An external examination of the perineum does not reveal ecchymosis; however, there is some blood at the urethral meatus. No vaginal bleeding is identified on internal examination.

You return to the head of the bed and with the help of an assistant maintain in-line stabilization and momentarily remove the cervical collar. You assess the patient's cervical spine for step-offs, deformity, or tenderness, and none are found. With further assistance and maintenance of in-line stabilization you log-roll the patient, remove the EMS spine board, and inspect the patient's back and buttocks for any signs of trauma. You palpate the thoracic and lumbar spine for any step-offs, deformities, or point tenderness. You find none on this patient. You perform a rectal examination with a lubricated finger and find good rectal tone with no gross blood. The patient is returned to the supine position and you are relieved to find distal motor function remains unchanged and intact after moving the patient. The nurse now requests a Foley catheter to be placed.

1. What does blood at the urethral meatus indicate and how is it managed?

2. What is the best imaging modality to assess for spinal injury?

Answers

1. Blood at the urethral meatus could suggest urethral or bladder injury.

2. While plain films were once the test of choice, CT scanning is much more detailed and can readily identify even small fractures.

The Secondary Survey—Perineum and Posterior

The secondary survey continues beyond the pelvis to include the perineum. If a pelvic injury is present, there may be ecchymosis of the perineal area. There is greater concern for associated injuries than just obvious external signs of trauma. A great amount of force is required to fracture the pelvis and this can be transferred to the internal organs it contains. Of greatest suspicion are bladder and urethral injuries, and in females, injuries to the reproductive organs.

Care should always be taken when manipulating a patient with suspected spinal injury to prevent further neurologic decline. The cervical spine should be evaluated for any deformity or step-off. If the patient is alert, communication about pain in a circumscribed area is helpful. The examination can be extended to the thoracic and lumbar spinal areas once the patient has been rolled onto his or her side. During the examination of the back one must be careful to inspect for any external wounds or penetrating trauma as well as spinal deformity. Once the patient is returned to the supine position, motor function should be reassessed to ensure there has been no deterioration of status, and findings of this examination should be documented.

A rectal examination is routinely performed on all trauma patients. Using a lubricated finger, sphincter tone is assessed by inserting a finger into the rectum and requesting the patient to bear down. This procedure demonstrates adequate tone and may be the only motor function present in a patient who has sacral sparing from a spinal cord injury. Once the finger is removed from the rectum, it can be inspected for gross blood, which if present may suggest traumatic injury to the rectum or colon.

In addition to CT imaging of the abdomen images are often taken down into the pelvis to assess the pelvic organs. Of interest in this patient with suspected pelvic injury is the potential for bladder and urethral injury in addition to any pelvic fracture that may be present. If blood is observed at the meatus, especially in the case of a patient with suspected pelvic injury, care should be taken not to immediately place a Foley catheter. The concern is that a urethral injury may be present and if a catheter is placed it could track into a false lumen and cause further morbidity. If urethral injury is suspected, a retrograde urethrogram should be performed (see Figure 25-3).

In most trauma cases a patient will receive imaging of the cervical spine to rule out fracture or dislocation. In the past a cervical spine series was routine in all trauma patients; however, with the increasing presence of CT scanners near the trauma bay, CT scanning of the cervical spine is considered far superior. Plain radiographs are very rarely ordered to assess for cervical fracture anymore. If the

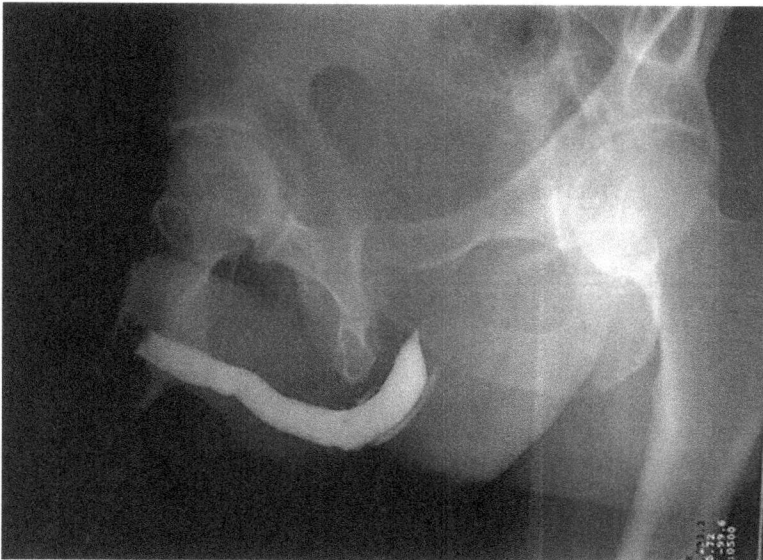

Figure 25-3. Positive retrograde urethrogram indicative of urethral injury. Adult male patient with straddle injury to perineum and blood at the urethral meatus. This positive retrograde urethrogram reveals extravasation in the bulbous portion of the urethra inducative of urethral injury. (Reproduced from Stone CK, Humphries RL. *Current Diagnosis & Treatment: Emergency Medicine.* 7th ed. New York: McGraw-Hill Professional; 2011. <www .accessemergencymedicine.com>. Copyright © The McGraw-Hill Companies Inc. All rights reserved.)

patient has thoracic or lumbar tenderness or signs of possible injury, images of these areas should also be performed. With most CT scanners the bony images can be pulled out if the patient has already received a CT scan of the chest and abdomen. If cervical spine injury is identified but no initial thoracic or lumbar films were obtained because the patient lacked pain in those areas, follow-up films should be obtained because the presence of one spinal fracture makes the presence of others far more likely. If a spinal fracture is found, emergent consultation with an orthopedic spine specialist or neurosurgeon is indicated. Some fractures are more stable than others, but definitive management should be left to the specialist.

The rectal examination has long been considered a component of a complete physical examination, especially in the setting of acute trauma. However, in recent years some studies have suggested that this test may provide little clinical information and may not need to be performed routinely. In the pediatric population this test is often deferred unless there is a high suspicion of rectal injury. Nevertheless, it is currently still an often-performed examination during the trauma evaluation.

Diagnostic Workup and Management

Once a retrograde urethrogram is performed and no urethral injury is identified, a Foley catheter may be placed carefully, usually by the urologist. If a bladder injury is suspected, a Foley catheter should be inserted to decompress the bladder and the patient will likely require operative repair. If injury to female reproductive organs is suspected, a gynecologist should be consulted to assist in the management of the patient.

If cervical, thoracic, or lumbar spine injury is suspected or confirmed on examination or radiologic studies, constant cervical spine immobilization should be maintained. The cervical collar should remain in place until the patient is evaluated by the orthopedist or neurosurgeon who will be caring for the patient. The patient should remain on bed rest and pain control achieved. If the injury is severe and unstable, the patient may require operative fixation. The treatment of a minor injury may be limited to an orthotic brace and limited activity.

PATIENT CASE RESOLUTION

This patient was the victim of a high-energy motor vehicle crash with multiple injuries. She was resuscitated in the trauma bay and found on CT imaging to have no significant intracranial, thoracic, or abdominal injuries. Her rapid pregnancy test was negative. Her tetanus status was updated and she was given antibiotic prophylaxis for her wounds. She was taken to the angiography suite where embolization of the pelvis was performed, which controlled her ongoing hemorrhage. Orthopedics placed an external fixation device with plans for open reduction and internal fixation of pelvic fractures. She was admitted to the intensive care unit for further observation. The chest tube placed was left to wall suction until after the scheduled surgery.

DISPOSITION

In most cases patients who are injured severely enough to present to a trauma bay will require further treatment and admission to the hospital. However, not all patients who present to the trauma bay will require admission. If the diagnostic workup does not reveal any injuries, the patient may be observed for a short time and then discharged home with follow-up. Factors that may affect this decision include the age and overall health of the patient, the mechanism of injury, pain control, ability to tolerate feeding, baseline functional status, and sobriety. Extremes of age are highly susceptible to poor outcomes from trauma and while no immediate injuries may be evident admission or short observation may be warranted. If the mechanism of injury was severe, patients, regardless of baseline health, may be kept for observation to ensure that their status does not deteriorate. Prior to leaving the hospital it is requisite that a patient has returned to baseline functional status, can mobilize with minimal assistance, and can perform activities of daily living. If patients live alone or are not able to care for themselves, they may require admission for physical and occupational therapy or placement into an acute rehabilitation facility. Many trauma patients have ingested alcohol or other intoxicating substances just prior to their arrival and these patients should be required to stay until they are clinically sober and safe to leave.

CERVICAL SPINE CLEARANCE

If a patient is deemed capable of being discharged home or has been admitted and has no obvious fracture of the cervical spine, the cervical collar can be considered for removal. However, even though there is no fracture there may still be ligamentous injury, which could cause cervical instability, and subsequent spinal cord injury. One way to determine that ligamentous injury is absent is to use NEXUS criteria (see Table 25-4). The NEXUS demonstrated that if a patient was sober without focal neurologic findings, was alert to person, place, and time, had no painful distracting injuries, and had no posterior midline cervical tenderness on palpation or full range of motion of the neck, then ligamentous injury was unlikely. Once patients are no longer intoxicated, they are questioned to see if they have received pain medications or have other painful injuries, which may distract them from feeling pain in their necks. If a patient denies any such distractions, the posterior portion of the cervical collar can be removed while leaving the front intact and the cervical midline palpated. If the patient has pain, the collar should be left in place. If there is no midline pain at rest, the anterior portion of the collar can be removed and the patient can be asked to bend the neck all the

Table 25-4. National Emergency X-radiography Utilization Study (NEXUS) Criteria for Omitting Cervical Spinal Imaging[a]

No posterior midline cervical spine tenderness
No evidence of intoxication
Alert mental status
No focal neurologic deficits
No painful distracting injuries

[a]Failure to meet any 1 criterion indicates need for cervical spine imaging.

Reproduced, with permission, from Tintinalli JE, Stapczynski JS, Cline DM, et al. *Tintinalli's Emergency Medicine: A Comprehensive Study Guide.* 7th ed. New York: McGraw-Hill Education; 2011 [Table 250-5].

way forward, then backward, and then to each side continually assessing for midline cervical pain. If the patient admits to pain, the collar should be replaced. If there is no pain, the collar can confidently be removed.

Patients who have persistent pain should remain in a cervical spine collar until a definitive study of ligamentous stability can be performed. This may include flexion–extension films of the neck or magnetic resonance imaging. The other option is to have the patient remain in the collar until outpatient follow-up at which time reexamination for midline pain can occur. If it persists, then further imaging may be warranted.

TRAUMA CLINIC

Another experience of being a member of the trauma team is caring for patients in the trauma clinic. Often these are patients who were admitted to the hospital for their injuries and are being followed in the outpatient setting to see that they are progressing well following discharge. Common injuries that will require follow-up include closed head injury, pneumothorax, rib fracture, and cutaneous injuries. Important factors to address with these patients include pain control, mobility, disability, and bladder function. Patients who underwent emergency stabilization in the operating room by exploratory laparotomy are routinely followed in the clinic.

Patients who experienced a closed head injury should be questioned regarding the presence of any neurologic symptoms. It is not uncommon to have a headache for sometime after a significant injury. Patients may also complain of an inability to focus or perform tasks that they were able to do prior to their injuries. If this is the case, referral to a neurologist or psychologist may be beneficial as the patient could require cognitive testing to track disability and subsequent progress.

Patients who experience closed chest trauma that resulted in a pneumothorax or rib fractures often experience significant pain following discharge from the hospital. In this population it is important to question respiratory status and identify what medications are being taken. If the patient is having difficulty breathing or shortness of breath, repeat imaging may be necessary to ensure there is not a recurrence of pneumothorax or that pneumonia has not developed due to decreased inspiratory force and atelectasis. If pain control is an issue, pain medication strength or frequency may need to be increased. Another option for pain control of rib fractures is a local anesthetic with lidocaine patches that can be placed daily at the site of the pain.

Patients will routinely follow up for suture or staple removal or chronic wound management following their traumatic injury. If sutures or staples are to be removed, the wound should first be assessed to see that it remains well approximated and there are no signs of infection such as redness, swelling, warmth, or draining purulence. If the wound appears well healed, the sutures or staples may be removed in an alternating fashion monitoring for wound dehiscence. If the wound does separate, it should be probed to ensure integrity of the underlying fascia. If the fascia is intact, the patient will only need more chronic wound follow-up with wet to dry dressing changes and return visits while the wound heals by secondary intention. If the fascia is not intact, the defect will have to be closed urgently. Trauma patients often experience severe cutaneous wounds that may heal poorly. These wounds may require skin grafts or vacuum dressings and will need to be routinely followed to ensure they are progressing. Referral to a plastic or reconstructive surgeon may be warranted.

Patients who underwent operative procedures during their admissions should receive routine postoperative visits with emphasis on posttraumatic care. Pain control should be addressed as described above. The patient should be assessed for adequate bowel and bladder function, especially while taking narcotic pain medication. If the patient underwent a splenectomy, immunization against encapsulated bacteria will be needed. Once trauma patients are felt to have recovered sufficiently from their wounds, their primary care physicians can continue to follow them.

TIPS TO REMEMBER

- Ensure an adequate airway prior to continuing your trauma evaluation.
- Maintain cervical spine precautions at all times.
- Perform an organized and stepwise trauma evaluation in order to identify all injuries.
- Continually reassess the patient during resuscitation.

COMPREHENSION QUESTIONS

1. A 25-year-old male presents to the trauma bay following a high-speed motor vehicle accident. He is alert and speaking clearly but is in obvious distress. Vital signs include heart rate 120, blood pressure 90/40, respiratory rate 30, and pulse oximetry 92% on 100% oxygen. You do not appreciate right-sided breath sounds. What is your first step in management of this patient?
   A. Endotracheal intubation
   B. Needle decompression
   C. Chest radiograph
   D. Chest tube insertion
   E. Intravenous crystalloid infusion

2. You perform the needed procedure and the patient's breathing improves. You decide to perform a chest tube thoracostomy. What is the proper location for placement of this tube?
   A. Second intercostal space midclavicular line
   B. Fourth intercostal space midclavicular line
   C. Fourth intercostal space midaxillary line
   D. Fourth intercostal space posterior axillary line
   E. Sixth intercostal space anterior axillary line

3. During your resuscitation this patient becomes unresponsive, only opening his eyes to painful stimuli and uttering incomprehensible words. He is exhibiting an abnormal flexion response in the upper extremities. What is your first step in management of this patient?
   A. Emergent CT scan of the head
   B. Naloxone
   C. Endotracheal intubation
   D. Elevation of the head of the bed
   E. Intravenous mannitol

4. As the resuscitation continues the only intravenous line is inadvertently pulled out. After 2 minutes and multiple failed attempts your nurses are unable to obtain intravenous access and the patient's blood pressure has now decreased to 70/40. What is your first step in the management of this patient?
   A. Attempt to place an intravenous line yourself.
   B. Place a subclavian triple lumen central line.
   C. Place an intraosseous line.
   D. Place a femoral introducer sheath.
   E. Perform a saphenous venous cutdown.

5. Once the patient is resuscitated, he has a prolonged stay in the intensive care unit. He is due to be transferred to an acute rehabilitation facility and would enjoy having his cervical collar removed. You review the cervical CT scan that shows no fracture. You recall which of the following as components of the NEXUS criteria used to clear his cervical spine and remove the collar? (Choose all that apply.)

        A. No posterior midline cervical tenderness
        B. Paraspinal tenderness
        C. No distracting injuries or neurologic deficit
        D. No recent intoxicants or pain medications
        E. GCS of 15

6. Which of the following actions are critical during the evaluation of every trauma patient? (Choose all that apply.)

        A. Maintenance of cervical spine precautions
        B. Routine pregnancy testing in all females of childbearing age
        C. Consideration of updating tetanus prophylaxis
        D. Analysis of hemoglobin concentration
        E. Rectal examination

Answers

1. B. This patient's presentation suggests tension pneumothorax. Needle decompression is the necessary immediate intervention. The airway appears intact at this time. Obtaining a chest radiograph and setting up a formal chest tube tray would be too time consuming. Eventually the patient will need volume resuscitation and a chest tube.

2. C. The correct location for chest tube thoracostomy is the fourth intercostal space in the midaxillary line. There are variations on placement; however, the second midclavicular space is reserved for needle decompression, and the sixth intercostal space is too inferior because it would risk inadvertent chest tube placement into the abdominal cavity.

3. C. It is imperative to continually reassess the trauma patient. This gentleman has had an abrupt onset of decreased mental status with a GCS of 8, which is an indication for immediate endotracheal intubation. CT scanning of the head will identify intracranial injuries; however, an airway must be secured first. Hyperventilation, head-of-bed elevation, and mannitol may be indicated if there is an intracranial process causing elevated ICP.

4. C. This patient is critically ill and needs immediate vascular access to continue volume resuscitation. Intraosseous access is quick and easily performed. Once intraosseous access is obtained, further options, such as an introducer, can be placed. A triple lumen central line does not provided adequate flow for trauma resuscitation.

5. A, C, D, and E. Paraspinal tenderness is not a component of the NEXUS criteria.

6. A, B, C, and E. The hemoglobin concentration is unreliable in the setting of acute trauma. Serial hemoglobin levels throughout hospital admission are more helpful.

SUGGESTED READINGS

Committee on Trauma, American College of Surgeons. *Advanced Trauma Life Support for Doctors.* 8th ed. Chicago: American College of Surgeons; 2008.
Tintinalli JE, Stapczynski JS, Cline DM, et al. *Tintinalli's Emergency Medicine.* 7th ed. New York: McGraw-Hill Education; 2011 [chapter 250].

Section IV.
The Intensive Care Unit

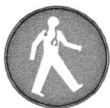

A New EM Resident Joins the ICU Team

Nicholas M. Mohr, MD, Joshua D. Stilley, MD, and Amy Walsh, MD

CASE DESCRIPTION

With emergency department (ED) rotations and the trauma rotation under your belt, you head off to the next challenge—the intensive care unit (ICU). By now, you are comfortable with long hours and sick patients, but you are about to be pushed even further.

1. Why is the ICU rotation important?
2. How is the ICU service different from ED months?

Answers

1. The ICU rotation provides a focused experience in the management of critically ill patients. It is the third pillar of EM education and is frequently reported to be the favorite of all the off-service experiences due the tremendous numbers of procedures and resuscitations the EM resident will perform during the rotation.

2. The ICU rotation provides a longitudinal view of the management of critically ill patients. Not only will you take over the care of acutely ill patients from the ED, but you will also receive transfers from outside hospitals and codes from the floor. You will also be responsible for managing acute complications in critically ill patients. Once stabilized, you will manage the patient to resolution.

INTRODUCTION TO THE ICU

Residency training in emergency medicine is a broad-based training experience where you will rotate both in the ED and on "off-service" rotations with faculty members from other departments. You will spend several months of your training rotating through ICUs to learn how to manage critically ill patients.

This experience is an important component to your emergency medicine training, because the resuscitation principles that you will learn in the ICU will apply directly to your patients in the ED. Furthermore, appropriate early management of these patients will determine their hospital trajectory, and likely will impact their survival.

Despite the importance of learning these principles, practicing in the ICU will be different from working in the ED. Your patient population will be slightly different, the day-to-day evaluation and management will be different, and your daily schedule will be different. Learning to function as an ICU resident will be an important aspect of learning how to resuscitate critically ill patients in the ED.

There are several principles for being successful on your off-service rotations that will apply to the ICU and other rotations:

- Be interested—Each rotation has something specific you must learn to apply to your patients in the ED. Engaging with your team, asking questions, and helping your co-residents will go a long way toward becoming part of the ICU team. Your supervising physicians are more likely to let you perform procedures and function independently if you are a team player who is working to get the team's work done.

- Have a good attitude—You will be working with trainees and faculty members from a variety of specialties. Think about what each of them can teach you. No one specialty is inherently more qualified to take care of critically ill patients than any other, but we all have different approaches, and we can learn from other providers' approaches and experience.

- Listen to your nurses—ICU nurses can be one of your greatest assets. They have often cared for many patients, and they will notice things that you do not. They spend more time at your patient's bedside than you do, and they will often be able to give you information you cannot get any other way. In addition to calling your supervising physicians for help, your ICU nurses can be a great resource for day-to-day critical care practice in your institution.

- Be on time with relentless attention to detail—The ICU is not the place for "gestalt medicine." It is important to show up early so that you can see each of your patients, and know their laboratory findings, fluid balance, and medical history. The well-prepared resident will be rewarded with more autonomy because the other team members will feel confident that (s)he is taking good care of his/her patients.

Before your first day, try to get a sign-out from the resident you are replacing so that you know which patients you are following. Find out what time rounds are held and what a normal daily schedule might be. Know what your call schedule will be so that you can be prepared. Learn how written notes are done, when they are expected, and if there is a computerized template that you should complete.

On your first day, arrive early to collect data and prepare presentations on each of your patients. When your supervising ICU physician arrives, introduce yourself, thank him/her for having you on the service, and ask about the expectations for your rotation. It can be helpful to have in mind specific skills that you would like to hone during your rotation.

Every day, arrive early enough to fully evaluate your patients. This includes:

- Physical examination.
- Talk with nurses and respiratory therapists to understand what happened overnight.
- Look at all the laboratory values, including the trends over the past several days.
- Know intake, output, and fluid balance over the past 24 hours.
- Read yesterday's note so that you know all the active issues, and review the recent notes of all consulting services.
- Develop a concise systems-based presentation, and have a definitive plan for your patient's care for the next 24 hours.
- If parts of your patient's course or care are unclear, make notes. Rounds are a good time to ask questions either about your patient or about general topics that pertain to critical care.

Be prepared on rounds with your presentation. Early in the course of your training, practice your presentation briefly before rounds start—you will appear much more prepared than if you were making it up "on the fly." Make a complete problem list, and organize yourself by systems so that you can plan your interventions systematically. Table 26-1 gives one method for organizing your presentation. *Have a plan* prior to staffing with your supervising physician. As you round and the team makes a plan, write a checklist of everything that the team is planning to do for the day: after rounds, you will be expected to call consults, order tests, confirm that interventions have occurred or are scheduled, and make sure that orders for tomorrow are correct.

When you are on call or admitting patients, remember that ICU care is complete care—your patient's write-up and workup cannot be constrained to only the admitting problem. You need to know about medical history, surgical history, and prior interventions.

You will be paged for patients in the ICU who have an acute problem. Commit yourself early in your training to personally evaluate every patient for which a nurse calls you. Even simple calls can be early warning of clinical changes, and you will only notice these changes if you go to the bedside to evaluate each patient. Your nurses will appreciate your care and attention, and you will provide superior care for your patients.

Finally, do not hesitate to call for help. This section was designed to cover some of the basic diseases and complications of ICU care, but it is not comprehensive. The most capable resident physicians are not necessarily the most intelligent; they are physicians who know best what their limitations are and strive actively to remediate gaps in knowledge and experience. When you see a patient who is decompensating, implement therapy and call your supervising physician for help.

Table 26-1. Organizing Your Presentation

Events from last 24 hours
Updates from consultants
Physical examination
ICU problem list
Systems-based presentation of assessment and plan:
Neuro
Respiratory
Cardiovascular
Renal/urology
Gastrointestinal
Infectious disease
Endocrine
Hematology
Fluids, electrolytes, and nutrition
Prophylaxis
Chest x-ray
Lines and tubes

When there is a significant change in a surgical patient, notify the surgical service. Call patients' families when you are making major changes. Take into consideration suggestions from all members of the health care team, including physicians, respiratory therapists, and nurses. Likely many of those professionals have been doing their jobs longer than you've been doing yours, and they may provide you with valuable insights.

Above all, remember that your rotation is not about you. Your rotation is about your patients: both the patients you care for in the ICU who deserve world-class medical care and your future patients in the ED for which your ICU rotation is preparing you. Be humble, ask questions, be attentive, and recognize that this is one more step in your ultimate development as an emergency physician.

GLOSSARY OF ICU ABBREVIATIONS

A/C: Assist/control
ALI: Acute lung injury
ARDS: Acute respiratory distress syndrome

BiPAP: Bilevel positive airway pressure (usually provided through a face mask)

CPAP: Continuous positive airway pressure (usually provided through a face mask)

CVL: Central venous line

Dialysis catheter: A large dual-lumen central venous line designed for use for temporary dialysis access (also called a Quinton™ catheter after an early nephrologist)

EMS: Emergency medical services

$EtCO_2$: End-tidal carbon dioxide concentration

EVD: External ventricular drain

FiO_2: Fraction of inspired oxygen

FFP: Fresh frozen plasma

G-tube: A tube inserted through the anterior abdominal wall to facilitate feeding

GJ: Gastrojejunal tube

I-time: Inspiratory time

IBW: Ideal body weight

ICP: Intracranial pressure

INR: International normalized ratio

NG: Nasogastric tube

NJ: Nasojejunal tube

P_{CO_2}: Partial pressure of carbon dioxide

P_{O_2}: Partial pressure of oxygen

PA catheter (Swan-Ganz catheter): Pulmonary artery catheter

PC: Pressure control

PCWP: Pulmonary capillary wedge pressure

PE: Pulmonary embolus

PEA: Pulseless electrical activity

PEEP: Positive end-expiratory pressure

PEEP valve: A device that can be connected to a bag-valve that can maintain PEEP in the endotracheal tube while providing positive pressure ventilation manually

PICC: Peripherally inserted central catheter

PPI: Proton pump inhibitor—a class of medications shown to decrease gastric acidity

PRBC: Packed red blood cells

PSV: Pressure support ventilation

SIMV: Synchronized intermittent mandatory ventilation

TACO: Transfusion-associated cardiopulmonary overload

Tracheostomy: A tube inserted through the anterior neck into the airway to provide long-term ventilatory support or airway maintenance

TRALI: Transfusion-associated lung injury

Trauma introducer: A large central venous line with a single lumen that can be used for large volume resuscitation, or occasionally for the introduction of a pulmonary artery catheter (also called a Cordis™ catheter after an early manufacturer)

VC: Volume control

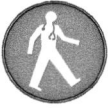

A 35-year-old Male on a Ventilator Develops Hypoxia

Joshua D. Stilley, MD and Nicholas M. Mohr, MD

CASE DESCRIPTION

Jonathan Bougie is a 35-year-old male, hospital day 3 status post blunt trauma from a motor vehicle collision. He suffered bilateral pulmonary contusions, a left-sided hemopneumothorax, an unstable pelvic fracture, and a nondisplaced parietal skull fracture without underlying intracranial hemorrhage. He is intubated and sedated with propofol and fentanyl infusions. He is ventilated on assist-control (pressure control) ventilation with PEEP of 5 cm H_2O, drive pressure of 10 cm H_2O, FiO$_2$ of 40%, and breathing at a rate of 15 with tidal volumes of 400 mL. He has been stable on the ventilator since admission. He has a left-sided chest tube to water seal, and an external fixation device on his pelvis.

You are the resident on call for the ICU and you are called to the bedside emergently to evaluate this patient. The nurse informs you that Mr Bougie's ventilator alarm began going off and his oxygen saturations have dropped to 80%. The patient's vital signs are BP 110/72, P 120, RR 16, pulse oximeter 80%, and T 37.2°C.

1. What is your differential diagnosis?

2. What are your initial steps of action?

3. What are your next steps?

Answers

1. The differential diagnosis of acute hypoxia of a patient intubated on mechanical ventilation can be remembered with the DOPE mnemonic: *d*isplacement of the endotracheal tube, *o*bstruction of the endotracheal tube, *p*neumothorax, and *e*quipment failure.

2. Begin your evaluation by looking for end-tidal carbon dioxide from the endotracheal tube (typically measured continuously from an adapter on the ventilator circuit) and confirm tube depth (measured at the level of the teeth) to rule out endotracheal tube dislodgement. Next, pass a suction catheter through the endotracheal tube to assess for tube patency and try to remove obstructing mucous. Listen for bilateral breath sounds as you think about the possibility of pneumothorax. Finally, remove the patient from the ventilator and provide manual bag-valve ventilation with 100% FiO$_2$. In this patient with a pneumothorax and a chest tube in place, assure that the chest tube is connected to suction.

3. Obtain a chest x-ray and call for assistance. You should be able to narrow the cause of your patient's decompensation to a problem with the (1) endotracheal tube, (2) lungs, (3) chest tube, or (4) ventilator using this algorithm.

COMPLICATIONS OF PATIENTS ON MECHANICAL VENTILATION

Discussion

There are many complications that can arise in a ventilated ICU patient, but through a systematic approach (DOPE mnemonic) the cause can usually be identified quickly. Taking your patient off the ventilator and using manual bag-valve ventilation will address equipment malfunction and can give you some important information. Is your patient easy to ventilate? If so, then your patient's problem is probably not endotracheal tube obstruction or tension pneumothorax. This can also be confirmed by endotracheal tube suction. If the suction catheter can pass to full depth, then you know your endotracheal tube is not obstructed.

Endotracheal tube dislodgement is a common cause of decompensation in the ICU. During patient transfers, it is easy for the endotracheal tube to get dislodged, and patients will often try to remove their endotracheal tubes even while in restraints. Verifying tube depth by the centimeters of depth at the teeth or gums is an easy way to ensure there has not been movement. End-tidal CO_2 capnometry is a great tool for ensuring that the tube is in the airway. Obtaining a chest radiograph can verify tube depth, airway patency, and lung expansion, but it cannot distinguish between endotracheal and esophageal intubation.

A pneumothorax can develop in a ventilated patient for multiple reasons. High transpulmonary pressure can lead to tissue injury, barotrauma, and pneumothorax. Often, ventilated patients have diseased lungs, which are more prone to barotrauma than are healthy lungs. Clinically, pneumothorax can be identified with asymmetric breath sounds, tracheal deviation, and/or subcutaneous emphysema, but clinical signs are insensitive in ruling out pneumothorax. The patient in this case has a chest tube already in place. Chest tubes can become occluded or disconnected, they can get lodged in a pulmonary fissure and stop draining, or the tubes can be disconnected from suction. Ensuring proper chest tube function is very important in this patient. A chest radiograph can be critical in ruling out significant pneumothorax. Ultrasound can also be utilized to look for characteristics of apposition of parietal and visceral pleura and can be used to rule out pneumothorax.

Equipment failure can be difficult to identify. Faults in the sensing, timing, or mechanical valves of the ventilator can all lead to the patient being inadequately ventilated. It is important to observe your patient breathing on the ventilator to be certain that the ventilator is working. Using bag-valve ventilation can also assure that hypoxia is not alleviated by bypassing the ventilator.

After you have worked through the DOPE mnemonic, you have most likely identified and corrected the problem, but there are a few other things to consider. Pulmonary embolism can occur in a patient who has been critically ill for even a short time. Pulmonary contusions and ARDS can lead to a rapid decline in the ability to ventilate and oxygenate the patient. Alternatively, a new onset of fever, oxygen desaturation, and increased tracheal secretions may suggest evolving ventilator-associated pneumonia. These patients should have blood and respiratory cultures sent and empiric antibiotic therapy should be considered.

Finally, don't be afraid to ask for help. Your respiratory therapist should always be available to help identify and correct problems any time you have a patient with oxygenation or ventilation problems. Other residents, fellows, or supervising physicians in the ICU should be called early if there is a change in your patient's condition. In many hospitals, anesthesia is on call for airway management problems and can be a valuable resource.

TIPS TO REMEMBER

- Remember the DOPE mnemonic (displacement, obstruction, pneumothorax, equipment failure).
- Manually ventilate the patient any time oxygen desaturation occurs.
- Use your resources liberally—patients with acute hypoxemia or ventilatory failure require a coordinated response to prevent decompensation and cardiac arrest.

COMPREHENSION QUESTIONS

1. What is the mnemonic to work through hypoxia on the ventilator and what does it stand for?

2. What is the sequence of actions for a mechanically ventilated ICU patient who has acute desaturation?

Answers

1. DOPE: displacement, obstruction, pneumothorax, and equipment failure.

2. Look for $EtCO_2$ and tube position, pass the suction catheter, listen for bilateral breath sounds, look for tracheal deviation, and take the patient off the ventilator to manually ventilate.

SUGGESTED READINGS

Kollef M, Isakow W. *The Washington Manual of Critical Care*. 2nd ed. Philadelphia: Lippincott Williams & Wilkins; 2011.
Marino PL. *The ICU Book*. 3rd ed. Philadelphia: Lippincott Williams & Wilkins; 2007.

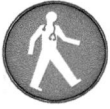

A 60-year-old Male With Fever and Hypotension

Nicholas M. Mohr, MD

CASE DESCRIPTION

Mac Burney is a 60-year-old man with a history of multiple abdominal surgeries after a gunshot wound to the abdomen 24 years ago. He has had multiple small bowel resections with resulting short gut syndrome and is dependent on total parenteral nutrition (TPN) through an indwelling peripherally inserted central catheter (PICC) for his nutrition. He was admitted to the surgery service 3 days ago for abdominal pain and high output from his colostomy, but last night had a fever of 39.8°C for which he was treated with acetaminophen 650 mg rectally. On rounds this morning, his blood pressure was 85/42 and he was transferred to the intensive care unit for closer monitoring and management.

You are the resident taking ICU admissions, and you are called to evaluate the patient on his arrival to the unit. As his bed is being wheeled into his room, the transferring nurse gives you a new set of vital signs: T 39.1°C, BP 72/36, P 137, RR 28, and O_2 saturation 92% (room air).

On your evaluation, the patient is sleepy, but can answer questions. He is somewhat tachypneic, but nonlabored, and he has a palpable radial pulse with delayed capillary refill. Shortly before transfer, the surgical resident sent a series of laboratory studies, and the results are just arriving as you are evaluating this patient:

WBC 23.4 / Hgb 18.2 / Plt 151 / Hct 53

Na	Cl	BUN	
146	109	49	Glu
4.5	18	2.1	241
K	HCO$_3$	Cr	

Arterial blood gas: pH 7.36, pco$_2$ 30, po$_2$ 123, HCO$_3$ 19

Lactate 5.8

1. What is your differential diagnosis for the patient's decompensation on the floor?

2. What therapy would you institute immediately?

Answers

1. Hypovolemic shock from high-output GI losses, gastrointestinal bleeding with hemorrhagic shock, primary myocardial infarction with cardiogenic shock, pulmonary embolus with right heart failure, pancreatitis, acalculous cholecystitis, urinary tract infection with septic shock, central line infection with septic

shock, adrenal crisis, *Clostridium difficile* infection with septic shock, and bowel perforation with septic shock.

2. Start aggressive crystalloid fluid resuscitation (20-30 mL/kg intravenous crystalloid bolus); think about sources of infection (urine, pneumonia, indwelling PICC line, intra-abdominal abscess, *C. difficile* colitis or enteritis) and get appropriate testing (blood cultures, urine culture, chest X-ray, *C. difficile* PCR, liver function testing, and lipase); start empiric broad-spectrum antibiotics; remove PICC line if this is a strongly suspected source of infection; place central venous line and consider vasopressor agents if hypotension persists.

SEPTIC SHOCK

Diagnostic Workup and Management

Shock is a life-threatening condition of global tissue hypoperfusion often characterized by hypotension, hemodynamic instability, organ failure, and death. Shock can be broadly divided into 4 categories (Table 28-1), and the physiology and treatment of each type are very different. Some shock states incorporate features of several types of shock. Rapidly elucidating the etiology of shock can save a patient's life.

Sepsis is a common cause of shock in the intensive care unit that carries with it a mortality of 20% to 50%. *Shock* is a state of global tissue hypoperfusion, and *septic shock* is the development of shock secondary to infection. Septic shock has complex physiology that incorporates features of several types of shock (hypovolemic, cardiogenic, distributive), which makes its treatment complicated. Appropriate aggressive protocolized treatment within the first 6 hours of sepsis resuscitation has been shown to improve 28-day survival. Sepsis is a broad continuum of disease that is characterized by a systemic inflammatory response secondary to a documented or suspected infection (Table 28-2).

Sepsis is a complex cytokine-mediated disorder that leads to capillary leak syndrome, organ failure (from hypoperfusion, direct cytokine effects, and microthrombus formation), distributive shock, and rapid death if left untreated. Hemodynamically, increased vascular permeability leads to third-spacing of intravascular volume and inadequate preload to maintain cardiac output (hypovolemic shock). Simultaneously, cytokine release contributes to systemic vasodilation and decreased vasomotor tone (distributive shock). Both of these mechanisms, along with direct myocardial depression (cardiogenic shock), lead to systemic hypotension, hypoperfusion, and lactic acidosis.

The tenets of sepsis therapy are based on early hemodynamic resuscitation, early broad-spectrum antimicrobial administration, and source control. The Surviving Sepsis Campaign has published guidelines for the timely resuscitation of patients hospitalized with suspected severe sepsis or septic shock.

Because septic shock is a disease of capillary leak, aggressive fluid resuscitation is required to restore adequate cardiac preload to maintain cardiac output.

Table 28-1. Types of Shock

Type	Physiology	Clinical Features	Treatment
Hypovolemic (diarrhea, poor oral intake)	Inadequate preload leads to decreased cardiac output; systemic vascular resistance increases to compensate and maintain blood pressure	Flat neck veins, poor skin turgor, delayed capillary refill, cool extremities, tachycardia, dry mucous membranes, orthostatic symptoms	Volume resuscitation (fluid bolus)
Cardiogenic (acute myocardial infarction, cardiac valve failure)	Inadequate cardiac output secondary to primary cardiac dysfunction leading to pump failure; systemic vascular resistance increases to compensate and maintain blood pressure	Distended neck veins and elevated jugular venous pressure, peripheral edema, dyspnea, rales on auscultation of lungs, delayed capillary refill, cool extremities	Revascularization if appropriate (in acute myocardial infarction), inotropic therapy, intra-aortic balloon pump, mechanical support (ventricular assist device, extracorporeal membrane oxygenation device)
Distributive (anaphylaxis, neurogenic)	Inadequate vascular tone (low systemic vascular resistance) leads to hypotension; cardiac output increases to compensate and maintain blood pressure	Warm extremities, normal capillary refill, bounding pulses	Vasopressor therapy
Obstructive (pulmonary embolus, cardiac tamponade, tension pneumothorax)	Inadequate cardiac output secondary to obstruction of blood flow; systemic vascular resistance increases to compensate and maintain blood pressure	Distended neck veins and elevated jugular venous pressure, peripheral edema, dyspnea, rales on auscultation of lungs, delayed capillary refill, cool extremities, pulsus paradoxus	Relieve obstruction (chest tube, pericardiocentesis, thrombolysis for pulmonary embolus)

Table 28-2. Diagnostic Criteria for Sepsis

Category	
Systemic inflammatory response syndrome (SIRS)	Must have at least 2 of the following: • Fever (T >38°C) or hypothermia (T <36°C) • Pulse >90 beats/min • Hyperventilation (respiratory rate >20 breaths/min) or hypocarbia (p_{CO_2} <32 mm Hg on an arterial blood gas analysis) • Leukocytosis (white blood cell count >12,000 cells/μL), leukopenia (white blood cell count <4000 cells/μL), or bandemia (immature white blood cells >10%)
Sepsis	Systemic response to infection (SIRS + documented or suspected source of infection)
Severe sepsis	Sepsis associated with acute organ dysfunction, hypoperfusion, or hypotension, which may include: • Respiratory failure • Acute kidney injury • Hepatic dysfunction • Circulatory failure (hypotension or direct myocardial depression) • Coagulation abnormalities (thrombocytopenia, coagulopathy, disseminated intravascular coagulation) • Encephalopathy • Elevated lactate
Septic shock	Sepsis-induced hypotension despite fluid resuscitation (30 mL/kg crystalloid fluid bolus) in addition to the presence of perfusion abnormalities (as described in "severe sepsis")

Data from Bone RC, Balk RA, Cerra FB, et al. Definitions for sepsis and organ failure and guidelines for the use of innovative therapies in sepsis. The ACCP/SCCM Consensus Conference Committee. American College of Chest Physicians/Society of Critical Care Medicine. *Chest.* 1992;101(6):1644–1655.

The Surviving Sepsis Campaign has identified resuscitation goals for preload (measured by central venous pressure through a central venous catheter), blood pressure, urine output, and central venous oxygen saturation ($ScVO_2$). Cardiac preload (left ventricular end-diastolic volume) can be very difficult to measure but is an important variable in optimizing cardiac output (Frank-Starling physiology). Clinicians often monitor the response of surrogate markers (central venous pressure, pulse pressure variation, thoracic bioimpedance or bioreactance, pulse contour analysis, pulmonary artery thermodilution) to sequential fluid boluses to establish a state of "volume responsiveness."

Once cardiac preload has been optimized, persistent hypotension is presumed to be secondary to peripheral vasodilation. Vasopressor agents (Table 28-3) can be used to increase the mean arterial pressure to a goal of 65 mm Hg. Typically, norepinephrine is used as a first-line vasopressor agent in septic shock, with secondary agents added when high doses of norepinephrine are required. With adequate preload indices and adequate blood pressure, $ScVO_2$ (a blood sample sent to the lab from a central venous catheter to measure oxygen saturation) can be used as a marker for the adequacy of cardiac output. According to the Fick principle, if the amount of oxygen required by the body is constant and the arterial blood is fully saturated with oxygen, then the oxygen concentration of venous blood will be directly related to the cardiac output (eg, decreased cardiac output will be associated with decreased $ScVO_2$). $ScVO_2$ <70% after fluid and vasopressor resuscitation should be optimized with either (i) blood transfusion (to increase the arterial oxygen content if the hematocrit <30%) or (ii) an inotrope (dobutamine, milrinone) to increase the cardiac output.

In conjunction with hemodynamic and volume resuscitation is treatment of underlying infection. Appropriate cultures (urine, blood, respiratory, cerebrospinal fluid, and/or wound cultures) should be obtained prior to the administration of antibiotics when possible, but cultures should not significantly delay indicated antimicrobial therapy. Empiric antibiotics should be administered against likely pathogens, including gram-positive bacteria, gram-negative bacteria, antibiotic-resistant (methicillin-resistant *Staphylococcus aureus*, *Pseudomonas* sp.) bacteria, and sometimes fungi. In some patients, empiric *C. difficile* therapy is appropriate. Good infection control practice requires that critically ill patients be initially treated broadly, and then antibiotic selection narrowed once a pathogen is identified (Figure 28-1). In an observational study, hospital mortality increased by 7% per hour of delay of appropriate antimicrobial therapy.

In addition to appropriate antibiotic selection is source control. *Source control* is the removal of the source of infection, when possible. For patients with device-associated infections (central catheter infections), the offending device should be removed as soon as possible. For patients with intra-abdominal abscess, severe *C. difficile* colitis, ischemic bowel, necrotizing fasciitis, wet gangrene, or other source of tissue infection, surgical removal or drainage of the source of sepsis is mandatory for survival.

Patients with severe sepsis often develop organ failure. Many patients will develop acute kidney injury and may require dialysis. Capillary leak that causes third-spacing of fluid peripherally may also affect the pulmonary system, and patients may develop noncardiogenic pulmonary edema and can require intubation and mechanical ventilation. Ileus, coagulopathy, electrolyte abnormalities, relative adrenal insufficiency, and liver dysfunction can occur, but most of these coincident organ failures improve with treatment of shock.

Table 28-3. Vasopressor Agents for Treating Sepsis-related Hypotension Not Responsive to Fluid Resuscitation

Medication (Dose)	Inotropy	Chronotropy	Arterial Vasoconstriction	Practical Uses
Norepinephrine 0.01–1.00 mcg/kg/min 8–30 mcg/min typical dosing	Yes	Yes	Yes	First line for many patients with severe sepsis or septic shock Significant vasoconstriction with inotropy that is helpful for patients with poor left ventricular reserve or sepsis-related cardiomyopathy
Dopamine 5–10 mcg/kg/min, increased chronotropy/inotropy >10 mcg/kg/min, predominant vasoconstriction, increased blood pressure	Yes	Yes	Yes	Randomized comparison to norepinephrine showed no significant differences in mortality, but *increased arrhythmias with dopamine* More tachycardia than with norepinephrine More potent inotrope than norepinephrine Differing effects at escalating doses with vasoconstriction at highest dose Available in premixed or preprepared bags and therefore can be initiated quickly
Phenylephrine 0.4–9.1 mcg/kg/min 0.2–1.0 mcg/kg/min typical dosing	No	No	Yes	Pure alpha vasoconstrictor Used primarily in sepsis in patients with excessive tachycardia or arrhythmias to avoid medications with chronotropic effect

Drug/Dose				Comments
Epinephrine 2-10 mcg/min	Yes	Yes	Yes	More recent data supporting its role in septic patients Increased production of lactate, especially gastrointestinal, as well as significant tachycardia has kept this a second-line medication
Vasopressin 0.01-0.04 U/min	No	No	Yes	Used due to relative depletion of vasopressin in sepsis Nonadrenergic vasoconstrictor *Should not be used as the sole vasopressor agent in sepsis*
Dobutamine 2.5-20.0 mcg/kg/min	Yes	Yes	Vasodilator	Used for patients exhibiting evidence of low-output state with sepsis due to underlying poor cardiac reserve or sepsis-induced cardiomyopathy Can lead to hypotension, and should be used with a vasoconstrictor initially if hypotension occurs due to vasodilatory effects

Adapted from Felner K, Smith RL. Sepsis. In: McKean SC, et al. *Principles and Practice of Hospital Medicine*. McGraw-Hill; 2012.

Broad-Spectrum Gram Negative Antibiotic (no *Pseudomonas* coverage)	Broad-Spectrum Gram Positive Coverage (MRSA Activity)	Anti-Pseudomonal Gram Negative Double-Coverage (neutropenia, strongly suspected pseudomonas infection, institutional practice)
• Third-generation cephalosporin (ceftriaxone, cefotaxime)		

OR

Broad-Spectrum Gram Negative Antibiotic (*Pseudomonas* coverage)	+	±
• Fourth-generation cephalosporin (cefepime) • Antipseudomonal β-lactam/β-lactamase inhibitor (piperacillin-tazobactam, ticarcillin-clavulanate) • Antipseudomonal carbapenem (meropenem, imipenem, doripenem) • Monobactam (aztreonam)	• Vancomycin • Linezolid	• Aminoglycoside (gentamycin, tobramycin, amikacin)

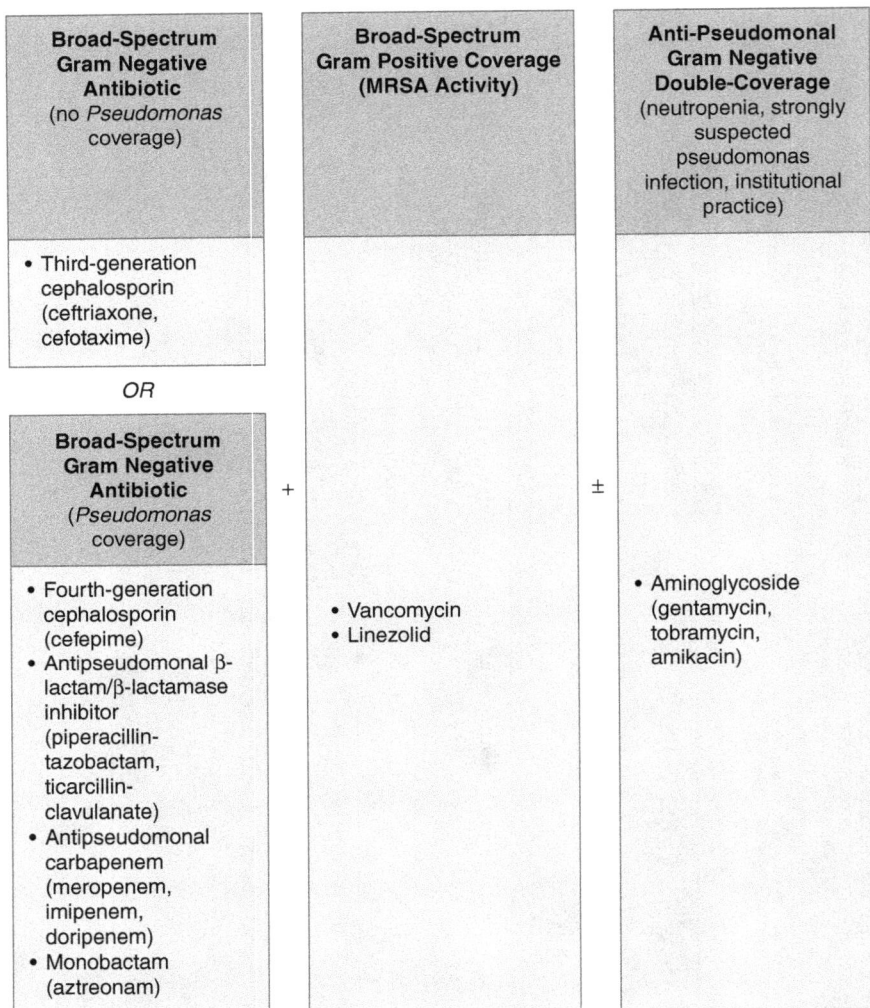

Figure 28-1. Antibiotic selection in severe sepsis and septic shock.

The patient described in the above vignette presents with shock, fever, leukocytosis, and lactic acidosis. He also has a suspected source of infection (long-standing PICC line for parenteral nutrition). With his fever, leukocytosis, and a suspected source, septic shock should be at the top of your differential diagnosis, and your initial therapy should consist of broad-spectrum antibiotics and fluid resuscitation. Subsequently, you should consider removing the PICC line for source control.

TIPS TO REMEMBER

● Severe sepsis and septic shock are critical illnesses associated with very high mortality.

● Aggressive resuscitation in the first 6 hours of management improves hospital survival.

● Early appropriate antibiotics and source control are 2 of the most important cornerstones of sepsis therapy.

COMPREHENSION QUESTIONS

1. Which of the resuscitation goals listed below are not among those to which the Surviving Sepsis Campaign recommends titrating hemodynamic resuscitation?
    A. Central venous pressure ≥8 mm Hg
    B. Mean arterial blood pressure ≥65 mm Hg
    C. Urine output ≥0.5 mL/kg/h
    D. Hemoglobin >12 g/dL
    E. ScVO$_2$ ≥70%

2. Which of the following has been *best* shown to improve survival in patients with septic shock?
    A. Blood product administration
    B. Timely administration of appropriate antibiotics
    C. Timely administration of parenteral nutrition
    D. Use of subcutaneous heparin for deep venous thrombosis prophylaxis
    E. Serial EKG monitoring and urgent cardiac catheterization for ischemic changes

3. Which of the following criteria is *not* part of the definition of septic shock?
    A. Respiratory rate >20 breaths/min
    B. Heart rate >90 beats/min
    C. Documented or suspected source of infection
    D. Signs of organ dysfunction (acute kidney injury, liver dysfunction, changes in mental status, elevation in serum lactate)
    E. Response to ACTH stimulation test

4. Which of the following vasopressor or inotrope doses would be an inappropriate infusion starting dose (doses in parentheses for non–weight-based dosing)?
    A. Norepinephrine 0.05 mcg/kg/min (5 mcg/min)
    B. Vasopressin 40 U/min
    C. Dopamine 5 mcg/kg/min
    D. Dobutamine 5 mcg/kg/min
    E. Phenylephrine 0.2 mcg/kg/min (200 mcg/min)

Answers

1. D. The Surviving Sepsis Campaign identifies a number of goals of resuscitation, including blood pressure, preload, urine output, and $ScVO_2$. For patients with low $ScVO_2$, a hematocrit of 30% (corresponding to hemoglobin concentration of 10 g/dL) is identified as an objective to try to optimize oxygen delivery.

2. B. Although the early goal-directed therapy algorithm includes many components, early appropriate antimicrobial therapy is best supported as impacting hospital survival.

3. E. Septic shock requires at least 2 of 4 of the SIRS criteria, a suspected or documented source of infection, evidence of at least 1 organ failure, and hypotension after an appropriate bolus of fluid. Response to the ACTH stimulation test is not part of the definition.

4. B. The appropriate dose of vasopressin when used as a vasopressor in septic shock is 0.04 U/min.

SUGGESTED READINGS

De Backer D, Biston P, Devriendt J, et al. Comparison of dopamine vs. norepinephrine in the treatment of shock. *N Engl J Med.* 2010;362:779–789.

Kollef M, Isakow W. *The Washington Manual of Critical Care.* 2nd ed. Philadelphia: Lippincott Williams & Wilkins; 2011.

Marino PL. *The ICU Book.* 3rd ed. Philadelphia: Lippincott Williams & Wilkins; 2007.

Rivers E, Nguyen B, Havsted S, et al. Early goal-directed therapy in the treatment of severe sepsis and septic shock. *N Engl J Med.* 2001;345(19):1368–1377.

Russell JA, Walley KR, Singer J, et al. Vasopressin versus norepinephrine infusion in patients with septic shock. *N Engl J Med.* 2008;358(9):877–887.

SAFE Study Investigators. A comparison of albumin and saline for fluid resuscitation in the intensive care unit. *N Engl J Med.* 2004;350(22):2247–2256.

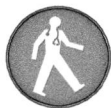

A 40-year-old Female With Headache

Amy Walsh, MD and Nicholas M. Mohr, MD

CASE DESCRIPTION

Argyll Robertson is a 40-year-old female with no past medical history who had the sudden onset of a severe headache behind her right eye about 3 hours ago. She immediately became nauseous and vomited in her bathroom. After about 5 minutes, her husband found her unresponsive on the bathroom floor. He called 911, who brought her to a local emergency department. A head CT was performed, and she was found to have "bleeding in the brain." She has normal coagulation studies. She was transferred by ambulance to your ICU for further management. On arrival, she is slightly sleepy, but interactive with the following vital signs: T 37.2°C, BP 187/110, P 92, RR 18, and O_2 97% (room air). She complains of persistent 10/10 headache.

1. What is the most likely diagnosis? What else is on your differential diagnosis?

You are reviewing her records and find her head CT (Figure 29-1). Diagnostic cerebral angiography is performed 6 hours after her arrival and reveals an 8-mm broad-based aneurysm of her anterior communicating artery, but no intervention was performed. Over the next 4 hours, she becomes progressively more somnolent. Repeat neurologic examination reveals that she is very sleepy, mumbling incomprehensibly, flexes to pain only, does not open her eyes, and is gurgling on her oral secretions.

2. What are your immediate diagnostic and management priorities?

Answers

1. Spontaneous subarachnoid hemorrhage (based on head CT). Other considerations by history are traumatic subarachnoid, subdural hematoma, epidural hematoma, intraparenchymal hemorrhage, meningitis, ischemic stroke, migraine headache, drug overdose, hypoglycemia, vertebral artery dissection, aortic dissection, ruptured ectopic pregnancy, or cardiac dysrhythmia.

2. Your first priority in this patient is securing her airway with endotracheal intubation (preferably by an experienced provider to limit the increase in intracranial pressure). The most likely causes of sudden neurologic deterioration early in the course of aneurysmal subarachnoid hemorrhage are: (i) obstructive hydrocephalus and (ii) rebleeding. A stat head CT should be performed immediately after endotracheal intubation. Empirically, you should administer

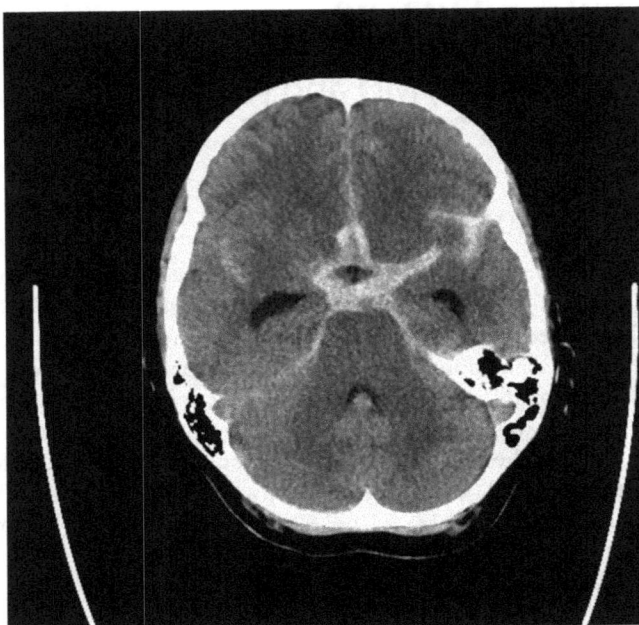

Figure 29-1. Head CT

an osmotic agent to lower intracranial pressure rapidly. Mannitol 0.5 to 1 g/kg or hypertonic saline 3% 250 mL may be given over 10 to 15 minutes (by institutional preference). More concentrated hypertonic saline (7.5%-23.4%) can be administered as well, but these formulations typically require central access and should be administered in consultation with your attending. If your patient has signs of hydrocephalus, an external ventricular drain (a catheter placed through a burr hole in the skull into the ventricle for drainage of cerebrospinal fluid) should be placed emergently.

SUBARACHOID HEMORRHAGE WITH ACUTE HYDROCEPHALUS

Diagnostic Workup and Management

The patient with subarachnoid hemorrhage can pose management challenges in the intensive care unit because of the wide variation in clinical presentation and the potential for rapid deterioration in clinical condition.

Spontaneous subarachnoid hemorrhage is a condition that results in 6700 in-hospital deaths annually, representing a mortality rate of almost 50%. Ruptured aneurysm is by far the most common cause, accounting for nearly 75% of all sub-arachnoid hemorrhage cases. Arteriovenous malformations and cerebral hemor-rhage account for about 10% of cases each, with the remainder occurring due to unknown causes. About 1% to 2% of the population has unruptured aneurysms, with larger aneurysms more likely to rupture spontaneously. Subarachnoid hem-orrhage is more prevalent in women than in men and increases in frequency with advancing age. Smoking, hypertension, and excessive alcohol intake increase the risk of subarachnoid hemorrhage.

Because these patients frequently present with altered mental status, airway management is a top priority. A patient who is unable to protect his/her airway should be intubated. Pretreatment with lidocaine and/or fentanyl prior to intuba-tion may attenuate the sympathetic response and a resultant increase in intracranial pressure, and should be considered for any patient being intubated for suspected intracranial hypertension. Patients may be sedated with etomidate (0.3 mg/kg), propofol (1-2 mg/kg), or versed (0.1-0.3 mg/kg), and paralysis for intubation may be provided using succinylcholine (1-1.5 mg/kg) or rocuronium (0.6-1.2 mg/kg). Hypotension and hypoxia must be avoided during airway management with use of vasopressor agents, preoxygenation and bag-valve-mask ventilation, and fluids. After securing the airway (and stabilizing breathing and circulation if necessary), the next important step is recognizing herniation and signs of increased intra-cranial pressure. Signs of increased intracranial pressure that should make you consider the need for osmotic therapy include decreasing level of consciousness, hypertension with bradycardia, pupillary response abnormalities, cranial nerve deficits, and respiratory abnormalities such as Cheyne Stokes breathing (periods of rapid breathing followed by periods of apnea).

One of the critical components of subarachnoid hemorrhage management is blood pressure control. Most patients with spontaneous subarachnoid hem-orrhage will be hypertensive after their hemorrhage occurs (regardless of base-line blood pressure). While the patient has an unsecured aneurysm (meaning a cerebral aneurysm that has not been treated with either endovascular coiling or surgical clipping), hypertension should be avoided and many centers lower mean arterial blood pressure empirically to try to prevent rebleeding. Providing analge-sic medications carefully can help attenuate hypertension, but one must be cau-tious not to mask ongoing neurologic assessment with sedating medications when possible. In cases of significant hypertension requiring antihypertensive therapy, arterial catheterization can facilitate continuous blood pressure monitoring, and can improve titration of antihypertensive agents. Although labetalol (10-20 mg IV) or hydralazine (10-20 mg IV) can be used acutely, maintaining blood pressure over time should use continuous infusions, such as nicardipine. Discuss blood pressure management with your neurosurgical consultant early so that your blood pressure management strategy is clear early in the course of care.

Several other early complications of subarachnoid hemorrhage can occur. Blood in the cerebrospinal fluid can make the brain very irritable, and seizure (both convulsive and nonconvulsive) is common after subarachnoid hemorrhage. Antiepileptic agents, such as levetiracetam, phenytoin, or others, may be used to reduce the incidence of early posthemorrhage seizures.

For patients being treated with anticoagulant medications (warfarin, dabigatran, etc) for other indications, anticoagulant activity should be reversed. Warfarin anticoagulation can be reversed with fresh frozen plasma, prothrombin complex concentrates, and/or vitamin K. Reversal for newer oral anticoagulants (ie, dabigatran) and antiplatelet agents (ie, aspirin, clopidogrel, dipyridamole) is controversial.

Several delayed complications of subarachnoid hemorrhage are common, and it is important for critical care physicians to monitor and treat these complications as they occur.

Vasospasm

Vasospasm refers to a phenomenon that occurs in patients after spontaneous subarachnoid hemorrhage whereby the large-capacitance cerebral arteries experience delayed narrowing, which can lead to ischemic brain injury. The highest risk period for onset is 3 to 5 days after the initial hemorrhage, and maximal narrowing occurs at 5 to 14 days. Symptomatically, these patients experience focal neurologic deficits, confusion, or increasing somnolence not explained by rebleeding or hydrocephalus, and approximately 20% experience stroke or death as a result of vasospasm.

There are data to support the use of nimodipine, statins, and some other pharmacologic agents for prevention of vasospasm in the window of peak incidence. Some centers screen for or diagnose vasospasm with transcranial Doppler (measuring velocity through cerebral blood vessels), cerebral angiography, or perfusion imaging. Therapy is directed at improving distal flow, and consists of hypertension therapy (using vasopressors), maintaining euvolemia, and in some cases local angioplasty or catheter-directed drug therapy.

Hydrocephalus

Acute hydrocephalus occurs within the first 24 hours after bleed. It is characterized by progressive onset of stupor and is treated with catheter drainage of the ventricular system (external ventricular drain). Delayed hydrocephalus can occur 10 days or more after initial symptoms, and if it is persistent may require placement of a ventriculoperitoneal shunt.

Rebleeding

Rebleeding occurs in 20% of patients with subarachnoid hemorrhage, and 70% of those who rebleed die. Most rebleeds occur within the first 2 weeks. Peak incidence occurs 24 to 48 hours after bleed and 7 to 10 days after initial bleed. Symptoms are similar to symptoms of the initial bleed such as severe headache, severe nausea and vomiting, change in level of consciousness, or a new focal neurologic deficit.

Hyponatremia

About 20% of patients with subarachnoid hemorrhage develop severe hyponatremia (Na <130 mEq/L). Hyponatremia does not correlate with site of aneurysm, but is more common after aneurysmal clipping or coiling. There are 2 primary clinical entities that result in hyponatremia in a subarachnoid hemorrhage patient: cerebral salt wasting (CSW) and syndrome of inappropriate antidiuretic hormone (SIADH). The classic presentation of SIADH involves decreasing sodium levels accompanied by decreasing BUN levels and urine output (free water overload). Key diagnostic criteria for SIADH include plasma osmolality <275 mOsm/kg, urine osmolality >100 mOsm/kg, urine sodium >40 mmol/L in the presence of normal dietary sodium, euvolemia, and exclusion of glucocorticoid and thyroid hormone deficiency.

CSW involves decreased sodium levels accompanied by hypovolemia with continuing diuresis and high levels of sodium excretion (wasting of sodium in urine). Differentiating the 2 entities is challenging because both are associated with hyponatremia with inappropriately sodium-rich urine, but can be simplified by carefully monitoring volume status (changes in BUN, blood pressure, and fluid balance).

Hyponatremia with subarachnoid hemorrhage can cause increased cerebral edema in an already injured brain, increasing the rate of delayed cerebral infarction by 3 times. Therapy for CSW and that for SIADH differ (sodium replacement vs fluid restriction), but fluid restriction is often difficult in patients at risk for cerebral vasospasm. In practice, hyponatremia is usually treated with sodium therapy (hypertonic saline therapy, oral sodium chloride tablets), taking care not to increase sodium level more rapidly than 0.5 mEq/h. In refractory cases, fludrocortisone, demeclocycline, or vasopressin receptor antagonists (eg, conivaptan, tolvaptan) can be used.

TIPS TO REMEMBER

- Acute changes in mental status should prompt urgent evaluation of the need for airway management and radiographic evaluation for rebleeding and hydrocephalus.
- Osmotic therapy should be given empirically for acute mental status changes based on physical examination findings rather than waiting for ancillary testing to confirm the diagnosis.
- Nicardipine is a reasonable infusion agent for blood pressure control in subarachnoid hemorrhage patients because it is short acting and titratable.
- There are many delayed complications in patients with subarachnoid hemorrhage that have significant effects on morbidity and mortality.

COMPREHENSION QUESTIONS

1. Name 4 symptoms that should make you consider administration of osmotic therapy.

2. When in the clinical course is it necessary to consider placement of an external ventricular drain?

3. What are the key clinical features that can help you distinguish CSW from the SIADH secretion?

Answers

1. Decreasing level of consciousness, hypertension with bradycardia, pupillary response abnormalities, cranial nerve deficits, and respiratory abnormalities.

2. When the patient's mental status is depressed to the point that physical examination can no longer be reliably used to monitor intracranial pressure, or when head CT shows signs of obstructive hydrocephalus.

3. Urine output (high in CSW, low in SIADH), blood pressure (decreasing in CSW, normal in SIADH), and BUN (high in CSW, normal in SIADH).

SUGGESTED READINGS

Connolly ES, Rabinstein AA, Carhuapoma JR, et al. Guidelines for the management of aneurysmal subarachnoid hemorrhage: a guideline for healthcare progessionals from the American Heart Association/American Stroke Association. *Stroke*. 2012;43:1711–1737.

Kollef M, Isakow W. *The Washington Manual of Critical Care*. 2nd ed. Philadelphia: Lippincott Williams & Wilkins; 2011.

Marino PL. *The ICU Book*. 3rd ed. Philadelphia: Lippincott Williams & Wilkins; 2007.

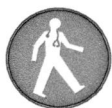

A 65-year-old Male With Hematemesis

Joshua D. Stilley, MD and Nicholas M. Mohr, MD

CASE DESCRIPTION

Paul Dieulafoy is a 65-year-old male with a history of alcoholic liver disease who presents to the emergency department with hematemesis. He first started vomiting earlier today, but 1 hour prior to presentation he had a large volume of blood in the emesis. His wife called 911 and he was brought to the emergency room. His initial vital signs are T 36.6°C, P 110, BP 110/60, R 20, and SpO_2 94%. Laboratory evaluation revealed hemoglobin of 6.5 mg/dL, platelets of $75 \times 10^3/\mu L$, and an INR of 1.5. One unit of packed red blood cells was transfused prior to admission to the intensive care unit. An NG tube is placed and a large volume of bloody fluid is suctioned.

On arrival to the intensive care unit, you are called to admit the patient. Your examination reveals a slightly anxious patient in no distress, NG tube still in place, and 1 peripheral IV.

1. What is the likely source of bleeding?

2. What are your priorities in management?

3. What complications should you watch for?

4. Should you correct his coagulopathy?

Answers

1. It is difficult to identify the cause of gastrointestinal (GI) bleeding prior to endoscopy, but the medical history can provide some clues. The most likely source of bleeding in this patient is esophageal varices. His known alcoholic liver disease puts him at risk for portal hypertension, varices, and upper GI bleeding. Gastric ulcers, duodenal ulcers, Mallory-Weiss tears, and aortoenteric fistulas should also be considered. Blood on NG tube aspiration can be helpful to confirm upper GI bleeding, but the absence of blood cannot rule out an upper GI source (postpyloric, clotted). Often the source cannot be identified until endoscopy.

2. Priorities for management are similar to all critically ill patients: airway, breathing, and circulation. Mr Dieulafoy is comfortable and in no distress, so he does not require airway management or breathing support. He requires 2 large-bore peripheral IVs (adequate resuscitation lines) or a large-bore central line

(a trauma introducer may be indicated for large-volume resuscitation). Serial hemoglobin measurements should be performed to monitor for ongoing bleeding (NG tube output is an unreliable screen for ongoing bleeding), and arrangements for endoscopy should be made.

3. Airway compromise should always be at the top of your risk assessment. Patients with GI bleeding can have large-volume bloody emesis and depressed mental status, and are at risk for aspiration. Patients who have already aspirated are at risk for respiratory failure from aspiration pneumonitis.

4. No. Platelets are not indicated unless the level is $<50 \times 10^3/\mu L$ except in special situations. Fresh frozen plasma (FFP) will not improve the INR below 1.5, so giving it to this patient is of no benefit.

UPPER GI BLEEDING

Diagnostic Workup and Management

As a resident in the ICU, your focus is trying to treat and anticipate life-threatening conditions. Patients with GI bleeding can have large-volume blood loss in a short amount of time, can decompensate and experience respiratory failure, and can develop profound hypotension. Serial hemoglobin/hematocrit levels should be ordered at a minimum of every 4 hours while the patient is hemorrhaging. Lactate levels can also be used to help measure peripheral oxygen delivery and adequacy of your resuscitation. Don't forget mental status and urine output as surrogate indicators for tissue perfusion for patients in shock. A type and screen should be performed to improve rapid access to blood products should they be emergently required.

Vascular access is an important part of resuscitation in patients with GI bleeding. Sometimes it is difficult to know whether patients are continuing to bleed until endoscopy is performed. In these cases, having adequate resuscitation access is critical. Resuscitation catheters are evaluated by their resistance to high-volume flow. Short, large-caliber catheters are the best lines to use for resuscitation; PICC lines (small caliber, very long catheter) are inadequate resuscitation lines. Large-bore peripheral IVs (minimum 2 IVs) are adequate for resuscitation. A peripheral IV can in some cases be "rewired" to a 6- to 8-French rapid infusion catheter for improved volume resuscitation access. In patients for whom large-bore peripheral access is not obtainable, central access should be sought. Patients for whom a central line is being placed for volume resuscitation should have a trauma introducer (or Cordis™ line) placed, because of its very large caliber and ability to introduce large volumes quickly. A standard triple-lumen or quad-lumen catheter is not preferred for volume resuscitation. Patients who are in hemorrhagic shock should be transfused with blood products, sometimes with the use of pressure bags or commercially available high-pressure rapid infusion devices (eg, Level One™ Rapid Infusion System).

Many GI bleeding patients have underlying liver disease, so they often have confounding factors of poor liver function and coagulopathy. Vitamin K can be given if the INR is elevated whether or not the patient is on warfarin, although it is unlikely to be very effective if warfarin is not the cause of the coagulopathy. FFP or prothrombin complex concentrates are used to correct an elevated INR acutely, but FFP will not correct the INR below 1.5, and its effect will only last for a few hours. Platelets need to be given if active hemorrhage continues and the platelets are below $50 \times 10^3/\mu L$, but there is little benefit for platelet counts above $50 \times 10^3/\mu L$. Cryoprecipitate (for fibrinogen levels below 100 mg/dL), recombinant factor VII, DDAVP (for patients with platelet dysfunction from significant renal disease), and other specific factors can also be used to correct coagulopathy.

One of the critical questions to answer in the face of GI bleeding is the source. Patients can have massive upper GI bleeding (eg, esophagus, stomach, duodenum) or can have massive lower GI bleeding (eg, colon, rectum). Predictors of upper GI bleeding include hematemesis, epigastric pain, a history of liver disease or varices, and previous upper GI bleeds. Identification of the source of bleeding based on melena alone is difficult if not impossible. Classically upper GI bleeding is taught to cause dark stools, while lower GI bleeding is described as a brighter red in the stool. The longer the blood is present within the GI tract, the more it will change from fresh-appearing blood with a bright red color to darker appearing. Unfortunately, brisk upper GI bleeding can appear very bright in the stool, while slower lower GI bleeds often will adopt a dark appearance.

Two of the standard medications used in upper GI hemorrhage include a proton pump inhibitor (PPI) and octreotide. PPIs (such as pantoprazole) are given as a bolus followed by an infusion during active bleeding. They help to promote gastric mucosa healing by decreasing clot fibrinolysis within the stomach and decrease rebleeding after endoscopy. Octreotide can also be given as a continuous infusion for patients with known or suspected portal hypertension to decrease portal venous pressures and decrease bleeding. The data supporting these medication's use is scant, so find out your institutional practice early in your rotation.

Definitive treatment for GI bleeding is procedural. Upper endoscopy is performed by a gastroenterologist and is often the only way to stop the bleeding. Endoscopy can control bleeding through placement of clips or bands, cautery, or injection of vasoconstrictors such as epinephrine. There are several challenges to endoscopy, though. Brisk bleeding can be difficult to localize, and clot burden can preclude definitive therapy. Occasionally, no bleeding is identified because bleeding has stopped prior to the procedure being performed.

Other adjunctive therapies exist for brisk bleeding. There are several devices (Minnesota tubes, Sengstaken-Blakemore tubes) that are balloon catheters that can be placed blindly and inflated in the esophagus to try to tamponade bleeding. Interventional radiology may be able to perform abdominal angiography to identify and embolize a source of bleeding. Occasionally, patients will require emergent transjugular intrahepatic portosystemic shunt placement to decrease portal pressures and stop bleeding. In some cases, surgeons will intervene to resect portions of stomach or intestine that are thought to be bleeding. These procedures are more often required with lower GI bleeding because endoscopic therapy is much more difficult.

GI bleeding is rarely an isolated disease. Among patients with cirrhosis, spontaneous bacterial peritonitis (SBP) can occur as either a cause or complication of upper GI bleeding. Antibiotic therapy has been recognized to be a useful adjunctive therapy in patients who present with upper gastrointestinal hemorrhage. Paracentesis and empiric antimicrobial prophylaxis are indicated in patients with cirrhosis and upper GI bleeding. Coverage for SBP often includes broad-spectrum antibiotic coverage for gram-positive cocci and gram-negative aerobes with an agent such as a third-generation cephalosporin. Antibiotic prophylaxis has been shown to prevent infections and reduce mortality, and is now recommended to be used uniformly in upper GI bleeding.

TIPS TO REMEMBER

- Closely follow markers of hemorrhage (hematocrit, vital signs) and aggressively replace blood products during episodes of bleeding.
- Involve consultants early to achieve definitive hemostasis in bleeding patients, communicate, and work together as a team. Use medical therapies to optimize your patient in preparation for definitive therapy.
- Vascular access is critically important in all hemorrhaging patients.

COMPREHENSION QUESTIONS

1. When giving FFP, what is your goal INR?

2. Why is vascular access important in GI bleed patients?

3. How often should you measure your patient's hematocrit?

Answers

1. 1.5. You will not be able to correct the INR below 1.5 with FFP alone.

2. The reason that your patient is in the intensive care unit is because he may need aggressive resuscitation for hemorrhagic shock. Not only is there a possibility of requiring a rapid crystalloid and blood resuscitation, but these patients also are treated with multiple medication infusions (PPI, octreotide, antibiotics). Having adequate vascular access is critical to preventing death, and the most opportune time to get adequate vascular access is before hemorrhagic shock ensues.

3. Measure serial laboratory studies as often as you need to adequately follow your patient's hemorrhage interventions. In actively bleeding patients, this may be every 2 hours (or every several units of blood transfusion). In a more stable patient every 6 to 8 hours may be appropriate.

SUGGESTED READINGS

Chavez-Tapia NC, Barrientos-Gutierrez T, Tellez-Avila Fl, Soares-Weiser K, Uribe M. Antibiotic prophylaxis for cirrhotic patients with upper gastrointestinal bleeding. *Cochrane Database Syst Rev.* 2010;9:CD002907.

Hebert PA, Walls G, Blajchman MA, et al. A multicenter, randomized, controlled clinical trial of transfusion requirements in critical care. *N Engl J Med.* 1999;340(6):409–417.

Kollef M, Isakow W. *The Washington Manual of Critical Care.* 2nd ed. Philadelphia: Lippincott Williams & Wilkins; 2011.

Marino PL. *The ICU Book.* 3rd ed. Philadelphia: Lippincott Williams & Wilkins; 2007.

SAFE Study Investigators. A comparison of albumin and saline for fluid resuscitation in the intensive care unit. *N Engl J Med.* 2004;350(22):2247–2256.

Villanueva C, Colorno A, Bosch A, et al. Transfusion strategies for acute upper gastrointestinal bleeding. *N Engl J Med.* 2013;368:11–21.

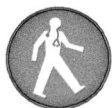

A 45-year-old Male With Abdominal Pain, Vomiting, and Altered Mental Status

Joshua D. Stilley, MD and Nicholas M. Mohr, MD

CASE DESCRIPTION

Mr. Sabino is a 45-year-old male with no past medical history who is admitted to the ICU from the ED with altered mental status, vomiting, and diffuse abdominal pain. He has been having increasing fatigue, polyuria, and polydipsia over the past 2 weeks, and vomiting started over the past 3 days. Today his wife found him stuporous in bed, and he was transported by ambulance to your ED. On arrival to the ICU, his vital signs are P 132, BP 112/75, R 22, and T 37°C. The critical care laboratory panels sent from the ED reveal a blood sugar of 794 mg/dL, sodium of 130 mEq/L, a potassium of 3.0 mEq/L, and a lactate of 7.0. Formal laboratory evaluation reveals a chloride of 100 mEq/L, a bicarbonate of 10 mEq/L, a BUN of 40 mEq/L, a creatinine of 2.0 mEq/L, and a beta-hydroxybutyrate of 9 mEq/L. Urinalysis is positive for ketones. The patient was transferred from the ED within 30 minutes of arrival, so no therapy was instituted.

1. What is your primary resuscitation fluid?

2. When should insulin be started?

3. What should you do about the potassium?

Answers

1. Normal saline is your primary resuscitation fluid. This patient is profoundly volume depleted, and will require volume resuscitation to stabilize.

2. Insulin can be started at any time. In some hospitals, insulin is started first with a bolus and then a continuous infusion, but it can also be started with just an infusion (without the bolus). Some authors advocate for knowing the potassium before the insulin is started.

3. The potassium is already low. Insulin will drive potassium back into the intracellular space, so with therapy for diabetic ketoacidosis (DKA), you would expect the potassium to drop rapidly. You should begin replacing potassium in this case immediately.

DIABETIC KETOACIDOSIS

Diagnostic Workup and Management

DKA is frequently encountered in the emergency department and in the intensive care unit. It affects not only known diabetics but also new diabetics as a frequent initial presentation. It is much more common for DKA to occur with type 1 diabetes mellitus, but it has been reported in type 2 diabetes as well. Acid–base disturbances, fluid management, and insulin therapy will be fundamental components of management of DKA patients.

Three criteria are required for the diagnosis of DKA: hyperglycemia (blood sugar >250 mg/dL), ketones (measured usually with the serum beta-hydroxybutyrate), and an anion gap metabolic acidosis. Alternative diagnoses include hyperglycemic hyperosmolar nonketotic state (HHS). HHS will present similarly with high blood sugar and very high serum osmolality, although there will be no acidosis. Treatment of these 2 conditions is very similar.

The most important factor to remember in these patients is that DKA is a disease of volume depletion. As patients become markedly hyperglycemic, they experience hyperglycemic diuresis, leading to polyuria. Volume resuscitation with normal saline is the first line of therapy, because it will not only help to rehydrate patients but also dilute the glucose and restore normal renal function. As patients' intravascular volume is restored, urine output returns and some of the excess glucose will continue to spill into the urine. Start your therapy with 1 L of normal saline per hour over the first 2 hours (more rapidly for patients in hypovolemic shock—to restore normal end-organ perfusion). You may then switch to 0.45% normal saline at 250 to 500 mL/h. When the serum glucose falls below 250 mg/dL, dextrose should be added to the intravenous fluid while the insulin drip is continued until the anion gap acidosis resolves.

Insulin is the second mainstay of treatment of DKA. It works to drive sugar into the cells and restore normal metabolic function. This therapy not only decreases the serum glucose but also begins to slow organic acid production. There are many varieties of insulin to select, but intravenous regular insulin is the mainstay of treatment. Long-acting insulin can be used for outpatient management, but it does not have a role in acute DKA management. Standard therapy is to start insulin 0.1 U/kg IV bolus followed by 0.1 U/kg/h. Some practitioners and hospitals do not use the initial bolus (data from pediatric patients suggest that bolus insulin is contraindicated in children) to assure a more gradual blood sugar reduction. During aggressive insulin management, it is important to monitor glucose levels every 1 to 2 hours to ensure that the patient does not become hypoglycemic. One standard algorithm for DKA management can be found in Table 31-1.

Patients with DKA will often be noted to be significantly hyperventilating. Because of the metabolic acidosis, normal patients will increase their minute ventilation to drive their p_{CO_2} to hypocapneic levels, improving the pH in a compensatory fashion. Patients with severe metabolic acidosis may have such severe

Table 31-1. Management of Diabetic Ketoacidosis

Fluid administration

1-2 L of normal saline over the first hour. Repeat if clinically significant volume contraction persists after the first hour

Change to half-normal saline, 500-1000 mL/h, depending on volume status. Continue for about 4 h. Decrease rate to 250 mL/h as intravascular volume returns to normal

Convert fluids to D_5W when plasma glucose falls to 250 mg/dL

Insulin

Administer 10-20 U of regular insulin IV

Mix 50 U of regular insulin in 500 mL of normal saline (1 U/10 mL). Discard first 50 mL of infusion to accommodate insulin binding to tubing. Administer through piggyback line along with parenteral fluids at a rate of 0.1 U/kg/h

Double the infusion rate after 2 h if there is no improvement in plasma glucose levels

Potassium

Administer supplemental potassium chloride once renal function is established; provide 20 mEq/L of fluids for patients who are initially normokalemic, 40 mEq/L for those who are hypokalemic at presentation. In the latter case, hold insulin until serum potassium levels begin to increase

Gauge subsequent replacement based on serum K^+ measurements at 2-h intervals

Bicarbonate

Sodium bicarbonate only for patients with blood pH less than 7.0

Add 1 ampule of sodium bicarbonate (44 mEq) to 500 mL of D_5W or half-normal saline. Administer over 1 h

Reproduced, with permission, from Gardner DG. Endocrine Emergencies. In: Gardner DG, Shoback D, eds. *Greenspan's Basic & Clinical Endocrinology.* 9th ed. New York: McGraw-Hill; 2011 (chapter 24).

altered mental status that they require intubation and mechanical ventilation, but one must be aware that hyperventilation must be continued via the ventilator to prevent severe acidemia and circulatory collapse. In most cases, patients will be able to correct pH on their own better than the ventilator can. As the metabolic acidemia resolves, respiratory effort and minute ventilation will normalize.

With hyperglycemia and acidosis, potassium moves into the extracellular space. Serum potassium will drop rapidly during initial insulin therapy due to a shift back into the intracellular space. Potassium should be measured every 4 hours during the initial treatment of DKA and replacement therapy should begin soon after initiation of insulin therapy. For patients with initial potassium levels in the low or normal range, potassium should be added to maintenance fluids to be continued during insulin therapy.

Careful monitoring and replenishment of other electrolytes may also be required. Phosphate and magnesium are often low, and repletion may be required. Although sodium bicarbonate therapy has been suggested to buffer the effect of the metabolic acidosis, it has not been shown to be beneficial in DKA.

Rapid alteration in electrolytes including glucose and sodium can have drastic effects on cellular physiology. DKA therapy induces osmotic gradients that can lead to cellular fluid shifts, including cerebral edema. Changes in mental status during DKA therapy should prompt rapid reevaluation of blood sugar and electrolytes, head CT, and empiric osmotic therapy (usually with mannitol) for suspected cerebral edema, because this can be a fatal complication of DKA (especially in children).

It is important to look for a reason for the patient to be in DKA. Patients with new-onset diabetes are insulin deficient, so DKA is a presenting syndrome. Established diabetics often have an inciting cause. Any condition that increases metabolic stress will increase insulin requirements. These conditions can include myocardial infarction, infection (often pneumonia or urinary tract infection), poor insulin compliance, or even hyperadrenalism. Optimal patient care requires identification and treatment of underlying conditions that lead to DKA.

TIPS TO REMEMBER

- Begin treatment with normal saline and replete volume aggressively for patients in shock.
- Regular insulin is dosed first with a bolus of 0.1 U/kg IV and then a drip of 0.1 U/kg/h IV.
- Monitor and replete potassium aggressively.
- Think about the cause of DKA (infection, myocardial infarction, insulin noncompliance).

COMPREHENSION QUESTIONS

1. What is your initial resuscitation fluid of choice for patients in DKA?

2. When should you begin replacing potassium?

3. What type of insulin do you use and what is your initial insulin dose?

Answers

1. Normal saline with 2 L administered in the first 2 hours.

2. Almost immediately, except in cases of hyperkalemia.

3. Regular insulin, 0.1 U/kg IV bolus and 0.1 U/kg/h.

SUGGESTED READINGS

American Diabetes Association. Hyperglycemic crises in diabetes. *Diabetes Care*. 2004;27:S94–S102.
Kollef M, Isakow W. *The Washington Manual of Critical Care*. 2nd ed. Philadelphia: Lippincott Williams & Wilkins; 2011.
Marino PL. *The ICU Book*. 3rd ed. Philadelphia: Lippincott Williams & Wilkins; 2007.

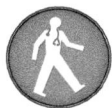

A 76-year-old Male With Dyspnea

Nicholas M. Mohr, MD

CASE DESCRIPTION

Mr Solis is a 76-year-old emaciated man with a history of severe chronic obstructive pulmonary disease (COPD) and a long history of tobacco abuse who is admitted from the emergency department with progressive dyspnea for 3 days. He has had a cough productive of a small amount of yellow sputum after a 1-day prodrome of mild rhinorrhea. He had been using his inhaler every 2 hours at home, but his son brought him to the hospital because he thought he was working harder to breathe. In the emergency department, he was given multiple doses of albuterol and ipratropium and was sent to the intensive care unit for further management.

You are the resident called to admit this patient. On your arrival, Mr Solis is breathing 32 times/min with intercostal retractions, has diffuse wheezing in all lung fields, and is able to speak in only 3 to 4 word phrases. His temperature is 36.7°C, pulse 116, BP 119/79, and oxygen saturation is 96% on 2 L oxygen by nasal cannula. A chest x-ray was performed in the emergency department (Figure 32-1), and his EKG was unchanged from his baseline.

Your patient is sleepy, but arousable and will answer questions. He denies chest pain, but does endorse dyspnea. His lung examination is notable for grossly diminished breath sounds in all lung fields with no audible wheezing. You ask your nurse to draw an arterial blood gas sample, which reveals the following results:

Arterial blood gas: pH 7.26; P_{CO_2} 70; P_{O_2} 94; HCO_3 34 (on 2 L oxygen by nasal cannula)

1. What is your differential diagnosis for this patient's admitting problem?

2. What therapy would you institute immediately?

3. Explain this patient's acid–base problem.

Answers

1. Exacerbation of COPD, asthma, pulmonary embolism, myocardial ischemia (anginal equivalent), congestive heart failure, right heart failure, pneumonia, and interstitial pulmonary fibrosis.

2. Inhaled beta-agonists (albuterol), inhaled anticholinergic medications (ipratropium), corticosteroids (methylprednisolone), consider testing for influenza, and noninvasive positive pressure ventilation.

3. Acute on chronic respiratory acidosis (note that bicarbonate level is elevated, and pH is less acidotic than would be expected for an acute P_{CO_2} of 70).

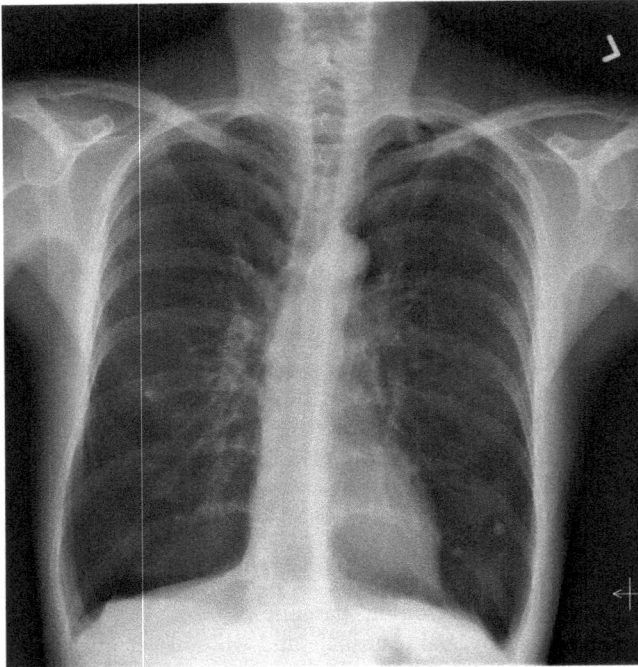

Figure 32-1. Chest x-ray.

COPD WITH RESPIRATORY FAILURE

Diagnostic Workup and Management

COPD is one of the most common causes of chronic respiratory failure in the United States, and is a significant cause of morbidity and mortality. It is an obstructive lung disease that is not fully reversible by bronchodilators, and is usually associated with chronic cigarette smoking (although some patients with COPD are lifelong nonsmokers). It is a heterogeneous disease often associated with chronic cough, dyspnea, sputum production, wheezing, and limitations in exercise.

Acute exacerbations are often triggered by upper respiratory infections (bacterial or viral) or environmental factors. Respiratory failure can ensue and rapidly progress to obtundation and death. Chest radiography is often performed because of the high rate of pneumonia in these patients when they present with respiratory distress. In evaluating these patients, establishing the severity of disease by asking about prior ICU admissions, prior intubations, recent corticosteroid use, recent hospitalizations, and recent pulmonary function testing can be helpful in predicting the clinical course.

Patients with COPD can present with worsening symptoms with or without significant hypoxemia. They can have diffuse wheezing on examination or the lung sounds can be coarse or relatively silent. The silent chest is an ominous finding, because it suggests that air movement is severely limited. Pulmonary embolism is also common in these patients, and must be considered in patients with atypical presentation or atypical response to typical therapy.

Treatments of choice for acute COPD exacerbations include bronchodilators and inhaled anticholinergics (albuterol, ipratropium), systemic corticosteroids, and antibiotics. These can be administered either by metered-dose inhaler or by nebulizer, but in critically ill patients, it can be difficult for patients to effectively use inhalers. Typical dosing is 2.5 to 5 mg albuterol nebulized every 1 to 4 hours as needed and 0.5 mg ipratropium nebulized every 4 hours. This dosing can be de-escalated as symptoms improve.

Corticosteroids are an important therapy to improve symptoms and decrease hospital length of stay. Oral and intravenous corticosteroids are equally effective, but most critically ill patients are treated with intravenous methylprednisolone 1 to 2 mg/kg in divided doses every 6 to 12 hours with rapid weaning to an oral taper (7-10 days) as symptoms improve.

Most patients with moderate–severe COPD exacerbations will warrant antibiotic therapy, especially when symptoms are associated with changes in sputum. Patients with a history of severe COPD, multiple recent courses of antibiotics, recent prior hospitalization, or prior *Pseudomonas* infection should be treated empirically for *Pseudomonas* (levofloxacin, cefepime, or piperacillin–tazobactam). Other patients may be treated with antimicrobials not active against *Pseudomonas* (levofloxacin, moxifloxacin, ceftriaxone, azithromycin, doxycycline).

In this patient, drowsiness and significant acute on chronic respiratory acidosis make him a candidate for noninvasive positive pressure ventilation (BiPAP). *BiPAP* stands for *bi*level *p*ositive *a*irway *p*ressure. This therapy can help to prevent intubation and help to offload respiratory effort while other therapies are being administered. BiPAP is positive pressure that is administered through a mask, and it can be titrated to the level of support required for the patient.

Any patient with acute respiratory acidosis on arterial blood gas analysis or significant respiratory distress can be treated with BiPAP (blood gas analysis is not required prior to starting therapy). In order to use BiPAP, a patient must be awake and cooperative, have an intact gag reflex, and preferably be able to manage his or her secretions without frequent suctioning.

Two pressure settings and an oxygen concentration setting are determined for patients being managed with BiPAP: the *e*xpiratory *p*ositive *a*irway *p*ressure (EPAP) and the *i*nspiratory *p*ositive *a*irway *p*ressure (IPAP). When the patient triggers a breath, the BiPAP machine pressurizes to IPAP, and then after inspiration, the pressure falls back to EPAP. Both pressures are indexed to zero pressure being atmospheric pressure (Figure 32-2). Fraction of inspired oxygen (FiO_2) can be adjusted from 21% (room air) to 100%.

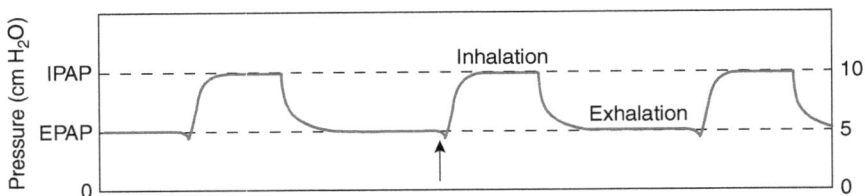

Figure 32-2. BiPAP diagram.

In BiPAP, the noninvasive ventilator machine cycles between 2 set pressures, the EPAP and the IPAP. When the patient takes a breath (arrow in Figure 32-2), the BiPAP machine senses the inspiration and cycles to the higher pressure, providing some ventilation support.

Typically, BiPAP is used with COPD for ventilatory support. Traditionally, the EPAP is left at 5 cm H_2O and the IPAP is set at 10 cm H_2O and titrated for tidal volume and patient comfort. Most BiPAP machines can measure tidal volume, and typically pressure will be adjusted for a tidal volume of 8 mL/kg (ideal body weight, calculated from patient height) and improvement in tachypnea and respiratory distress. A respiratory therapist will help you adjust BiPAP to titrate to your patient's comfort.

Some patients will continue to deteriorate despite optimal BiPAP support. These patients will have worsening arterial blood gas values and worsening mental status, and they will require endotracheal intubation and mechanical ventilation.

TIPS TO REMEMBER

- COPD is a chronic disease associated with frequent exacerbations and significant morbidity and mortality.
- Moderate–severe COPD exacerbations should be treated with beta-agonists, inhaled anticholinergics, corticosteroids, antibiotics, and noninvasive ventilation as necessary.
- BiPAP can be titrated to patient comfort as an alternative to endotracheal intubation.

COMPREHENSION QUESTIONS

1. COPD is primarily an obstructive lung disease that is not fully reversible with bronchodilator agents. True/false?

2. Severe COPD exacerbations should be treated with inhaled bronchodilators, inhaled anticholinergics, inhaled corticosteroids, and intravenous or oral antibiotics. True/false?

3. A patient with a normal blood gas should never be placed on noninvasive ventilation. True/false?

4. IPAP should be set such that the tidal volume exceeds 10 mL/kg of actual body weight. True/false?

5. BiPAP settings for this patient are set at EPAP 5, IPAP 15, and FiO_2 50%. On reassessment 1 hour later, the following arterial blood gas is available: pH 7.18, P_{CO_2} 80, P_{O_2} 115, and HCO_3 35. His clinical status has not significantly changed. The most appropriate next intervention is which of the following?
   A. Increase the IPAP to 20 cm H_2O.
   B. Decrease the FiO_2 to 40%.
   C. Increase the EPAP to 10 cm H_2O.
   D. Proceed with endotracheal intubation.
   E. Continue with current settings and wait for other therapies (bronchodilators, corticosteroids, antibiotics) to take effect.

Answers

1. True. COPD is an obstructive lung disease with varying degrees of reversibility with bronchodilator therapy.

2. False. Systemic corticosteroids should be used.

3. False. Severe respiratory distress is an indication for noninvasive ventilation regardless of blood gas analysis.

4. False. 8 mL/kg of ideal body weight.

5. D. Patients who fail noninvasive ventilation should be intubated for more aggressive ventilatory support.

SUGGESTED READINGS

Kollef M, Isakow W. *The Washington Manual of Critical Care.* 2nd ed. Philadelphia: Lippincott Williams & Wilkins; 2011.

Marino PL. *The ICU Book.* 3rd ed. Philadelphia: Lippincott Williams & Wilkins; 2007.

Plant PK, Owen JL, Elliott MW. Early use of non-invasive ventilation for acute exacerbations of chronic obstructive pulmonary disease on general respiratory wards: a multicenter randomized controlled trial. *Lancet.* 2000;355(9219):1931–1935.

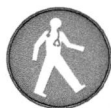

A 70-year-old Male With Altered Mental Status

Amy Walsh, MD and Nicholas M. Mohr, MD

CASE DESCRIPTION

Mr Justin Thyme is a 70-year-old male who presents to the emergency department with altered mental status. He was scheduled to attend a primary care appointment today, but he called his physician's office to cancel because he was "too weak" to get to the office. His primary care provider was concerned and called an ambulance to bring the patient in. On arrival in the ED, Mr Thyme is confused and ill-appearing. His only complaint currently is nausea. PMH is remarkable for diabetes mellitus, chronic obstructive lung disease, coronary artery disease, and chronic renal insufficiency. You get an EKG, shown in Figure 33-1.

On laboratory evaluation, your patient has a K^+ of 7.7 and creatinine of 5.5 (up from a baseline of 2.0).

1. What are the first therapeutic steps in the management of hyperkalemia?

2. What are the indications for emergent dialysis?

Answers

1. An acronym that can help you remember the components for management of acute hyperkalemia is:

  C: Calcium gluconate (1 g [10 mL] by peripheral IV over 5 minutes)

  B: Bicarbonate, sodium (1 ampule [44.6 mEq])

  I: Insulin, regular (10 U IV)

  G: Glucose (1 ampule of D50 [25 g dextrose])

  K: Kayexalate™ (sodium polystyrene, 30 g)

  DROP: Diuretics (furosemide), dialysis

  Please see the discussion for more information on the appropriate use of these agents.

2. Indications for dialysis:

  A: Acidosis

  E: Electrolytes (usually potassium)

  I: Ingestion (lithium, iron, ethylene glycol, and others)

  O: Overload (meaning fluid overload)

  U: Uremia (this is an indication for dialysis, but unlikely to require emergent dialysis)

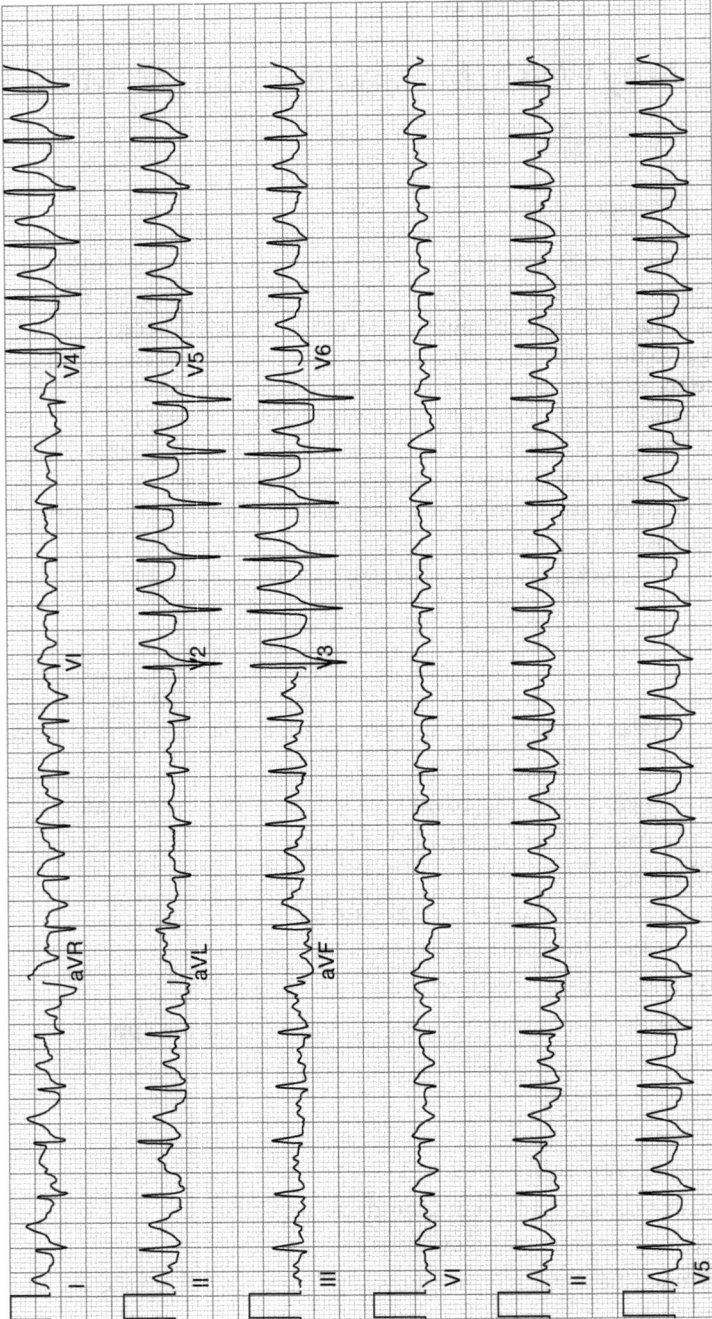

Figure 33-1. Electrocardiogram.

HYPERKALEMIA

Diagnostic Workup and Management

Because this patient has EKG changes typically associated with hyperkalemia, calcium gluconate should be immediately considered. Calcium works rapidly by stabilizing the cardiac membrane to prevent progression to cardiac dysrhythmia while other medications drive potassium intracellularly. In patients with hyperkalemia thought to be secondary to laboratory error (hemolysis), the EKG should be normal.

Secondary therapies are used to move potassium from the extracellular space to the intracellular space. Intravenous regular insulin (10 U IV) is a very effective therapy for this purpose, and it can be given with a source of glucose (dextrose D50, 1-2 ampules [25-50 g]) in patients who are not hyperglycemic. Sodium bicarbonate has been used in patients with significant acidosis, and high-dose albuterol (20 mg nebulized) has been used in some circumstances.

A third line of therapy is used to eliminate potassium from the body. Sodium polystyrene (Kayexalate™) is a cation exchange resin that has been used historically as a substance that binds potassium in the gastrointestinal tract. Recent studies have questioned its utility, but sodium polystyrene is still used in many centers as a temporizing agent in patients with anuria. Patients who have intact renal function can be given furosemide for hyperkalemia. Furosemide is a loop diuretic that increases renal potassium loss. The final method of potassium removal is dialysis, which can rapidly remove potassium from body stores. As the potassium level falls, electrocardiographic manifestations of hyperkalemia should resolve (Figure 33-2).

The EKG series shown in Figure 33-2 represents electrocardiographic manifestations of hyperkalemia in a single patient. Classically, hyperkalemia findings include: (a) peaking of the T-wave, (b) loss of the p-wave, and (c) widening of the QRS before deteriorating into the sinusoidal morphology classically associated

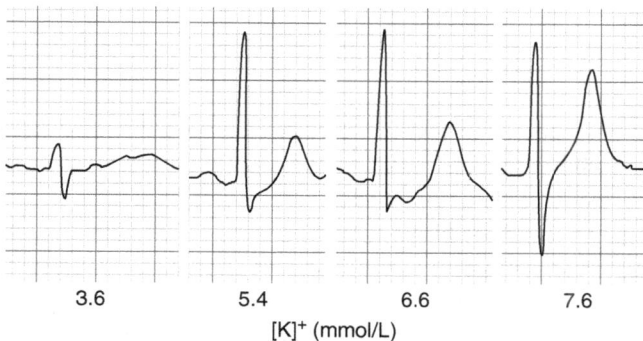

3.6   5.4   6.6   7.6

[K]$^+$ (mmol/L)

Figure 33-2. Images of progression of EKG changes in hyperkalemia.

with hyperkalemic cardiac arrest. The serum potassium at which these changes occur, and the order in which EKG manifestations are recognized, can be variable See Figure 33-2.

Acute kidney injury is often detected as an incidental finding on laboratory analysis secondary to another acute illness. Signs of acute kidney injury may include oliguria or anuria, nausea and vomiting, or symptoms of volume overload (dyspnea, jugular venous distension, pulmonary edema, peripheral edema). Acute kidney injury can be divided into 3 categories: prerenal kidney injury, intrarenal kidney injury, and postrenal kidney injury.

Prerenal kidney injury is caused by poor perfusion of the kidneys due to poor cardiac output (CHF), hypovolemia, or systemic hypotension and hypoperfusion (severe sepsis, for instance). It is suggested by a BUN:creatinine ratio >20, elevated urine specific gravity or urine osmolality, or a low fractional excretion of sodium (FeNa, or alternatively by urine sodium <15). Typically these patients rapidly recover renal function when renal perfusion improves (due to fluid resuscitation, inotropes, or vasopressors depending on the cause of the hypoperfusion).

Intrarenal kidney injury can be caused by many conditions, all affecting the kidney directly, such as acute tubular necrosis (often from prolonged prerenal physiology), renal vascular disease, glomerulonephritis, hemolytic uremic syndrome, thrombotic thrombocytopenic purpura, interstitial nephritis, rhabdomyolysis, vasculitis, or toxic alcohol ingestion. Intrarenal causes usually have an elevated FeNa, can have a BUN:creatinine ratio <20, and are often elucidated in consultation with a nephrologist.

Postrenal kidney injury is caused by urinary obstruction. The urinalysis is usually normal. Obstruction can be evaluated by renal ultrasound and placement of a Foley catheter.

After Mr Thyme's initial interventions, his potassium has improved to 6.6, with improvement of EKG findings (Figure 33-2). His mental status is somewhat improved. Foley catheter was placed, but he is anuric. His wife arrives and notes that he has been home with diarrhea and vomiting for the past 2 to 3 days, and has been unable to eat or drink.

TIPS TO REMEMBER

- For high potassium with EKG changes, administer calcium gluconate immediately to stabilize the myocardial membrane and prevent degeneration into a malignant ventricular dysrhythmia.

- Insulin, glucose, sodium bicarbonate (for acidosis), and albuterol can be used as temporizing measures.

- Definitive therapy should always be pursued (diuretics, dialysis). Consider emergent dialysis for patients with severe hyperkalemia and compromised renal function.

COMPREHENSION QUESTIONS

1. Would you order dialysis for Mr Thyme? Why or why not?

2. What type of acute kidney injury is this?

Answers

1. Probably. Mr Thyme's potassium has been temporarily forced into the intracellular space because of the interventions you have performed, but it will gradually be released back into the serum. Because of his underlying renal disease and his anuria, it is likely that his renal function will be slow to normalize, if it recovers. This patient should be immediately given several liters of normal saline volume resuscitation and his urine output should be monitored. You should consult nephrology in preparation for possible hemodialysis, and he will need to have a temporary dialysis catheter placed. While this is occurring, if his urine output improves with volume resuscitation and his potassium falls, you may be able to avoid hemodialysis. If his renal output does not improve with volume resuscitation alone, dialysis will be his only definitive option.

2. His acute kidney injury most likely started as prerenal kidney injury complicated by his baseline renal insufficiency. After a prolonged period of prerenal kidney injury, however, acute kidney injury can evolve into intrarenal physiology (acute tubular necrosis).

SUGGESTED READINGS

Kollef M, Isakow W. *The Washington Manual of Critical Care*. 2nd ed. Philadelphia: Lippincott Williams & Wilkins; 2011.
Marino PL. *The ICU Book*. 3rd ed. Philadelphia: Lippincott Williams & Wilkins; 2007.

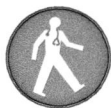

An 84-year-old Female With Cough and Fever

Joshua D. Stilley, MD and Nicholas M. Mohr, MD

CASE DESCRIPTION

Mrs. Sutton is an 84-year-old female nonsmoker resident of a nursing home. She has a history of mild hypertension and lives in the nursing home for 24-hour care and mobility assistance. Three days ago she developed a cough and fever. She was admitted to an outside hospital, diagnosed with pneumonia, and was started on antibiotic treatment with azithromycin and ceftriaxone. She did well for 24 hours, but last night she had worsening respiratory failure. She was intubated at the outside hospital and transferred to your ICU. On arrival her vital signs are BP 110/60, P 110, R 24, T 39°C, SpO_2 92%, weight 90 kg, and height 5'5". The ventilator is set on assist-control volume control mode with a rate set at 16, tidal volume of 450 mL, positive end-expiratory pressure (PEEP) of 5, and fraction of inspired oxygen (FiO_2) 60%. This gives a peak pressure of 30 cm H_2O and a plateau pressure of 22 cm H_2O. She is overbreathing the ventilator at a rate of 19. You obtain laboratory studies including blood cultures that show WBC 18.5, Hgb 13.0, Plt 203, Na 136, K 4.0, Cl 110, HCO_3 18, BUN 20, Cr 1.0, and glucose 110. Arterial blood gas analysis shows pH 7.35, p_{CO_2} 32, p_{O_2} 100, and HCO_3 16. Her chest x-ray is shown in Figure 34-1.

1. What likely pathogens need to be covered?

2. What antibiotics should be used?

3. How do you interpret the ABG?

4. How reliable will the cultures obtained in the ICU be?

Answers

1. The guidelines for antimicrobial therapy for pneumonia recommend that antibiotic therapy be directed at likely pathogens based on health care exposures. Although her initial therapy would be appropriate for community-acquired pneumonia, her residence in a nursing facility puts her at risk for health care–associated pneumonia. Health care–associated pneumonia requires coverage for *Streptococcus pneumoniae*, *Staphylococcus aureus* (including methicillin-resistant *S. aureus* [MRSA]), and *Pseudomonas aeruginosa* (depending on local infection and resistance patterns).

2. There is a range of antibiotics that may be appropriate. Gram-negative and gram-positive agents should be used with specific coverage for MRSA and for

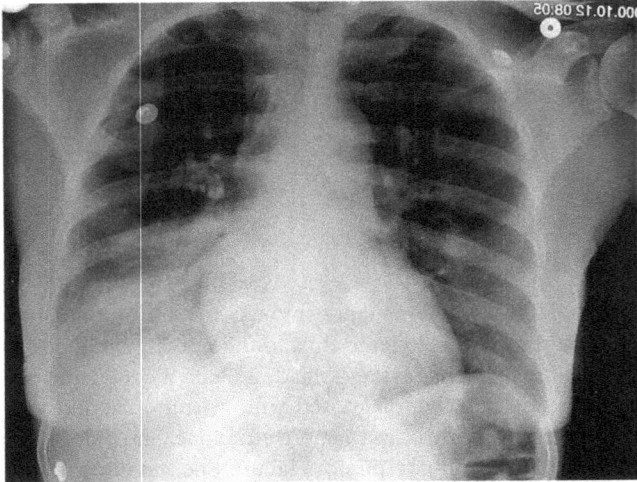

Figure 34-1. Chest x-ray. (Reproduced, with permission, from Stone C. Respiratory Distress. In: Humphries RL, Stone C, eds. *Current Diagnosis & Treatment Emergency Medicine.* 7th ed. New York: McGraw-Hill; 2011 [chapter 13].)

Pseudomonas. Common agents for gram-negative and pseudomonal coverage include a beta-lactamase penicillin (piperacillin/tazobactam), an antipseudomonal cephalosporin (cefepime), or a carbapenem (imipenem, meropenem). MRSA is usually covered by adding vancomycin, although newer agents, such as linezolid, also have MRSA activity.

3. The ABG shows a compensated metabolic acidosis.

4. You are unlikely to obtain an organism from the cultures if the patient is already on antibiotics active against the pathogen. However, if the organism was not covered by the antibiotics or if the infection is virulent, you may have a positive culture. Blood cultures are recommended for ICU patients with pneumonia, and respiratory cultures (either from quantitative bronchoalveolar lavage or from tracheal aspirate, depending on your local customs) can be helpful in subsequently narrowing antibiotic spectrum.

PNEUMONIA

Diagnostic Workup and Management

Patients with pneumonia resulting in respiratory failure will be frequently encountered in the intensive care unit. Treating these patients requires a combination of respiratory support (mechanical ventilation) and antimicrobial therapy.

Ventilators have various modes, types of breaths, and types of triggers. The most common controlled mode used in critically ill patients is assist/control. In assist-control mode, every breath delivered is the same—whether the patient triggers the breath or the ventilator delivers the breath with no respiratory effort from the patient, the same type of breath is delivered.

The 2 types of ventilator breaths that can be delivered are either volume-directed or pressure-directed breaths. Under volume-directed ventilation, the ventilator is set to deliver a determined volume with each breath. Under pressure-directed ventilation, the ventilator delivers a specific pressure for a given amount of time. Under either volume-directed or pressure-directed ventilation, lung compliance can be measured as it changes during a patient's course. In volume-directed ventilation, worsening lung compliance will be apparent with an increase in the pressure required to deliver the same volume. In pressure-directed ventilation, worsening lung compliance will be apparent with a decrease in the tidal volume delivered with a given drive pressure.

The third factor influencing mechanical ventilation is the type of triggering. Ventilators will deliver a breath when 1 of 2 events occurs: either (i) your patient tries to take a breath and the ventilator senses that she is trying to breathe or (ii) your patient does not take a breath in a specified period of time, so the ventilator delivers a breath to ventilate her. In assist-control ventilation, the ventilator responds in exactly the same fashion when either of these events occurs.

PEEP is the amount of pressure the ventilator maintains at expiration. The utility of PEEP is that it can help to prevent collapse of alveolar subunits. When alveoli collapse, they contribute to an intrapulmonary shunt, meaning that sections of lung are not ventilated, but are still perfused. This blood dilutes oxygenated blood in the pulmonary venous system and contributes to systemic hypoxemia. PEEP can range anywhere from 0 to 28 cm H_2O, but a good starting point is 5 cm H_2O, and most patients are ventilated with PEEP between 5 and 12 cm H_2O.

When a patient is ventilated, it is important to protect the lungs. Ventilator-induced lung injury is thought to be secondary to the fact that high-tidal-volume ventilation induces and worsens a pathologic injury to the lungs. Lung-protective ventilation is described as mechanical ventilation that limits tidal volume to 6 mL/kg of ideal body weight. The pressure with which lungs are ventilated is also important to prevent barotrauma. Plateau pressure is the pressure measured in the airways during an inspiratory hold maneuver (meaning with no air flow during the end of inspiration), and approximates the pressure experienced at the level of the alveolus. This pressure should be limited to 30 cm H_2O to limit lung injury. Expectedly, lung-protective ventilation may limit your ability to fully ventilate your patient, so these patients are allowed to become moderately hypercapnic (pH ≥7.20) to facilitate protective ventilatory strategies (permissive hypercapnia). Low-tidal-volume, low-pressure ventilation has been shown to improve outcomes in acute respiratory distress syndrome and is now recommended as a routine practice to prevent ventilator-induced lung injury in all critically ill patients.

In adjusting your ventilator for blood gas results, tidal volume and respiratory rate will influence ventilation (minute ventilation = tidal volume × respiratory rate), and the FiO_2 and PEEP will influence oxygenation. Maintaining lung-protective ventilation requires that tidal volume be limited, but respiratory rate can be increased (for hypercapnic respiratory acidosis) or decreased (for hypocapneic respiratory alkalosis) to change the respiratory component of acid–base balance. The minute ventilation will be determined by your patient's actual respiratory rate, so if respiratory effort exceeds the minimum set rate on the ventilator, your ability to slow your patient's breathing will be limited (consider analgesia in patients with pain or agitation). Hypoxia can be treated by increasing the oxygen (FiO_2), PEEP, or both. Oxygen saturation should be maintained at greater than 90% to 92%, and arterial p_{O_2} should be maintained at greater than 55 to 60 mm Hg.

Pneumonia can be divided into 3 categories: community-acquired, health care–associated, and hospital-acquired. In community-acquired pneumonia, coverage for *S. pneumoniae*, *Haemophilus influenza*, and *Mycoplasma pneumoniae* is important. This can generally be accomplished with a third-generation cephalosporin alone in combination with a macrolide such as azithromycin. Health care–associated pneumonia recognizes that patients who live in a nursing facility, receive hemodialysis, have been hospitalized in the last 90 days, or have home infusion therapy have infections that more closely resemble hospital-acquired pathogens. Hospital-acquired pneumonia is defined as a patient developing pneumonia after 48 hours in the hospital. The most common infections in health care–associated pneumonia and hospital-acquired pneumonia include *S. aureus*, and gram-negative infections such as *P. aeruginosa*, *Klebsiella pneumoniae*, *Escherichia coli*, and *Acinetobacter* sp. Antibiotics that typically cover *Pseudomonas* include aminoglycosides (gentamicin, tobramycin), beta-lactamase penicillins (piperacillin/tazobactam), carbapenems (imipenem, meropenem, doripenem), monobactams (aztreonam), fluoroquinolones (ciprofloxacin), and antipseudomonal cephalosporins (cefepime, ceftazidime). Vancomycin or linezolid is required for MRSA coverage.

TIPS TO REMEMBER

- Ventilate with a lung-protective ventilatory strategy.
- Ensure adequate antibiotic coverage.

COMPREHENSION QUESTIONS

1. What bacteria are responsible for community-acquired pneumonia?

2. What bacteria are responsible for health care–associated or hospital-acquired pneumonia?

3. What antibiotics treat *Pseudomonas*?

Answers

1. *S. pneumoniae*, *H. influenza*, and *M. pneumoniae*.

2. *S. pneumoniae*, *S. aureus*, and *P. aeruginosa*.

3. Aminoglycosides (gentamicin, tobramycin), beta-lactamase penicillins (piperacillin/tazobactam), carbapenems (imipenem, meropenem), monobactams (aztreonam), fluoroquinolones (ciprofloxacin), and antipseudomonal cephalosporins (cefepime, ceftazidime).

SUGGESTED READINGS

Acute Respiratory Distress Syndrome Network. Ventilation with lower tidal volumes as compared with traditional tidal volumes for acute lung injury and the acute respiratory distress syndrome. *N Engl J Med.* 2000;342(18):1301–1308.

American Thoracic Society, Infectious Diseases Society of America. Guidelines for the management of adults with hospital-acquired, ventilator-associated, and healthcare-associated pneumonia. *Am J Respir Crit Care Med.* 2005;171:388–416.

Chastre J, Wolff M, Chevret S, et al. Comparison of 8 vs 15 days of antibiotic therapy for ventilator-associated pneumonia in adults: a randomized trial. *JAMA.* 2003;290(19):2588–2598.

Kollef M, Isakow W. *The Washington Manual of Critical Care.* 2nd ed. Philadelphia: Lippincott Williams & Wilkins; 2011.

Mandell LA, Wunderink RG, Anzueto A, et al. Infectious Diseases Society of America/American Thoracic Society consensus guidelines on the management of community-acquired pneumonia in adults. *Clin Infect Dis.* 2007;44:S27–S72.

Marino PL. *The ICU Book.* 3rd ed. Philadelphia: Lippincott Williams & Wilkins; 2007.

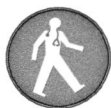

A 32-year-old Male With Multi-system Trauma

Nicholas M. Mohr, MD

CASE DESCRIPTION

Mr Cowley is a 32-year-old gentleman admitted from the operating room after having had emergent exploratory laparotomy for gunshot wounds to the abdomen. He was shot 4 times and sustained injuries to his liver, inferior vena cava, colon, stomach, and a segment of small bowel. He was intubated in the emergency department and arrived to the operating room significantly hypotensive. His liver injury was oversewn, he had segments of colon and small bowel removed, his bowel was left in discontinuity, and his inferior vena cava was repaired. His abdomen was packed with sponges and the fascia was left open with a vacuum dressing before he was urgently transferred to the intensive care unit for continuation of his resuscitation.

On arrival to the ICU, his vital signs are T 34.9°C, HR 136, BP 80/41 (mean arterial pressure 54), RR 16 (on ventilator), and oxygen saturation 94%. Most recent laboratory studies from the operating room show hemoglobin 6.4 (hematocrit 19%), platelets 85,000/μL, international normalized ratio 1.9, and PTT 51. His arterial blood gas shows a pH of 7.25, p_{CO_2} 30, p_{O_2} 196, and HCO_3 12. Your physical examination shows a young man who is intubated, with a midline abdominal incision with a vacuum dressing and blood in the vacuum tubing, and he moves all extremities spontaneously. He has no rashes.

1. What is your differential diagnosis of this patient's hypotension?

2. What is your resuscitation fluid of choice? Do you provide any blood products at this point, and if so, which ones?

3. What is the triad of conditions that contributes to death in traumatic patients with hemorrhagic shock?

The next morning, he is requiring 100% FiO_2 and his oxygen saturation is 90%. He has bilateral pulmonary edema on his chest x-ray.

4. What is his diagnosis?

5. How might you change his ventilator to improve his oxygenation?

Answers

1. Hemorrhagic shock, septic shock (though this would still be early in a trauma patient), neurogenic shock (less likely since he is neurologically intact), anaphylactic shock, and postoperative sedation.

2. This is a patient in hemorrhagic shock. The treatment for hemorrhagic shock is blood replacement therapy. At this point, packed red blood cells, fresh frozen plasma, and platelets should be given to resolve his coagulopathy, while at the same time you are treating his hemorrhagic shock.

3. Hypothermia, coagulopathy, and metabolic acidosis. These 3 factors contribute to the others (hypothermia and acidosis contribute to coagulopathy, bleeding contributes to acidosis and hypothermia, and shock leading to death is the result).

4. Overnight, he likely had a very aggressive resuscitation including blood products. He has acute respiratory distress syndrome (ARDS) or transfusion-associated lung injury (TRALI), but the treatment for both is the same.

5. The only intervention shown to improve mortality in patients with ARDS is low-tidal-volume (6 mL/kg ideal body weight) ventilation with adequate levels of PEEP and avoidance of unnecessary transfusion of blood products.

COMPLICATIONS OF MAJOR TRAUMA AND HEMORRHAGIC SHOCK

Diagnostic Workup and Management

Hemorrhagic shock is a disease characterized by global tissue hypoperfusion secondary to blood loss. It can be a complication of traumatic injury, gastrointestinal bleeding, and even from scheduled surgical interventions. The management of hemorrhagic shock has changed over the past 5 decades, primarily from lessons learned by military physicians worldwide.

The cornerstone of management for hemorrhagic shock is blood replacement therapy. Packed red blood cells have been used for a generation to restore circulating blood volume. The problem with isolated red cell replacement is that the blood being lost as a result of a traumatic injury contains both red cells and coagulation factors. Furthermore, factors necessary for a clot to form (coagulation factors, platelets, fibrinogen) begin to deplete as large clots are forming.

The pathophysiology of hemorrhagic shock is central to understanding balanced trauma resuscitation. Trauma victims who have had significant blood loss present to the hospital with acquired coagulopathy (from bleeding), metabolic acidosis (from shock), and hypothermia (from exposure and bleeding). All of these 3 factors are interdependent: acidosis and hypothermia contribute to coagulopathy; continued bleeding contributes to worsened shock and acidosis, which worsens coagulopathy and contributes to continued bleeding. The natural course of this disease is that hemorrhagic shock results in global tissue hypoperfusion (shock), organ dysfunction, and death.

The understanding of this disease has led to some new interventions aimed at arresting the progression of shock. The first concept is *damage control surgery*. Damage control surgery is the concept that early surgical intervention need not repair all the injuries—it is intended only to temporize the bleeding patient to allow resuscitation (and in some cases, evacuation to a different hospital) to occur. The patient in this vignette was taken emergently to the operating room and the bleeding was controlled. He was not subjected to a prolonged surgery for definitive repair of his injuries, but rather his bleeding was controlled; his abdomen was packed and a vacuum dressing was applied. He will be taken back to the operating room in the next 24 to 48 hours for definitive management once his resuscitation is complete, his acidosis is resolved, and he is warmed. At that point, his tissue will be more amenable to repair and he will no longer be in the fatal spiral of hemorrhagic shock.

The second concept that has changed trauma care is the concept of the *hemostatic resuscitation*. Partly due to recognition that coagulopathy is life-threatening, centers have begun to use fresh frozen plasma and platelets empirically with packed red blood cells to replace the blood volume of a hemorrhaging patient. In most centers, this protocol is called the "massive transfusion protocol" and is instituted when a patient's blood loss is expected to be 1 complete blood volume (approximately 10 U packed red blood cells for an adult). Each hospital has a different ratio of blood components, but most hospitals use a ratio of 1:1 to 2:1 (PRBC:FFP) with platelets being included for every 4 to 8 U of PRBCs. Most ratios try to replicate a resuscitation ratio similar to that of warm fresh whole blood.

In patients for whom massive transfusion is being used, several factors need to be considered. First, massive transfusion is not a therapy for surgical bleeding—patients with surgical injuries still require operative repair, and no quantity of coagulation factors will stop the bleeding. Second, significant metabolic derangements can occur that require monitoring and therapy. Hyperkalemia and hypocalcemia are very common (hyperkalemia from lysis of blood cells in the blood storage process and from acute kidney injury, hypocalcemia from chelation with citrate in banked blood), and require treatment as they develop. Coagulation studies should be measured, and significant coagulopathy may require treatment in addition to that prescribed for the standard resuscitation formula. Transfusion reactions can occur, immune suppression is ubiquitous with blood transfusion, and there remains a small risk of infectious complications secondary to transfusion.

One of the principal complications that occurs secondary to massive transfusion is lung injury. ARDS is characterized by noncardiogenic pulmonary edema, hypoxic respiratory failure, and bilateral edema on chest x-ray. It is likely a cytokine-mediated inflammatory disease of the lung. It remains difficult to distinguish clinically ARDS from TRALI, but the treatment for both conditions is identical.

Another complication of massive transfusion is *abdominal compartment syndrome*. The inflammatory response apparent in the lungs also occurs in other body compartments, and the abdomen is one that can cause complications. For patients who have not had their abdominal fascia left open, edema and fluid can increase the intra-abdominal pressure to impair venous drainage of intra-abdominal organs. Urine output falls, intrathoracic pressure rises, and bowel ischemia, acute kidney injury, and death can occur. Several temporizing measures exist, but definitive therapy requires laparotomy for abdominal decompression.

Hypoxia in the ICU should be approached with a standardized algorithm, but in patients for whom ARDS remains the appropriate diagnosis, only 2 methods exist to improve oxygenation with a standard mechanical ventilator: increasing the fraction of inspired oxygen or increasing the mean airway pressure.

ARDS is a heterogeneous disease: some sections of lung are affected while others are not. Those sections that are affected become collapsed and atelectatic. Deoxygenated pulmonary blood flow that passes through these regions does not participate in oxygen exchange, so it mixes with oxygenated pulmonary venous blood and creates relative hypoxemia, or physiologic shunt. The only method currently available to "recruit" these regions of diseased lung is increasing mean airway pressure, which helps to stent these alveoli open and recruit them to participate in gas exchange.

Mean airway pressure is the primary determinant of *lung recruitment*, and can be increased either by increasing the PEEP or by increasing the inspiratory time (in pressure control ventilation). Figure 35-1 shows how an increase in inspiratory time can increase the mean airway pressure. Other rescue strategies for severe lung injury exist (placing patients in a prone [face-down] position, high-frequency oscillatory ventilation [HFOV], airway pressure release ventilation, inhaled epoprostenol or nitric oxide), but most patients can be maintained on standard mechanical ventilation with careful attention to the pressure–volume relationship of the diseased lung.

The only therapy shown consistently to improve survival in patients with ARDS is low-tidal-volume ventilation. This treatment probably works by avoiding overdistension of nondiseased alveolar subunits by limiting tidal volume, which can reduce inflammation and protect the healthy lung from further injury. Patients with severe ARDS should be ventilated with a tidal volume of 6 mL/kg ideal body weight and a plateau pressure of no more than 30 cm H_2O. Furthermore, titrating mean airway pressure (PEEP) to markers of physiologic shunt fraction (such as hypoxia) can help to maintain open lung physiology while healing occurs.

In this patient, hypotension could be related to several causes. The most common cause of hypotension in the acutely injured patient is bleeding (hemorrhagic shock). For those patients with spinal cord injuries, neurogenic shock is

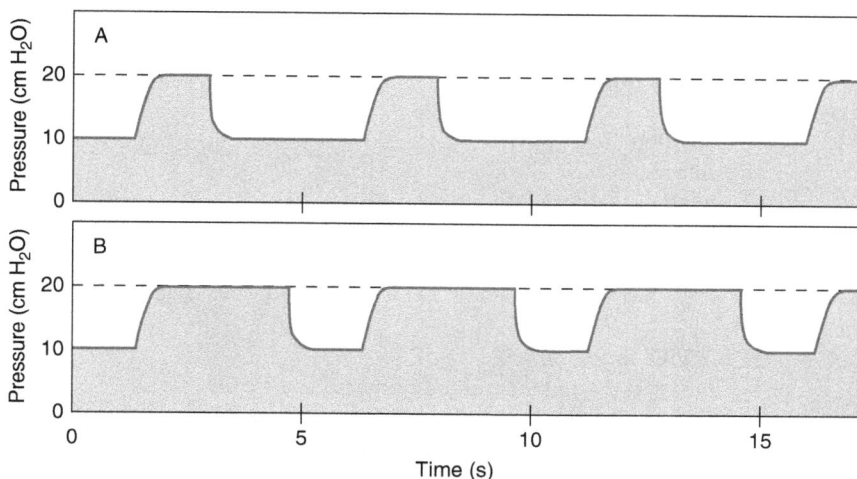

Figure 35-1. Inspiratory time can be used to increase mean airway pressure. Mean airway pressure is the primary determinant of lung recruitment. It can be estimated by looking at the ventilator pressure tracing. In both scenarios in the figure, a patient is being ventilated with pressure control ventilation with PEEP 10 cm H_2O and drive pressure 10 cm H_2O (peak airway pressure 20 cm H_2O) with rate 12. In *Scenario A*, the ratio between the inspiratory time and the expiratory time (I:E ratio) is 1:2, while in *Scenario B*, the I:E ratio has been reversed to 2:1. The area under the pressure curve (shaded) is significantly greater in scenario B, so the mean airway pressure (area under pressure curve/time) is increased, lung recruitment is improved, and less physiologic shunt (hypoxemia) and improved oxygenation would be expected.

another etiology, but typically this diagnosis is made after ruling out sources of bleeding. In this patient, aggressive resuscitation from hemorrhagic shock can be lifesaving.

TIPS TO REMEMBER

- The triad of coagulopathy, metabolic acidosis, and hypothermia contributes to death from hemorrhagic shock in traumatically injured patients.

- Damage control surgery and hemostatic resuscitation are 2 strategies for arresting progression of hemorrhagic shock and improving survival.

- One of the complications of massive resuscitation is ARDS. Oxygenation can be improved by increasing mean airway pressure (PEEP) and increasing FiO_2, but the only therapy shown to improve survival is low-tidal-volume ventilation.

COMPREHENSION QUESTIONS

1. Which of the following components is *not* part of the lethal triad of hemorrhagic shock?

    A. Coagulopathy
    B. Anemia
    C. Metabolic acidosis
    D. Hypothermia

2. Which of the following criteria is *not* required for the diagnosis of ALI/ARDS?

    A. p_{O_2}/FiO_2 ratio <300
    B. Chest x-ray with bilateral pulmonary edema pattern
    C. Absence of volume overload (pulmonary capillary wedge pressure <18, no clinical signs of volume overload)
    D. FiO_2 must be greater than 60%

3. Which of the following interventions has been best shown to improve survival in patients with ALI/ARDS?

    A. High levels of PEEP
    B. Low-tidal-volume ventilation
    C. Empiric antibiotic therapy
    D. Prone positioning
    E. HFOV
    F. Endotracheal pulmonary surfactant
    G. Early tracheostomy

4. Which of the following complications of massive transfusion resuscitation is most important to diagnose?

    A. Hypokalemia
    B. Hypomagnesemia
    C. Hypocalcemia
    D. Immune-mediated platelet destruction
    E. Volume overload

Answers

1. B. Coagulopathy, hypothermia, and metabolic acidosis comprise the lethal triad of shock. Anemia often develops after blood loss, but it does not contribute to the development of the other 3 conditions.

2. D. There is no absolute value for FiO_2 that is required for the diagnosis of ARDS. The other criteria are required to make this diagnosis, however.

3. B. Low-tidal-volume ventilation is the only intervention listed that consistently has been shown to decrease mortality in ARDS.

4. C. Although several of these complications can occur with massive transfusion, hypocalcemia can lead to worsened hypotension and low cardiac output. Intravenous calcium replacement therapy (usually 1-2 g intravenous calcium chloride or calcium gluconate) can be effective in these cases at restoring cardiac output and blood pressure.

SUGGESTED READINGS

Acute Respiratory Distress Syndrome Network. Ventilation with lower tidal volumes as compared with traditional tidal volumes for acute lung injury and the acute respiratory distress syndrome. *N Engl J Med.* 2000;342(18):1301–1308.

Bickell WH, Wall MJ, Pepe PE, et al. Immediate versus delayed fluid resuscitation for hypotensive patients with penetrating torso injuries. *New Engl J Med.* 1994;331(17):1105–1109.

Kollef M, Isakow W. *The Washington Manual of Critical Care.* 2nd ed. Philadelphia: Lippincott Williams & Wilkins; 2011.

Marino PL. *The ICU Book.* 3rd ed. Philadelphia: Lippincott Williams & Wilkins; 2007.

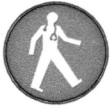

A 77-year-old Male Status Post Coronary Artery Bypass Graft

Nicholas M. Mohr, MD

CASE DESCRIPTION

Adolph Fick is a 77-year-old man with a history of coronary artery disease who presents to the hospital with progressive exertional chest pain for 2 weeks. He is unable to walk up a flight of stairs without having severe pain, and he has to stop to rest. His EKG showed nonspecific T-wave inversions during pain, and he was admitted to the cardiology service for workup 3 days ago.

During his hospital stay, he underwent cardiac catheterization and was found to have critical stenosis of his left main coronary artery, so he was referred to cardiac surgery for operative revascularization. This patient was scheduled for 2-vessel coronary artery bypass grafting (CABG) on cardiopulmonary bypass, which was performed this morning. You are the resident admitting this patient to the surgical intensive care unit from the operating room.

On arrival, your patient is intubated and sedated (assist-control volume-control, respiratory rate 12, PEEP 5, tidal volume 500 mL, FiO_2 50%). He has a pulmonary artery catheter in place with pulmonary pressure of 41/18 mm Hg, a central venous pressure of 10 mm Hg, a cardiac index of 2.5 L/min/m², and a mixed venous oxygen saturation (SvO_2) of 69%. He also has atrioventricular epicardial pacing leads, and his pacemaker is set with a rate of 92 beats/min (his pulse is 92 beats/min with good pacemaker capture). He is on dobutamine 5 mcg/kg/min and norepinephrine 6 mcg/min (0.07 mcg/kg/min), and his blood pressure is 110/48 (mean arterial pressure 68 mm Hg).

1. What is your intended postoperative course of action for a postcardiac surgery patient in the intensive care unit?

2. What are common complications to consider for cardiac surgery patients in the postoperative period?

After 3 hours, the patient's bedside nurse calls you to say that his blood pressure and urine output are falling. His norepinephrine requirement (goal mean arterial pressure 65 mm Hg) has increased to 12 mcg/min (0.14 mcg/kg/min) and the output from his mediastinal chest tube has fallen to almost none. In the last hour, his urine output has fallen to less than 10 mL/h. You ask for a new set of hemodynamic parameters and his nurse tells you that his blood pressure is 98/30 (mean arterial blood pressure 52 mm/Hg), heart rate is 125 beats/min, pulmonary pressure is 44/28 mm Hg, central venous pressure is 26 mm Hg, cardiac index is 1.4 L/min/m², and SvO_2 is 48%.

3. What diagnosis are you concerned your patient may have and what workup and therapy would you consider immediately?

Answers

1. The first step to managing the cardiac surgery patient is to communicate with the surgical team. It can be extremely helpful to know the preoperative condition of the patient, complications during surgery, post–cardiopulmonary bypass cardiac function, and concerns about bleeding. The normal course of a cardiac surgery patient depends on your understanding of these factors, and then making a postoperative plan with your cardiac surgeon and your critical care team as to the goals of your patient's postoperative care.

   Often, a patient who does not have ongoing bleeding, who had an uncomplicated surgery, who has good cardiac function, and who was a good preoperative surgical candidate can be extubated once he awakes from his anesthesia. One would expect that bleeding from chest tubes will decrease over the first several hours and vasopressor agents can be weaned. Inotropic agents are used for support of the post-bypass heart (usually the right ventricle specifically), so these are typically weaned in a scheduled iterative fashion with careful attention to hemodynamics to evaluate tolerance to weaning. Cardiac surgery patients are placed on beta blocking medications, but only after inotropes have been fully weaned. Nearly all cardiac surgery patients will have epicardial pacing leads, but the requirement for cardiac pacing is greatest initially, and most patients are able to be weaned from their pacemaker and have the pacemaker wires removed after the first few days. If no complications occur, many patients will be in the intensive care unit for 1 to 2 days before being transferred to a cardiac surgery floor.

2. Atrial fibrillation, ventricular tachycardia, postoperative hypothermia, epicardial pacemaker malfunction (failure to capture), volume overload, electrolyte abnormalities (potassium, magnesium, calcium), cardiac tamponade, stroke, heparin rebound (development of "rebound" coagulopathy from heparin given during the operative case), bleeding from chest tubes, right heart dysfunction or failure, acute kidney injury, failed extubation, and nosocomial infections.

3. Cardiac tamponade—this patient requires immediate operative reexploration and clot evacuation, so you should immediately call your attending intensivist and the cardiac surgeon on-call. Temporizing measures include volume loading to optimize preload, avoidance of positive pressure ventilation if your patient is not currently intubated, avoidance of excessive sedation, and inotropic agents (in some circumstances). Patients who decompensate will require bedside sternotomy in the intensive care unit. Equivocal cases may be evaluated with echocardiography (often transesophageal if available) by an experienced echocardiographer, because postoperative tamponade may not have a typical echocardiographic appearance like chronic pericardial effusion might. Furthermore, tamponade after cardiac surgery can be localized, so some of the typical hemodynamic and imaging characteristics may be missing, although this patient does exhibit the classic "equalization of pressures" where all the diastolic pressures equilibrate with tamponade physiology.

CARDIAC SURGERY COMPLICATIONS

Diagnostic Workup and Management

Cardiac surgery patients are very complex, and they are likely a population of patients that you have not been exposed to prior to your critical care rotation. Because of that, these patients often provoke a great deal of anxiety and uncertainty among trainees. You are not alone.

Part of the complexity stems from the impressive physiologic response to cardiopulmonary bypass. When patients are placed on bypass and the heart is arrested, a variety of pathologic changes occur to the peripheral vasculature and to the myocardium. The hours following return of circulation are often characterized by instability, and although these procedures are frequently done very successfully, complications can occur. Furthermore, many of these patients are being treated with devices that are not commonly used outside of cardiothoracic surgery (ie, epicardial pacemakers, ventricular assist devices, intra-aortic counterpulsation balloon pumps, etc), causing titration of these therapies to be unfamiliar.

The most important component of caring for postcardiac surgery patients is to establish strong communication with your staff intensivist and your cardiac surgeon. Changes in clinical course can have medical causes or surgical causes, but in the first 12 hours after surgery, many of the early complications will be related to surgery.

As discussed in the question above, the most serious postoperative complication is cardiac tamponade. Tamponade can lack some of the typical findings you might expect in noncardiac surgery patients because the bleeding and clot can be localized, compressing only a portion of the right atrium or the right ventricle. Hallmarks include hypotension (or increasing vasopressor requirements), decreased cardiac output, or cardiopulmonary collapse. Workup may include echocardiography, but patients with a convincing clinical picture will go to the operating room for surgical exploration. Cardiac surgery patients who have abrupt clinical decompensation may require emergent sternotomy at the bedside to temporize for operative repair.

In addition to forming collections of blood and clot around the heart, the existence of bleeding will be another very important consideration. A postoperative chest x-ray should be reviewed to assure that pleural chest tubes and mediastinal chest tubes (tubes placed in the pleura and mediastinum, respectively, for draining postoperative bleeding) are positioned correctly, that the lungs are inflated, that blood is not collecting, and that the pulmonary artery catheter is positioned correctly. The output from each of these tubes will be recorded carefully and should be reviewed—the chest tube output should be falling. The threshold for operative reexploration may differ between surgeons and procedures, but generally, chest tubes should drain less than 500 mL/h in the first hour and decrease proportionally such than no more than 300 mL/h for 3 hours or 200 mL/h for the first 6 hours is exceeded. Increased bleeding should be discussed with your cardiac surgeon, as significant bleeding in the absence of significant coagulopathy likely suggests surgical bleeding.

Patients after cardiac surgery have many reasons to continue bleeding. Cardiopulmonary bypass requires large doses of heparin, and although protamine is used intraoperatively to reverse coagulopathy, a "heparin rebound" effect may occur in which the heparin effect may last longer than the protamine and the PTT may rise again. In this case, additional protamine is often given. Significant platelet dysfunction and thrombocytopenia can occur from the surgery itself, and platelet transfusions may be required to keep the platelet count above $50 \times 10^3/\mu L$. In patients with brisk bleeding, fibrinogen may also be depleted and contribute to coagulopathy, so cryoprecipitate may be required to restore normal coagulation function. These patients will also require frequent reassessment and blood transfusion as appropriate.

Postoperative myocardial dysfunction is very common. Most patients will require inotropic support after coming off cardiopulmonary bypass. Although many patients requiring cardiac surgery have some preoperative cardiac dysfunction, the time during which the heart is arrested causes stunning to the myocardium. Because of the inability to completely protect the heart, right ventricular dysfunction is common, so inotropic support to the recovering right ventricle is often required. Some patients may even require right ventricular afterload reduction (with inhaled pulmonary vascular vasodilators such as nebulized epoprostenol or nitric oxide) to promote adequate cardiac output. The cardiac output of the left ventricle can never exceed that of the right ventricle (because the RV and the LV are in series), so supporting right ventricular function helps to preserve end-organ function. Often, these inotropes are weaned slowly to assure that the recovering heart can continue to provide adequate cardiac output without ongoing support.

In addition to the myocardial effects of cardiac surgery, cardiopulmonary bypass also causes an inflammatory state that can resemble the systemic inflammatory response syndrome (SIRS). Capillary leak can occur and organ dysfunction is not rare. These features typically resolve over the course of hours to days and patients are able to be weaned from supportive therapies.

Cardiac dysrhythmia is very common after cardiac surgery. Atrial fibrillation is a common dysrhythmia, and stable patients can be treated with amiodarone, magnesium, beta blockade, calcium channel blockade, or electrical cardioversion. Unstable patients will require sedation and electrical cardioversion. Maintaining potassium levels and magnesium levels will help to keep the myocardium polarized and may prevent dysrhythmia from occurring. The postoperative myocardium has sustained significant operative injury, so cardiac serum markers are rarely indicated in managing these patients.

Many patients after cardiac surgery will have pulmonary artery catheters in place. The pulmonary artery catheter, in conjunction with an arterial catheter, is a useful monitoring device that can provide information about cardiac filling

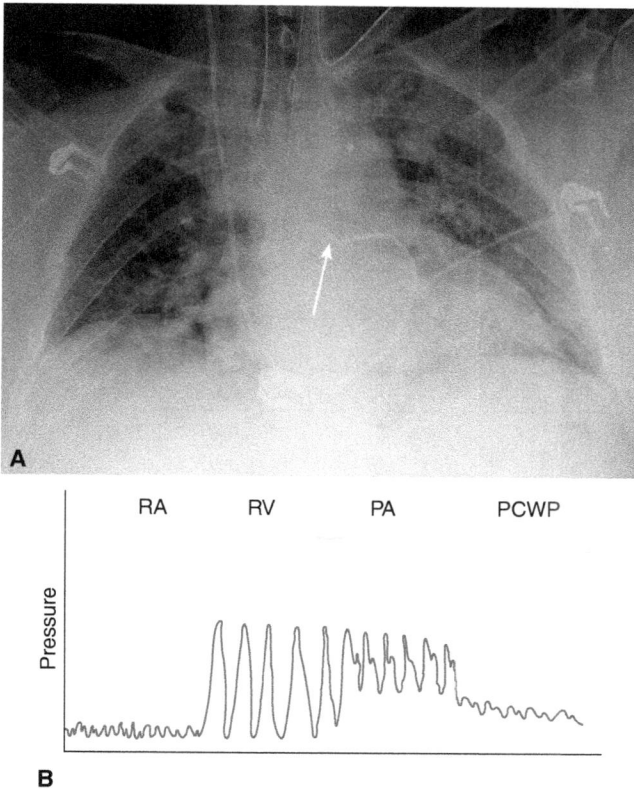

Figure 36-1. Pulmonary artery waveform and normal pressures. Pulmonary artery catheters are becoming less common in clinical practice. (A) Normal positioning of a pulmonary artery catheter in the main pulmonary artery. (B) Normal pulmonary artery catheter waveform morphology. (Modified, with permission, from Crossno, Jr. JT. Procedures in pulmonary medicine. In: Hanley ME, Welsh CH, eds. *Current Diagnosis & Treatment in Pulmonary Medicine.* New York: McGraw-Hill; 2003 [chapter 5].)

pressures and cardiac function. The catheter (Figure 36-1) directly measures pressures by waveform analysis (at the level of the right atrium and pulmonary artery) that can give a measure of both right ventricular preload and right ventricular afterload. Inflating the balloon with a small amount of air will change the pulmonary arterial waveform to a pulmonary capillary wedge pressure ("wedge"), which theoretically stabilizes a column of static blood through the pulmonary vasculature with the left atrium. This pressure will give an approximation of the left ventricular preload, and the arterial blood pressure (from the arterial line) will give an approximation of left ventricular afterload. In patients with normal pulmonary

Table 36-1. Normal Values for Many of the Hemodynamic Parameters Used in Clinical Practice and their Clinical Significance

Parameter	Normal Value	Clinical Significance
Central venous pressure (CVP)	0–6 mm Hg	Right ventricular end-diastolic pressure
Right ventricular systolic pressure	20–30 mm Hg	Right ventricular afterload
Pulmonary artery occlusion pressure (PAOP/PCWP)	6–12 mm Hg	Approximates left ventricular end-diastolic pressure
Cardiac output (CO)	4–6 L/min	Systemic blood flow
Cardiac index (CI)	2.5–3.5 L/min/m²	Cardiac output standardized to patient size
Stroke volume (SV)	40–80 mL/beat	Blood volume per cardiac cycle
Systemic vascular resistance (SVR)	800–1400 dynes × sec/cm⁵	Systemic resistance (LV afterload)
Pulmonary vascular resistance (PVR)	100–150 dynes × sec/cm⁵	Pulmonary resistance (RV afterload)
SvO_2 (mixed venous O_2 sat)	60–75%	Measures systemic oxygen extraction
Mean arterial blood pressure	75–100 mm Hg	Normal systemic blood pressure

Data from Alarcon LH. Physiologic monitoring of the surgical patient. In: Billiar TR, Dunn DL, eds. *Schwartz's Principles of Surgery*. 9th ed. New York: McGraw-Hill; 2010 [chapter 13].

vascular resistance, the pulmonary arterial diastolic pressure will often approximate the wedge pressure.

Additional information obtained from the pulmonary artery catheter includes the cardiac output (using a thermodilution curve—a computer measures the temperature on a thermistor on the tip of the catheter after injecting cold saline on a proximal port and approximates the cardiac output) and the SvO_2 (Table 36-1). The SvO_2 can be measured directly on some catheters or can be obtained from sending a pulmonary arterial blood sample to the laboratory for measurement of the oxygen saturation. Assuming that arterial blood is fully saturated with oxygen ($SaO_2 = 100\%$) and assuming that the total body oxygen consumption is constant, changes in SvO_2 correlate closely with cardiac output and/or hemoglobin concentration. This can be a very useful number, and is often one of the first indices to fall during significant bleeding or dropping cardiac output according to the following relationship:

$$\text{Oxygen delivery} = \text{Cardiac output} \times \text{oxygen extraction}$$

$$\text{Oxygen extraction} = \text{Arterial oxygen content} - \text{mixed venous oxygen content}$$

$$\begin{aligned} \text{Oxygen content (arterial/venous)} = &(\text{Hemoglobin} \times 1.36 \\ &\times \text{oxygen saturation [arterial/venous]}) \\ &+ (p_{O_2} \text{ [arterial/venous]} \times 0.0031) \end{aligned}$$

Because the p_{O_2} is a small component of the oxygen content, oxygen delivery can be reduced to the following equations. A decrease in SvO_2 can be explained by decrease in arterial oxygen saturation, decrease in cardiac output, or decrease in hemoglobin.

$$\frac{\text{Oxygen delivery (constant)}}{\text{Cardiac output}} = \text{Hemoglobin} \times 1.36 \times (\text{arterial oxygen saturation [100\%]} - SvO_2)$$

$$\frac{\text{Oxygen delivery (constant)}}{\text{Cardiac output} \times \text{hemoglobin} \times 1.36} = \text{Arterial oxygen saturation [100\%]} - SvO_2$$

Patients who have undergone cardiopulmonary bypass usually will have epicardial pacemaker leads placed. Those leads are placed on the heart and are brought out through the skin and connected to an external temporary pacemaker. Many patients will have abnormalities of their conduction system postoperatively and require pacing to maintain normal cardiac depolarization. For most patients, the pacemaker can be placed in a backup mode later during the postoperative recovery period and the wires can be removed, but acutely, the pacemaker can be used to set a rate that optimizes cardiac output.

$$\text{Cardiac output} = \text{Stroke volume} \times \text{heart rate}$$

As patients recover from cardiac surgery, a number of other physiologic complications can occur, including acute kidney injury and stroke. Patients should be monitored carefully for these complications.

TIPS TO REMEMBER

- Maintain frequent open communication among the members of the care team.
- Think about cardiac tamponade on every patient with evolving hypotension, oliguria, and low cardiac output.
- Monitor closely bleeding, coagulopathy, and anemia, and treat dysrhythmia.
- Postoperative cardiac surgery patients have unique monitoring and treatment, and they afford the learner a perfect opportunity to better understand cardiovascular physiology.

COMPREHENSION QUESTIONS

1. A 53-year-old man is transferred to the ICU after having a bioprosthetic aortic valve replacement. He does well and is extubated postoperatively, but 8 hours postoperatively he becomes hypotensive with low urine output. You give him 500 mL of lactated Ringer's and 20 minutes later he suffers cardiac arrest with pulseless electrical activity (PEA). The appropriate definitive treatment is which of the following?

        A. 1 L bolus of normal saline

        B. Calcium chloride 1 g intravenously

        C. Emergent transfer to the operating room for surgical exploration

        D. Starting epinephrine at 0.1 mcg/kg/min

        E. Emergency bedside sternotomy in the ICU performed by cardiac surgery

2. Your postoperative cardiac surgery patient has a sudden onset of atrial fibrillation with rate 165 and BP 110/71. Which of the following drug–dose combinations would be the most appropriate intervention?

        A. Digoxin 125 mg PO

        B. Amiodarone 150 mg IV bolus over 10 minutes, followed by 1 mg/min

        C. Metoprolol 50 mg PO

        D. Diltiazem 90 mg IV every 6 hours

        E. Amiodarone 300 mg IV bolus

3. Which of the following etiologies would *not* explain a decrease in the SvO_2?

        A. Tension pneumothorax

        B. Starting dobutamine at 5 mcg/kg/min

        C. 500 mL of blood lost to a bleeding gastric ulcer, followed by replacement with 500 mL of albumin (colloid volume replacement)

        D. Cardiac tamponade

        E. Worsening lung injury with a drop in the arterial oxygen saturation from 100% to 88% by pulse oximetry

Answers

1. E. Immediately after cardiac surgery, rapid progression of shock to cardiac arrest must be considered to be rapidly developing cardiac tamponade. The therapy for cardiac tamponade is rapid surgical decompression. Although several of these therapies may be attempted while definitive decompression is performed, only relieving the mechanical pressure will restore perfusion. This clinical situation is emergent—one must not wait for transfer to the operating room.

2. B. Intravenous medications will be most rapid-acting and effective for atrial fibrillation with rapid ventricular response. Amiodarone, metoprolol, or diltiazem would all be appropriate choices, but only answer B offers the correct intravenous dose.

3. B. SvO$_2$ should decrease with decreased cardiac output, decreased systemic oxygen saturation, or decreased hemoglobin concentration. Dobutamine infusion would be expected to increase cardiac output.

SUGGESTED READINGS

Kollef M, Isakow W. *The Washington Manual of Critical Care*. 2nd ed. Philadelphia: Lippincott Williams & Wilkins; 2011.
Marino PL. *The ICU Book*. 3rd ed. Philadelphia: Lippincott Williams & Wilkins; 2007.

Section V.
Emergency Ultrasound

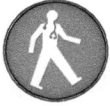

A New EM Resident Is Asked to Perform a Bedside Ultrasound

Jonathan dela Cruz, MD, RDMS

CASE DESCRIPTION

During your first shift in the ED, a 23-year-old female presents with left-sided pelvic pain. The pregnancy test is positive, and the attending asks you to perform an ultrasound (US) to determine if an intrauterine pregnancy (IUP) is present. You have not had any prior US experience.

1. Why should the EM physician use bedside US?
2. How does bedside US in the ED differ from diagnostic US (performed by radiology)?
3. How will I learn US?

Answers

1. Bedside US is an extension of the physical examination, and the ED is a time-critical venue in which the rapid acquisition of clinical information can mean the difference between life and death. An EM physician experienced in US can quickly acquire additional information about a patient that may be lifesaving in an emergency. All EM training programs have an US curriculum.

2. An EM physician performs a bedside US to answer a specific clinical question such as, "Does this hypotensive patient with abdominal pain have fluid (presumably blood) in the peritoneal space?" A diagnostic US is often ordered to answer a specific clinical question, but the test is a more comprehensive survey of the area in question. For example, a bedside US for a patient with lower abdominal pain in the first trimester of pregnancy will often look for the presence of an IUP, whereas a diagnostic US will survey the entire area and may find an adnexal mass or ovarian torsion.

3. The first step is learning the basics. Operation of the machine is sometimes referred to as "knobology." Next you will learn the basic steps of each of the EM applications for US. Finally, you will need to practice. There is no substitute for practice on real patients with real-time feedback from EM physicians experienced in US.

INTRODUCTION TO EMERGENCY ULTRASOUND

Technologic advances in the field of ultrasonography have increased the portability and availability of US machines across all specialties in medicine. This has enabled health care providers to perform impromptu imaging of their patients while simultaneously correlating their clinical findings to confirm a working diagnosis and develop an appropriate treatment plan. No field of medicine has been impacted more by this technology than EM. Emergency bedside ultrasonography aids the ED provider in making a rapid and efficient disposition and also provides assistance in performing invasive emergent procedures in a safe and timely fashion. Emergency medicine has embraced ultrasonography and it is now part of the core curriculum of all US emergency medicine training programs. The growth of emergency US as a subspecialty can be seen from the increase from 6 fellowships in 2002 to the >80 fellowships listed in 2012. Familiarity with emergency bedside ultrasonography is a requirement, as this technology becomes more and more a part of the ED physicians' everyday practice. This chapter provides an overview of the scope of practice of emergency bedside ultrasonography, the core emergency bedside US applications taught in EM residency training, and US basics.

SCOPE OF PRACTICE

The emergency US examination performed by emergency physicians is distinctly different from the evaluations of other specialties (see Table 37-1). It is usually performed at the bedside simultaneously with the clinical examination, resuscitation, or procedure. It has been typically described as an extension of the palpating hand and a "visual" stethoscope during the physical examination. ED US provides both anatomical and functional information complementary to the routine physical examination. The bedside examination, which is performed by the emergency physician, usually attempts to answer a single, focused clinical question within minutes. This is analogous to the use of ECG, point-of-care laboratory assays, nasolaryngoscopy, and the slit lamp examination in the hands of emergency physicians; these processes similarly extend bedside diagnostic capabilities. A comparison of the differences between traditional ultrasonography and emergency bedside ultrasonography can be seen in Table 37-1.

Table 37-1. Comparison of Traditional Ultrasonography and Emergency Bedside Ultrasonography

Traditional Ultrasonography	Emergency Bedside Ultrasonography
• Scheduled examination for formal evaluation	• Bedside examination for emergent evaluation
• Utilized for complete evaluation of an anatomical region	• Utilized for focused examination of a single organ or organ system
• Lengthy examination needed for full diagnostic assessment	• Rapid examination to answer a single clinical question

Table 37-2. Emergency Bedside Ultrasound Applications (ACEP 2008 Policy Statement)

Core EMBUS Applications	Emerging EMBUS Applications
Trauma	Advanced echo
Intrauterine pregnancy	Transesophageal echo
AAA	Bowel (including intussusceptions, appendicitis, pyloric stenosis, diverticulitis, SBO)
Cardiac	Adnexal pathology
Biliary	Testicular
Urinary tract	Transcranial Doppler
DVT	Contrast studies
Soft tissue/musculoskeletal	
Thoracic	
Ocular	
Procedural guidance	

The American College of Emergency Physicians (ACEP) updated their policy statement on emergency bedside ultrasonography in 2008. In the document, ACEP gives guidelines on 11 core emergency bedside US applications ED physicians should be familiar with and commented on 7 other emerging applications at the time the policy was written (see Table 37-2).

ULTRASOUND BASICS

It is important for every sonographer to have a strong understanding of US physics and human anatomy. They are the basis of translating how an US machine can create an anatomical image and how that image can be interpreted to depict a clinical picture. For the novice emergency ultrasonographer, there are a few US basics one should be familiar with when first learning how to perform and obtain sonographic images.

The Ultrasound Machine

Each US machine can be separated into 2 major systems: the computing/display system and the US probe. There are a variety of different computing/display systems each made by their respective manufacturers. Each computing/display system has different attributes based on its manufacturer's desired audience. For example, certain computing/display systems may emphasize computing resources toward smoother movement and temporal resolution, therefore catering to a cardiology audience interested in seeing cardiac movement. Another manufacturer may choose to emphasize computing resources toward higher resolution images at the expense of smoother movement to better visualize still images, therefore catering to a musculoskeletal specialist. Nonetheless, the job of the computing/display system is to take information from the US probe and translate it to information that can be used by the end user or sonographer. How this information is displayed depends on the interpretation mode that will be discussed later.

In the same fashion, there are different types of US probes that are used to obtain better information for specific anatomical examinations. For the novice emergency ultrasonographer, there are 4 probes that are commonly used in the ED. Table 37-3 lists these common probes including their specific characteristics and common uses.

Ultrasound Modes

As mentioned earlier, the information gathered from an US probe can be translated by the computing/display system to information useful for the sonographer to interpret. There are 3 major US modes that are commonly used in the ED: brightness mode (B-mode), motion mode (M-mode), and Doppler mode (D-mode).

B-mode is the most commonly used and the one most people associate with when thinking about US. It translates information from the US probe into a grayscale image. This is the mode employed to visualize specific anatomical regions. Images are presented in a fashion such that objects of high echogenicity, meaning highly reflective of sound waves, are displayed brighter or along the white spectrum of the gray scale. Objects of lower echogenicity, meaning more likely for sound waves to pass through, are displayed darker or along the black spectrum of the gray scale. Echogenicity is directly proportional to density; therefore, bone has high echogenicity and shows up white. Blood being much less dense shows up black. This mode is the usual default mode of most machines. Figure 37-1 is an example of a B-mode image of a heart.

M-mode is a graphical presentation of a single "beam of sound" over time. It is commonly employed to calculate changes in a structure sequentially. In the emergency department this mode is commonly used to calculate fetal heart rate. Basically the sonographer chooses a single "beam of sound" and that "beam of sound" is graphed. On the x-axis of the graph is time and the y-axis of the graph is a graphical representation of the single "beam of sound" according to depth. Figure 37-2 is an example of an M-mode image calculating the fetal heart rate of a fetus.

D-mode displays velocities of objects as they move toward and away from the US probe. The object being measured most commonly in the ED is blood. This

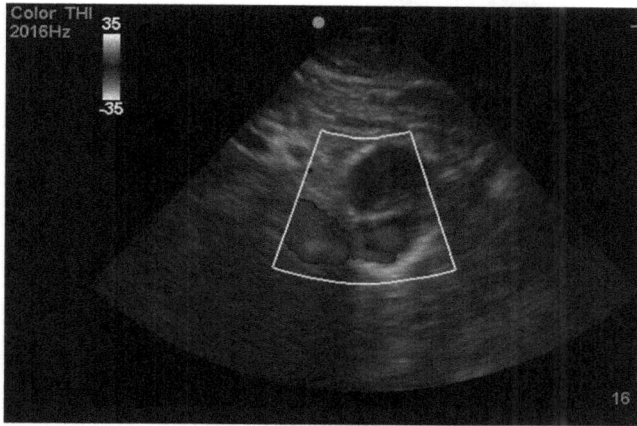

Figure 37-3. D-mode (color Doppler of abdominal vessel).

stepwise fashion to help the novice emergency sonographer understand probe placement and orientation while giving them skills in image acquisition and interpretation.

SUGGESTED READINGS

ACEP. Emergency ultrasound guidelines. Dallas, TX: American College of Emergency Physicians; 2008. <http://www.acep.org/workarea/downloadasset.aspx?id=32878>.

Blaivas M, Theodoro DL, Sierzenski P. Proliferation of ultrasound fellowships in emergency medicine: how do we ensure future experts are expertly trained? *Acad Emerg Med.* 2002;9(8):863–864.

Stone CK, Humphries RL. *Current Diagnosis and Treatment: Emergency Medicine.* 7th ed. New York: McGraw-Hill Education; 2011.

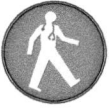

A 30-year-old Patient Status Post Motor Vehicle Crash

Jonathan dela Cruz, MD, RDMS

CASE DESCRIPTION

A 30-year-old male presents to the emergency department status post rollover motor vehicle crash. He was a restrained driver, and was hit at 70 mph on the driver's side. He presents tachycardic, hypotensive, and with abdominal pain. He is tender to palpation diffusely.

1. What are your next steps in managing this patient?
2. What clinical decision pertaining to patient disposition needs to be answered on this patient immediately?
3. What emergency ultrasound examination can be performed to expedite the care of this patient?
4. What will you be looking for on your emergency ultrasound examination?

Answers

1. Airway, breathing, and circulation assessment along with obtaining 2 large-bore IVs, supplemental oxygen, and continuous cardiac monitoring.
2. Does this patient need immediate surgical intervention?
3. *F*ocused *a*ssessment with *s*onography in *t*rauma.
4. Intraperitoneal fluid.

CASE REVIEW

Evaluation of a trauma patient is always done in an algorithmic fashion. The reason for this is to systematically address the most emergent conditions of the patient while at the same time fully evaluating the patient for all injuries. This approach is outlined in detail in Section III. However, all trauma evaluations start with an assessment of the patient's ABCs as well as obtaining the safety net for therapeutic intervention and monitoring (the EM mantra of IV, O$_2$, monitor). In this particular scenario intervention of the patient's circulatory status is needed. While the patient is actively being resuscitated, identifying a cause of the patient's tachycardia and hypotension is of paramount importance. A lengthy differential presents itself in a trauma situation; however, the abdominal pain and tenderness begs the question, "Does this patient have an intra-abdominal injury that requires immediate surgical intervention?"

FOCUSED ASSESSMENT WITH SONOGRAPHY IN TRAUMA

Prior to the advent of emergency ultrasonography, identification of intra-abdominal injury was commonly performed through diagnostic peritoneal lavage (DPL). This procedure required sampling the intraperitoneal space with a catheter and looking for evidence of blood. The procedure is quite lengthy and its sensitivity was not always the best. With the advent of computer tomography (CT) these patients instead underwent radiographic imaging with contrast enhancement to identify any injuries. Although less invasive than DPL, logistically moving the patient to the CT scanner to get it performed used up precious time of the "golden hour" of treatment. Emergency ultrasonography by use of the FAST examination can be performed at the bedside, therefore decreasing wait times for definitive treatment. Times as short as 2.1 minutes have been reported for a FAST examination evaluation. Assessment with the FAST examination can visualize as little as 100 mL of intraperitoneal fluid indicating possible intraperitoneal hemorrhage. It also has a reported sensitivity in the high 90s. Bedside ultrasonography is very user dependent; however, the most experienced ultrasonographers can identify intra-abdominal injury with fairly high confidence.

BASIC IMAGE ACQUISITION

Axis Orientation

Performing the FAST examination entails obtaining 4 different windows in B-mode using either a curved linear abdominal probe or phased array probe to assess for free fluid (and therefore possible hemorrhage). The examination should begin by assessing for pericardial effusion in the subcostal view of the heart. When obtaining ultrasound images in general, one can think of the ultrasound as a means of obtaining cross-sectional views of the body. One can imagine a fan coming out of the ultrasound probe with 1 end of the fan lining up with the probe indicator (Figure 38-1). The fan represents the "slice of the body" you are obtaining. When acquiring an image in which the fan cuts the body in a top half and bottom half, it is called a short-axis view of the body. When the fan cuts the body perpendicular to this plan (ie, a front half and back half, or left half and right half), it is called a long-axis view of the body. Any cut of the body that is at a diagonal or a combination of a short- and long-axis view is considered an oblique view. What can be confusing at times is when the axis of view is referring to a specific organ rather than the body. For example, the axis of the heart is diagonal to the axis of the body. Therefore, a long-axis view of the heart represents an image that is more of an oblique-axis view of the body (Figure 38-2).

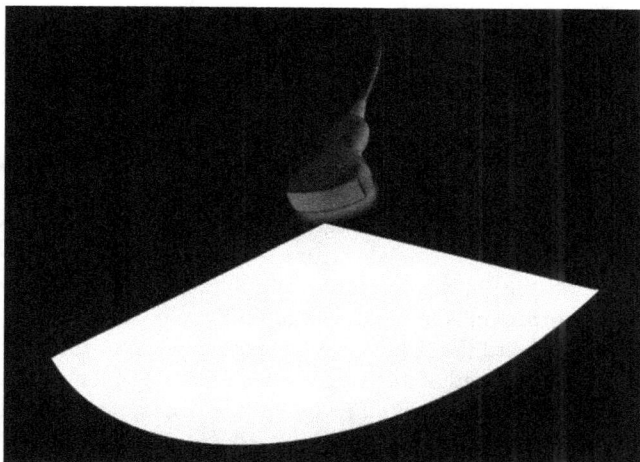

Figure 38-1. Ultrasound probe "fan-slice" orientation.

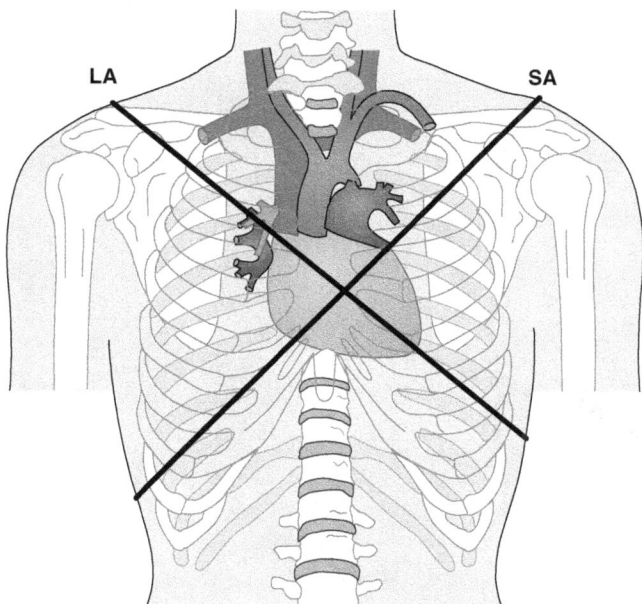

Figure 38-2. Cardiac axes. (Reproduced from Ma OJ, Mateer JR, Blaivas M. *Emergency Ultrasound.* 2nd ed. <www.accessemergencymedicine.com>. Copyright © The McGraw-Hill Companies Inc. All rights reserved.)

Probe Indicator and Image Orientation

The subcostal view of the heart requires placing the probe in the epigastric region pointing toward the patient's left shoulder and with its indicator (represented by a bump, dot, groove, or line located on the side of the probe) pointed toward the right side of the patient's body (Figure 38-3). The subcostal view of the heart done in this fashion obtains a long-axis view of the heart showing its 4 chambers. When looking at the ultrasound display screen in general, the image you see shows the "fan slice" of the body you have obtained (Figure 38-4). When looking at the screen, it is important to note the dot that is traditionally placed on the top left corner of the screen. This dot corresponds to the indicator on the ultrasound probe that traditionally is pointed toward the right side of the patient when obtaining a short-axis view of the body, or the head of the patient when obtaining a long-axis view of the body. This orientates the ultrasound image on the display screen to show either

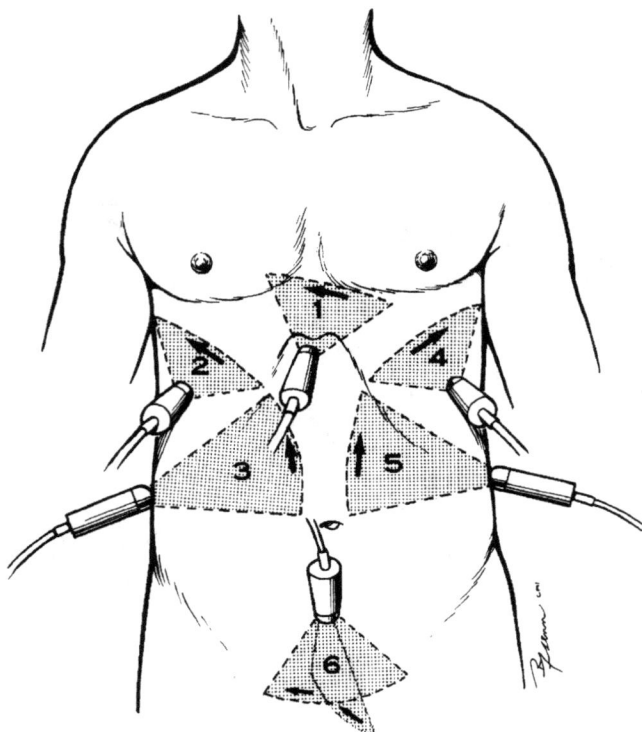

Figure 38-3. Probe placement for FAST examination. (Reprinted with permission from Ma OJ, Mateer JR, Ogata M, et al. Prospective analysis of a rapid trauma ultrasound examination performed by emergency physicians. *J Trauma.* 1995;38:879–885.)

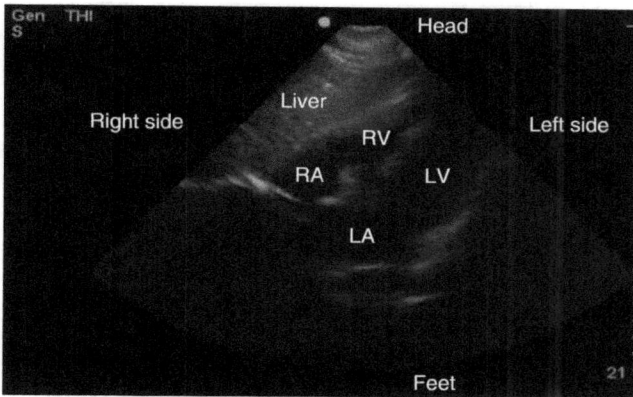

Figure 38-4. Subxyphoid 4-chamber view.

the right side of the patient or the head of the patient on the left side of the screen respective to axis. For your purposes always orientate your probe and display screen in the traditional manner in which the indicator dot on the display screen is on the top left corner of the screen. The subcostal view of the heart done during a FAST examination is not a formal echocardiography study; therefore, traditional ultrasound orientation is used and the dot is on the left side of the display screen.

The second view obtained is of the right upper quadrant (RUQ), assessing for fluid in Morison's pouch. This view is the most sensitive for identifying intraperitoneal fluid. This view is obtained by placing the probe along the midaxillary line on the right side of the patient's body right underneath the rib cage. The probe indicator should be pointing toward the patient's head (long-axis view of the body). Three structures need to be identified in this view: the diaphragm, the liver, and the right kidney (Figure 38-5).

The third view or left upper quadrant (LUQ) view, assessing for fluid in the splenorenal space, is obtained in a similar fashion. The probe is usually placed slightly more posteriorly along the posterior axillary line, underneath the rib cage, and with the probe indicator pointed toward the head of the patient. The probe needs to be more posterior because the left kidney usually sits more posterior in the body. Again, 3 structures need to be identified for a quality view: the diaphragm, the spleen, and the kidney. Depending on patient position and anatomy sometimes the stomach can obscure the image (Figure 38-6). Air is the enemy of ultrasound. It can scatter sound waves, therefore returning false information back to the ultrasound probe. Because of air in the stomach, artifact can be seen in the LUQ view at times. To combat this, moving the patient onto his or her right side can sometimes move the stomach out of view from the ultrasound probe, therefore improving image quality.

The final view obtained is that of the pelvis/bladder. The bladder is first identified in the long axis (with the probe indicator pointing toward the patient's

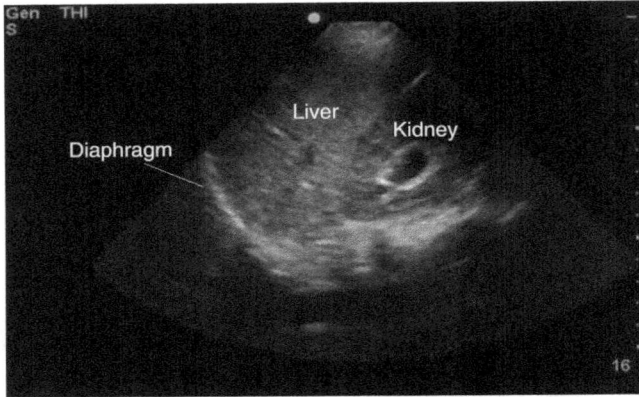

Figure 38-5. RUQ view FAST examination.

head) with the probe placed in the suprapubic region. The bladder is identified as a large anechoic structure in the pelvis. A short axis can then quickly be obtained by rotating the probe counterclockwise with the probe indicator to the right side of the patient's body. Fanning the probe up and down allows for full evaluation of the pelvic space looking for fluid above or behind the bladder (Figure 38-7).

BASIC IMAGE INTERPRETATION

Assessing for free fluid is performed by identifying any areas of anechoic space in between tissue planes. As discussed, blood transmits sound waves very freely to the point it is essentially anechoic and shows up black in B-mode. Any anechoic areas on an ultrasound can be useful to identify blood vessels or fluid-filled

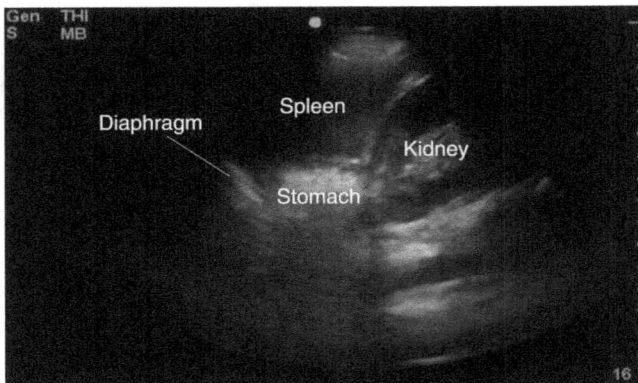

Figure 38-6. LUQ view FAST examination.

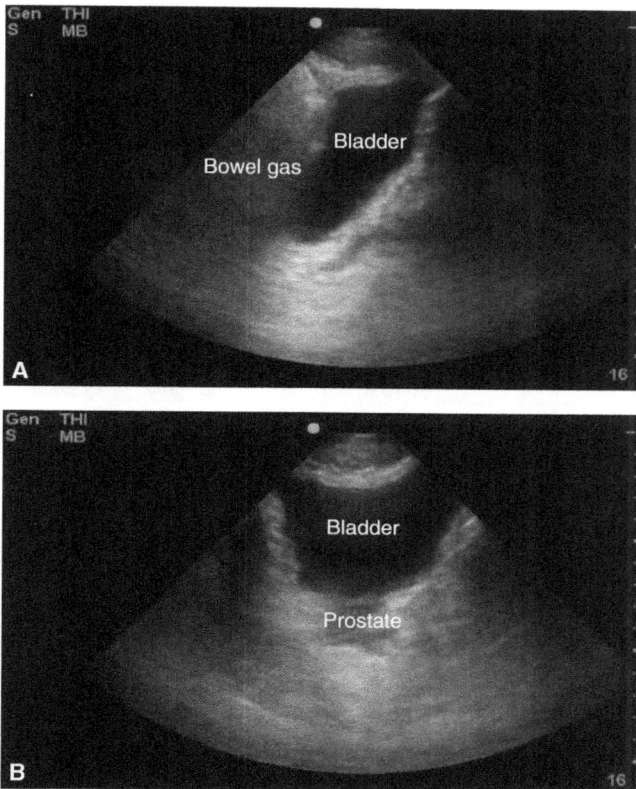

Figure 38-7. (A) Pelvic/bladder (male) long-axis view FAST examination. (B) Pelvic/bladder (male) short-axis view FAST examination.

structures such as the bladder or gallbladder. Pathology is always suspected when sharp anechoic areas are seen in between tissue planes. This may be a result of hemorrhage or, in the right clinical scenario, ascites. (See Figure 38-8 for examples of positive FAST examination windows.)

TIPS TO REMEMBER

- Initial assessment of any trauma patient should involve assessment of the ABCs as well as obtaining IV access, oxygen supplementation, and cardiac monitoring.

- Abdominal pain in the hemodynamically unstable patient is highly suspicious for intra-abdominal hemorrhage that needs immediate surgical intervention.

- The FAST examination can help expedite decisions for immediate need for surgical intervention in the trauma patient.

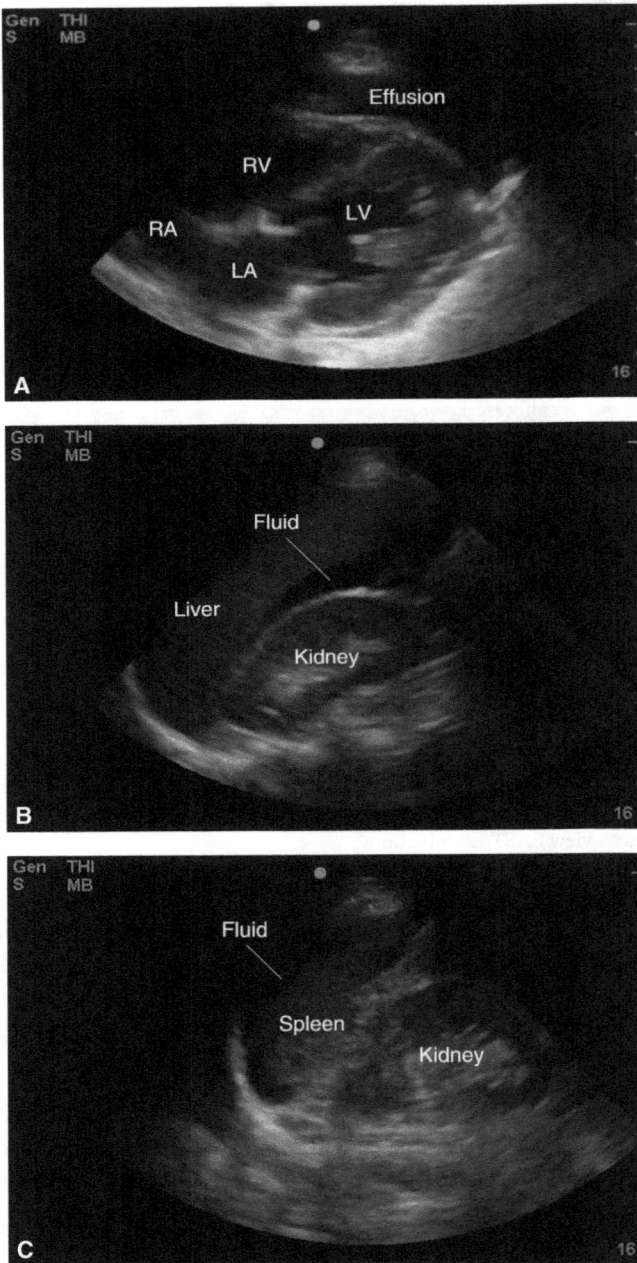

Figure 38-8. (A) Positive FAST pericardial effusion. (B) Positive FAST fluid in Morison's pouch. (C) Positive FAST subcapsular hematoma of the spleen.

COMPREHENSION QUESTIONS

1. All of the following are windows of the FAST examination *except*?
    A. Cardiac
    B. RUQ
    C. Retroperitoneal
    D. LUQ
    E. Pelvic/bladder

2. With the display indicator dot placed on the top left corner of the screen, where should your probe indicator be placed to obtain a long-axis view of the RUQ?
    A. Left side of the patient
    B. Right side of the patient
    C. The patient's left elbow
    D. The head of the patient

3. What is your diagnosis on the following FAST image?

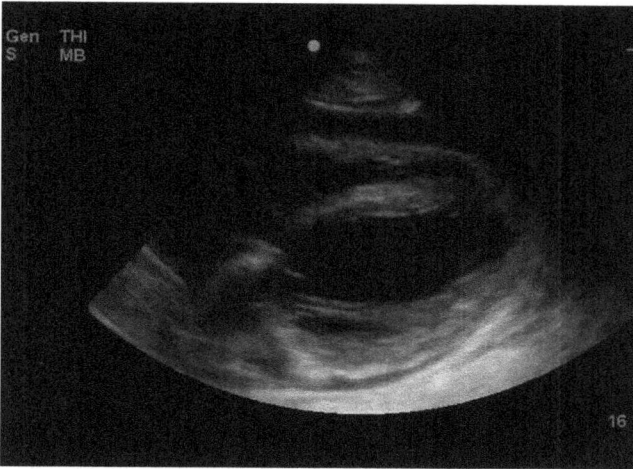

A FAST image

    A. Fluid in Morison's pouch
    B. Pericardial effusion
    C. Fluid behind the bladder
    D. A normal window of the FAST examination

Answers

1. C. Retroperitoneal is not a view obtained during the FAST examination.

2. D. Pointing the indicator to the head of the patient is the proper orientation.

3. B. This image is a subcostal cardiac view. A sharply demarcated anechoic space can be seen suggesting a pericardial effusion.

SUGGESTED READINGS

Ma OJ, Mateer JR, Blaivas M. *Emergency Ultrasound*. 2nd ed. China: McGraw-Hill; 2008. <www.accessemergencymedicine.com>.

Ma OJ, Mateer JR, Ogata M, et al. Prospective analysis of a rapid trauma ultrasound examination performed by emergency physicians. *J Trauma*. 1995;38:879–885.

Thomas B, Falcone RE, Vasquez D, et al. Ultrasound evaluation of blunt abdominal trauma: program implementation, initial experience, and learning curve. *J Trauma*. 1997;42:384–388.

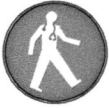

A 27-year-old Female With First Trimester Vaginal Bleeding

Jonathan dela Cruz, MD, RDMS

CASE DESCRIPTION

A 27-year-old female G1P0 presents complaining of vaginal bleeding. The patient states she is 9 weeks pregnant. She states she has some abdominal cramping. She denies any trauma. On examination she is in no acute distress with no abdominal tenderness. Your pelvic examination is remarkable for a trace amount of blood in the vaginal vault. Her cervical os is closed. She is hemodynamically stable with normal vitals.

1. What is your differential diagnosis?

2. What labs do you want to order?

3. What emergency ultrasound examination can be performed to expedite the care of this patient?

4. What will you be looking for on your emergency ultrasound examination?

Answers

1. Threatened abortion, ectopic pregnancy, and normal pregnancy.

2. CBC, blood type and Rh, and quantitative beta-hCG.

3. A transabdominal or transvaginal emergency ultrasound.

4. Assessment for a live interuterine pregnancy.

CASE REVIEW

Most first trimester women with vaginal bleeding who present to the emergency department hemodynamically stable can be placed into 3 categories: abnormal pregnancy (ie, miscarriage/threatened abortion, molar pregnancy), ectopic pregnancy, and normal pregnancy. Technically a patient with first trimester vaginal bleeding cannot be diagnosed with a normal pregnancy until the follow-up appointment with an obstetrician because of the unexplained bleeding. Thus, evaluation in the ED for these patients is directed toward ruling out an ectopic pregnancy and gathering lab workup results for follow-up evaluation.

The lab workup commonly performed on these patients includes a CBC, blood type and Rh status, and a quantitative beta-hCG. A CBC is usually performed to assess for any blood loss. Finding out if the patient is Rh (−) is important to make sure she does not need protection with RhoGAM to prevent antibody formation against future pregnancies. A quantitative beta-hCG is useful for follow-up evaluation of the patient. If an abnormal pregnancy is suspected, a doubling beta-hCG in 48 hours would be helpful in identifying a viable pregnancy. Quantitative beta-hCG in some institutions has been used as a discriminatory test for identifying patients in which ultrasound can visualize a fetus. Cutoffs of 1600 to 2000 mIU/mL have been employed at some institutions. However, Kohn et al found that patients presenting to the ED with first trimester vaginal bleeding having a beta-hCG less than 1500 mIU/mL had a higher likelihood of ectopic pregnancy. Cutoffs such as those suggested above could make physicians to miss assessing these patients for ultrasonographic signs supporting an ectopic diagnosis.

The use of emergency ultrasonography in this scenario is to identify risk for ectopic pregnancy. Contrary to what is initially thought by most novice emergency sonographers, risk for ectopic pregnancy is not revealed by identifying a pregnancy outside the uterus, but rather ruling in a live intrauterine pregnancy (LIUP). If a LIUP is visualized, an associated ectopic or heterotopic pregnancy has a prevalence of around 1 in every 10,000. Identifying a LIUP essentially rules out an ectopic pregnancy.

FUNDAMENTALS OF EMERGENCY ULTRASOUND EVALUATION FOR LIUP

Emergency ultrasound assessment for LIUP can be performed either transvaginally with an endocavitary probe or transabdominally with a curved linear abdominal probe or phased array probe. The transvaginal approach goes beyond the scope of this book and is used when assessing pregnancies of very early gestation. The use of an endocavitary probe allows for close contact with the uterus, therefore increasing visualization. The transabdominal approach allows for rapid assessment by the emergency medicine provider. Two views are traditionally used, the long-axis and short-axis views of the pelvis.

When performing a transabdominal pelvic ultrasound, it is important to perform it when the patient has a full bladder. Having a full bladder allows the emergency sonographer to have an "echogenic" window from which to view the uterus. Because fluid allows for sound waves to pass so freely, having a distended bladder gives the ultrasound a medium by which to transmit sound waves. With a contracted bladder sound waves from the probe have a high chance of being absorbed, deflected, or scattered while passing through tissue rather than fluid.

LIUP evaluations are traditionally performed in the long axis of the body. Obtaining a long-axis view is performed similar to that of the bladder window of the FAST examination. The bladder is best identified in the long axis (with the probe indicator pointing toward the patient's head) with the probe placed

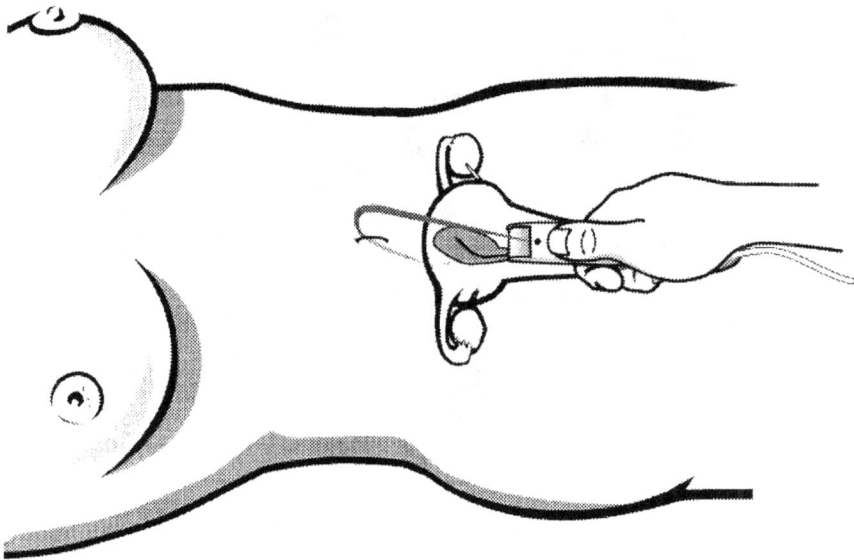

Figure 39-1. Probe placement for evaluation of LIUP. (Reproduced from Ma OJ, Mateer JR, Blaivas M. *Emergency Ultrasound.* 2nd ed. China: McGraw-Hill; 2008. <http://www .accessemergencymedicine.com>. Copyright © The McGraw-Hill Companies Inc. All rights reserved.)

suprapubically (Figure 39-1). With the bladder identified the uterus can be visualized posterior to it. The uterus is best visualized by first identifying the cervical stripe and following posterior to the uterus. The probe is then fanned from left to right to assess the lateral poles of the uterus for a pregnancy (Figure 39-2).

INTERPRETATION FOR LIUP AND ECTOPIC PREGNANCY

Assessment for LIUP by the novice emergency ultrasonography should concentrate on identifying fetal cardiac activity in the uterus. More advanced sonographers can identify IUP by identifying yolk sacs and fetal poles at very early gestations with correlating measurements; however, learning about these techniques is best left until after becoming comfortable with identifying intrauterine cardiac activity. The first step in identifying such cardiac activity is identifying a gestational sac within the uterus. A gestational sac is best described as a round anechoic structure. Within that anechoic structure should lay an isoechoic structure representing the fetal pole. Using transabdominal techniques a fetal pole can first be visualized at 7 to 10 weeks gestation. Evaluation with transvaginal ultrasound can increase visualization to as early as 5 weeks. Cardiac

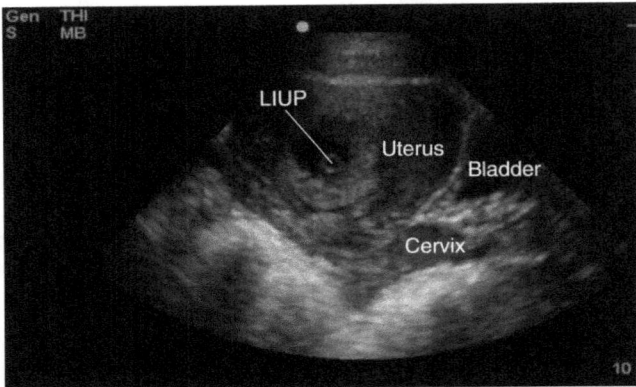

Figure 39-2. Transabdominal long-axis evaluation for LIUP.

activity, however, isn't visualized until 6 weeks. Within the fetal pole should be a "flickering" of the fetal heart. Once this is visualized, the emergency ultrasound evaluation is sufficient for identifying a LIUP. Calculations to determine fetal gestational age can be performed through use of M-mode but at this point are more academic than clinically necessary.

When fetal heart activity or a fetal pole is not identified, suspicion should increase for an ectopic pregnancy. Other signs supporting this on ultrasound include any complex masses viewed when fanning the lateral sides or adnexa of the uterus, or pelvic free fluid (identified similar to that in the FAST examination) suggesting rupture.

TIPS TO REMEMBER

- Evaluation of first trimester vaginal bleeding in the ED involves ruling out ectopic pregnancy and setting up appropriate follow-up.
- The emergency ultrasound evaluation for LIUP can help expedite care of these patients.

COMPREHENSION QUESTIONS

1. Emergency ultrasound evaluation for ectopic pregnancy involves:
   A. Identifying a pregnancy outside the uterus
   B. Evaluation for pelvic free fluid
   C. Evaluation for presence of a LIUP
   D. A and B
   E. B and C

2. At what gestational age can transabdominal emergency ultrasound first visualize the fetus?

    A. 3 weeks

    B. 5 weeks

    C. 7 weeks

    D. 12 weeks

3. A quantitative beta-hCG of greater than 1500 mIU/mL puts a first trimester bleeder at greater risk for ectopic pregnancy.

    A. True

    B. False

Answers

1. **B.** Identification of a LIUP essentially rules out ectopic pregnancy. Free fluid can support the diagnosis in light of no LIUP.

2. **C.** Transabdominal emergency ultrasound can best first visualize the fetus at 7 to 10 weeks.

3. **B.** A lower beta-hCG in light of first trimester vaginal bleeding puts you at higher risk for ectopic pregnancy.

SUGGESTED READINGS

Kohn MA, Kerr K, Malkevich D, O'Neil N, Kerr MJ, Kaplan BC. Beta-human chorionic gonadotropin levels and the likelihood of ectopic pregnancy in emergency department patients with abdominal pain or vaginal bleeding. *Acad Emerg Med.* 2003;10(2):119–126.

Ma OJ, Mateer JR, Blaivas M. *Emergency Ultrasound.* 2nd ed. China: McGraw-Hill; 2008. <www.accessemergencymedicine.com>.

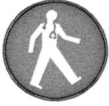

A 60-year-old Male With Flank Pain

Jonathan dela Cruz, MD, RDMS

CASE DESCRIPTION

A 60-year-old male presents to the ED with flank pain, which he states came on suddenly. In the ED he is initially hypertensive; however, his blood pressure starts to fall. He is in moderate distress with tenderness to palpation of his abdomen. He has also started to develop numbness in his lower extremities.

1. What are your next steps in managing this patient?
2. What life-threatening condition could this patient have?
3. What emergency ultrasound examination can be performed to expedite the care of this patient?
4. Who needs to be notified immediately?

Answers

1. ABCs, IV, O_2, and monitor.
2. Ruptured abdominal aortic aneurysm (AAA).
3. Emergency ultrasound for evaluation of ruptured AAA.
4. Vascular surgery for immediate surgical intervention.

CASE REVIEW

Ruptured AAA is a life-threatening condition associated with a high rate of morbidity and mortality. Although the classic presentation is an elderly patient with a history of hypertension with severe abdominal pain and hypotension, it should at least be part of the differential of patients presenting to the ED with flank pain. Other associated findings include a pulsating abdominal mass, decreased lower extremity pulses, and extremity numbness due to either ischemia of the lower extremities or ischemia of the spinal cord secondary to an associated dissection involving the tributaries to the thoracic spine (neurologic deficits above and below the diaphragm associated with abdominal or chest pain are very suspicious for aortic dissection). Serious morbidity and mortality can best be avoided by rapid recognition, diagnosis, and mobilization of the surgical team for emergent intervention.

Stabilization and resuscitation efforts in the ED are of paramount importance as these patients can rapidly decline with acute rupture. Obtaining the ED safety net and expediting mobilization of blood products (by early type and crossmatch or ordering of unmatched universal donor blood) is helpful in preparing for impending vascular compromise due to uncontrolled intraperitoneal hemorrhage.

Emergency ultrasound for evaluation of AAA can aid in early detection of this condition and reduce mortality. Prior to the advent of bedside ultrasonography, computer tomography was employed in those patients who presented hemodynamically stable. Transportation times and the possibility of vascular compromise in radiology put these patients at high risk for poor outcomes. Identifying an aortic aneurysm or evidence of intraperitoneal rupture and hemorrhage through a screening bedside ultrasound is now becoming the standard of care.

FUNDAMENTALS OF EMERGENCY ULTRASOUND EVALUATION FOR AAA

Emergency ultrasound assessment for AAA is performed with the abdominal curved linear probe or phased array probe. The aorta is traditionally assessed in the short axis of the body. A short-axis view of the aorta is performed by placing the probe in the epigastric region with the probe indicator pointed toward the right side of the patient's body and following it down to the bifurcation into the iliac arteries past the umbilicus (Figure 40-1). The first landmark to be identified

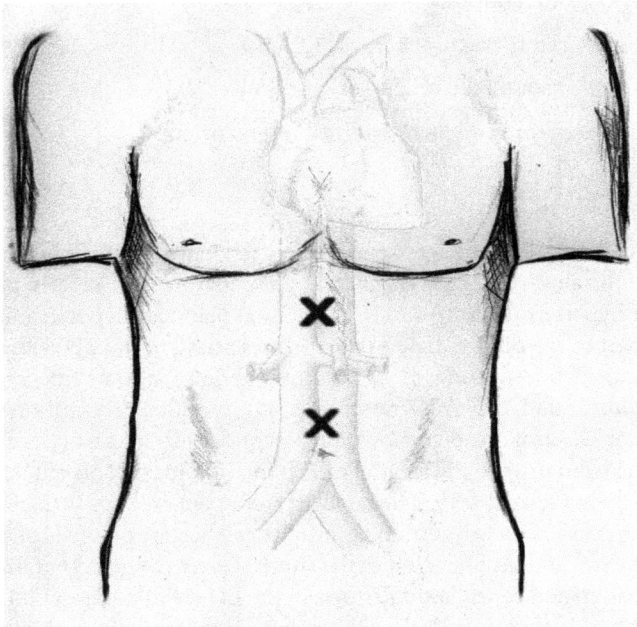

Figure 40-1. Probe placement for aorta evaluation. (Reproduced from Ma OJ, Mateer JR, Blaivas M. *Emergency Ultrasound*. 2nd ed. China: McGraw-Hill; 2008. <http://www .accessemergencymedicine.com>. Copyright © The McGraw-Hill Companies Inc. All right reserved.)

is the vertebral spine shadow. This is best described as a curved hyperechoic structure with associated anechoic shadow posterior to it. In normal anatomy the aorta can be seen as a pulsating circular anechoic structure found just to the right part of the display screen. If unable to visualize, the culprit is usually scattering of the sound waves from the probe by bowel gas. This is best combated by increasing downward pressure on the probe, therefore pushing bowel and gas to the sides of the display screen and giving sound waves a direct path to the aorta (Figure 40-2A).

The short-axis view is continued by following the aorta inferiorly with the ultrasound probe. As the sonographer moves the probe inferiorly, the celiac trunk can sometimes be visualized exiting the aorta and bifurcating into the hepatic and splenic arteries. This is often called a "seagull sign" (Figure 40-2B). The superior

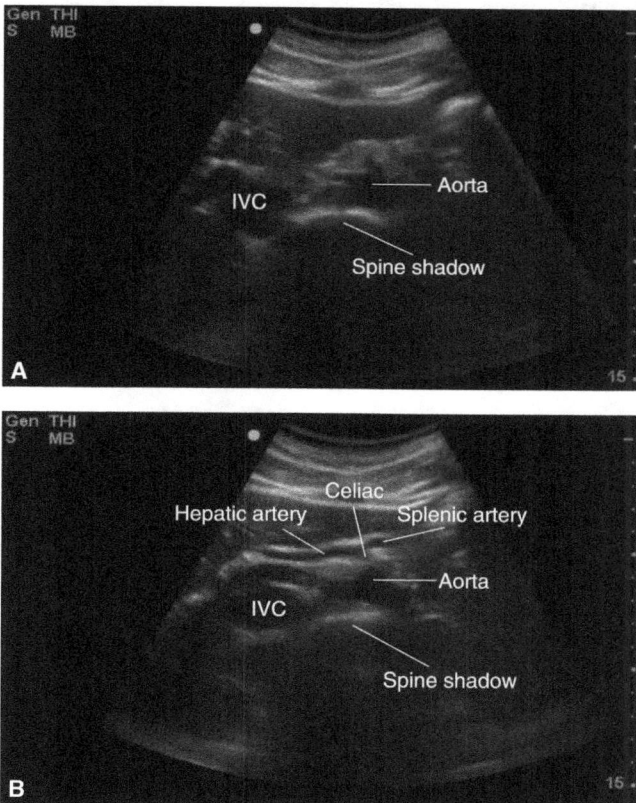

Figure 40-2. (A) Short-axis aorta examination (identifying the spine shadow). (B) Short-axis aorta examination (level of the celiac trunk). (C) Short-axis aorta examination (level of the superior mesenteric artery). (D) Short-axis aorta examination (level of the bifurcation).

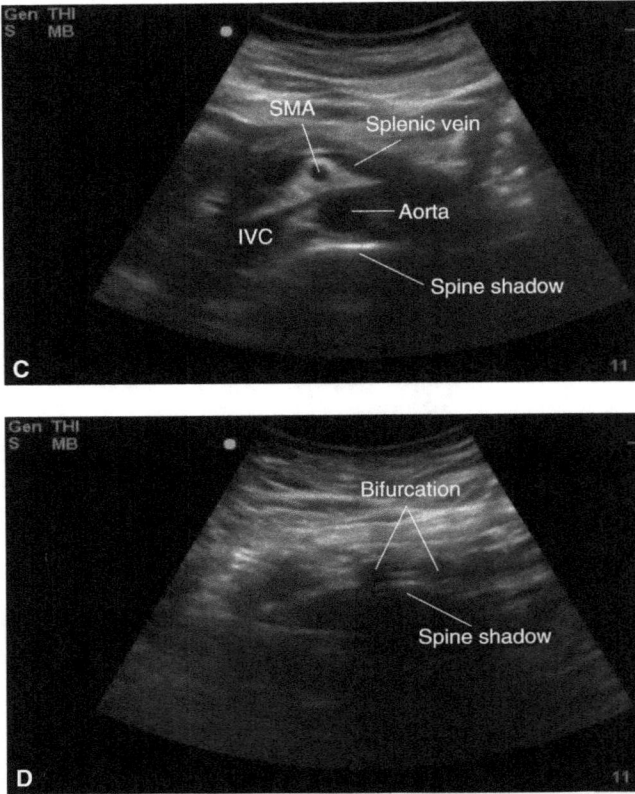

Figure 40-2. (*Continued*).

mesenteric artery and left renal vein are next visualized moving more inferiorly (Figure 40-2C). The aorta is then followed down inferiorly until the bifurcation into the iliac vessels (Figure 40-2D).

INTERPRETATION FOR AAA

Assessment for AAA is done by first measuring the caliber of the aorta at its largest diameter. This is usually performed in the short-axis view. An aorta larger than 3 cm in diameter is suggestive of AAA. In addition, when visualizing the aorta, one should look for an intimal flap or intraluminal hematoma that may point toward signs of dissection or impending rupture. When rupture has occurred, performing a FAST examination may be helpful in identifying intra-peritoneal hemorrhage.

TIPS TO REMEMBER

- AAA should always be in the differential for patients presenting with flank pain.
- A patient with abdominal pain and hypotension should have a bedside FAST and aortic ultrasound.

COMPREHENSION QUESTIONS

1. Signs suggestive of AAA or ruptured AAA include:
    A. Flank pain
    B. Neurologic deficits
    C. Hemodynamic instability
    D. All of the above

2. The first landmark used to identify the aorta on emergency ultrasound examination is:
    A. IVC
    B. Vertebral spine shadow
    C. Bladder
    D. Liver

3. An AAA is suspected with a diameter cut off of:
    A. 2 cm
    B. 3 cm
    C. 5 cm
    D. 6 cm

Answers

1. D. All of these findings can suggest AAA or ruptured AAA.

2. B. The vertebral spine shadow is the first landmark used to help identify the aorta that is commonly then seen to the right of it on the display screen.

3. B. A cutoff of 3 cm for AAA has good sensitivity and specificity.

ADDITIONAL ULTRASOUND INDICATIONS IN THE ED

Emergency Echocardiography

The evaluation of cardiac arrest and shock mandates assessment for the presence of cardiac activity and pericardial effusion. Pulseless electric activity may actually be a low myocardial flow state, amenable to therapy. Signs and symptoms for significant pericardial effusion, or tamponade, such as Beck's triad, are often nonspecific or lacking in critical patients. There is no alternative test to emergency echocardiography for detecting cardiac mechanical activity or pericardial effusion.

Indications for emergency echocardiography include suspicion of pericardial effusion or for detection of cardiac activity, usually in the hemodynamically unstable or symptomatic patient. Emergency echocardiography is usually performed by the transthoracic method. Common views include the subcostal, apical, and parasternal.

With more advanced training and clinical experience emergency bedside ultrasound can be utilized in consultation with a cardiologist to evaluate for general wall motion abnormalities of the heart when suspicion of ongoing myocardial ischemia is suspected in the critically ill patient.

Hepatobiliary Ultrasound

Indications for hepatobiliary ultrasound include the suspicion of a biliary etiology for epigastric, abdominal, flank, or right shoulder pain. The gallbladder is visualized to detect echogenic material that may produce shadowing suggestive of cholelithiasis. A thickened gallbladder wall diameter (greater than 0.3 cm) or presence of fluid around the gallbladder suggests cholecystitis. The abnormal size of the common bile duct (greater than $0.6 + 0.1 \times$ [no. of decades above the age of 60]) suggests choledocholithiasis. This procedure may be performed separately or as a view of the upper abdomen in combination with other indications as noted. Limitations include contracted gallbladder, nonvisualization because of bowel gas, difficulty imaging common bile duct stones, and other pathology in the local right upper quadrant anatomy (liver, lung, or ribs).

Urinary Tract Ultrasound

Indications for ultrasound of the urinary system include assessment for hydronephrosis manifested by costovertebral pain, flank pain, or abdominal pain with vomiting; or bladder distension manifested by lower abdominal pain, urinary incontinence, or urinary retention. Both kidneys should be visualized from upper to lower pole in coronal/long and transverse planes for detection of hydronephrosis and echogenicity suggestive of stones with or without shadowing. Both kidneys can be imaged to exclude ureteral obstruction. The bladder should be visualized in 2 planes to assess for obstruction of residual volumes.

Deep Vein Thrombosis

Indications for ultrasound of the lower extremities for deep vein thrombosis include extremity pain and swelling. The use of emergency ultrasound for detection of DVT is centered on the use of multilevel compression ultrasound on deep veins at the levels of significant bifurcations and anastomoses. This includes an abbreviated visualization covering 5 cm below the level of the proximal femoral vein and 5 cm below the popliteal region. Inability to compress venous structures correlates with obstruction by a clot. This abbreviated study has been shown to have good sensitivity with finding DVTs when used in conjunction with outpatient follow-up formal examination requiring compression of all venous structures of the lower extremity.

Soft Tissue/Musculoskeletal Ultrasound

Indications for ultrasound in regard to the soft tissue and musculoskeletal system include assessment for cellulitis, abscess, effusion, or foreign bodies. Images can promptly be obtained by probing the area in question. Quick identification of the offending pathology will help aid the emergency physician in finding a patient's next course of treatment.

Thoracic Ultrasound

Emergency thoracic ultrasound focuses on prompt evaluation of pleural effusion or pneumothorax manifested by symptoms of chest pain or shortness of breath. Images of the chest should be obtained with assessment for, but not limited to, "sliding sign," comet tail artifact, and A-lines. Absence of proper lung–chest wall interface movement suggests air in the pleural space and pneumothorax. Fluid in the pleural space can be identified with pleural effusion.

Ocular Ultrasound

Indications for ocular ultrasound include assessment for posterior chamber or orbital pathology manifesting in loss of vision. The orbit should be evaluated in 2 anatomical planes assessing for retinal detachment, vitreous hemorrhage, and dislocation or disruption of any ocular structures.

Procedural Ultrasound

Ultrasound can be a helpful adjunct in the performance of a wide variety of procedures. It can assist the emergency physician when there are issues of localization of abnormalities, localization of normal structures, and absence of body landmarks attributable to body habitus, condition, or ongoing care. Sonographic guidance can improve the speed and accuracy of performance of procedures in addition to reducing associated complications. Ultrasound may localize the percutaneous insertion/incision site before the procedure, or may provide real-time guidance of the procedure with needle, catheter, or other device.

All of the following are approved procedures in the department of emergency medicine. These are typically performed in a blind fashion and ultrasound should be considered an additional tool to provide better localization for successful completion of the procedure:

- Intravenous lines
- Regional anesthetic blocks
- Lumbar puncture
- Bladder size and aspiration
- Abscess location and aspiration
- Arthrocentesis, thoracentesis, and paracentesis
- Foreign body localization, including pacemaker visualization, intrauterine device location, soft tissue foreign bodies
- Emergency temporary pacemaker insertion
- Emergency pericardiocentesis
- Soft tissue and musculoskeletal evaluation

SUGGESTED READINGS

Harris LM, Faggioli GL, Fiedler R, Curl GR, Ricotta JJ. Ruptured abdominal aortic aneursyms: factors affecting mortality rates. *J Vasc Surg.* 1991;14:812–818.

Ma OJ, Mateer JR, Blaivas M. *Emergency Ultrasound.* 2nd ed. China: McGraw-Hill; 2008. <www.accessemergencymedicine.com>.

Plummer D, Clinton J, Matthew B. Emergency department ultrasound improves time to diagnosis and survival of abdominal aortic aneurysm. *Acad Emerg Med.* 1998;5:417.

Section VI.
Emergency Medical Services

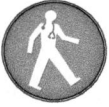

A 54-year-old Male With Chest Pain

Rebecka R. Lopez, MD and
Ryan N. Joshi, DO, EMT-P

CASE DESCRIPTION

The 911 dispatcher receives a call describing a 54-year-old male with complaints of new-onset chest pain for approximately 15 minutes. After verifying the location of the patient, emergency medical services (EMS) personnel are dispatched. After calming the caller, the dispatcher learns that the patient is having difficulty breathing but remains coherent.

1. How is it decided what services will be dispatched to meet this patient?

2. What additional treatments and/or workup can this patient receive in the field?

3. Should this patient be transferred to a hospital? If so, which one?

Answers

1. The 911 dispatcher follows a protocol for deciding what services a patient will likely require. Depending on the regional protocol, this patient with chest pain and difficulty breathing will likely be met by ACLS-trained emergency medical technicians (EMTs).

2. EMTs will determine if any treatment or additional workup is needed to stabilize a patient. However, any additional treatment should not delay definitive care. Treatment will depend on the service level of the responder.

3. This patient likely needs to be transferred to a hospital for definitive care. However, transfer depends on many factors including the patient's consent and stability. Once stabilized, the patient will, with few exceptions, be transferred to the nearest center.

THE EMS SYSTEM

As you prepare to embark on the career of emergency medicine it is crucial that you understand the EMS system and what your responsibilities as an EM physician entail. An EMS experience is incorporated into all EM residencies. Most commonly, EM residents will complete ambulance ride-alongs, communicate with EMS over the radio, provide education for EMS personnel, and assist in the development of EMS protocols. In addition, EM residency will likely include experience in disaster planning and patient transfer.

The formal organization of the EMS system in the United States began in 1968 with the release of the National Highway Traffic Safety Administration's study, "Accidental Death and Disability: The Neglected Disease of Modern Society." This study showed that many preventable deaths were occurring daily in the United States and that prevention could be accomplished through a collaboration of community education, higher safety standards, and improved prehospital care. A focused effort to improve and advance prehospital care began. It was during this time that Dr R. Adams Cowley created the United States' first statewide EMS program in Maryland, the Maryland Division of EMS. In the early 1970s, the states of California, Washington, Virginia, Oregon, Pennsylvania, and Florida began to train paramedics for the EMS system. Over the next decade, with the help of government and private entities, as well as popular television shows such as *EMERGENCY!*, the training of paramedics and the expansion of EMS services in the United States were dramatic.

National EMS standards for the United States are determined by the US Department of Transportation and adjusted by each state's Department of EMS. The National Registry of Emergency Medical Technicians was created in 1970 after President Nixon proposed the idea in order to provide a nationally recognized certification for providers and to establish their scope of practice.

EM Physician Role

As an EM physician, you may have various roles in the EMS system. When working in the emergency department, your role is to provide medical direction for those crews that are transporting patients to your facility. You will be tasked with interpreting radio reports of patients and giving additional orders if needed to those crews. You may also be involved in off-line medical control as a medical director with an EMS agency. Your job will be to establish training and written protocols for crews to follow when treating patients in the field. Your most common interaction with EMS crews will be when they are presenting patients to you in the emergency department. Remember that the EMS provider is the only other person in the medical field who is faced with the same decisions as you. The EMS provider is the first person to assess the critically ill or injured patient and must provide immediate care. Providers do not have the resources that you have in the hospital. They typically have only 1 other person to assist them. You also must keep in mind that sometimes patients must be packaged and loaded into their units in very difficult situations. Providers must then obtain vitals, start IVs, obtain EKGs, or perform airway management interventions before they can even begin to transport patients. Please keep these things in mind when you receive radio reports or in-room presentations from ED crews. They are your eyes, ears, and hands in the field.

THE 911 SYSTEM

The 911 emergency service is the first point of contact between a patient and the EMS system. From the public safety answering point (911 center) an emergency medical dispatcher is responsible for acquiring information and determining the appropriate response to a stated complaint. Most dispatchers utilize a finite list of chief complaints, each with its own algorithm, to determine severity and the appropriate response. Dispatchers also provide instructions (CPR, hemorrhage control, etc) to the caller for any critical conditions noted prior to EMS arrival as a way of decreasing the time of onset of potentially life-sustaining treatments. Of the 911 calls made, few are true medical emergencies, many do not require treatment, and even fewer require actual transfer to a hospital for further care. Just as in the ER itself, some patients will refuse medical care and it is the job of the EMT to determine decisional capacity and even require the patient to sign out AMA if needed. Signatures of refusal are similar to an AMA form in the hospital with small changes, including a "refusal of transport" component.

At any time, EMTs may contact the base station (in a centralized system) or the accepting hospital (in a decentralized system) for additional guidance. The base station is staffed by nurses or physicians and is the most direct way hospital-based personnel can partake in patient care prior to arrival at the hospital. This component of EMS is referred to as direct medical control (DMC). Those responsible for DMC must have a broad knowledge of EMS protocols, EMT capabilities, and medical formularies in order to function within the confines of field medicine. In these scenarios it is very clear how EMS functions as an extension of the emergency department and how invaluable communication between EMTs and emergency department staff is for patient care.

After the 911 dispatcher makes the radio call, the closest available unit will respond to the location. This unit, or person, is otherwise known as a first responder. First responders can provide the most basic services in response to a radio call, namely, crowd control and occasionally CPR. Examples of first responders include police officers, fire fighters, and even a trained layperson already at the scene. The next level of EMS personnel are EMTs, who are generally divided into 3 different sublevels: EMT-B (Basic), EMT-I (Intermediate), and EMT-A (Advanced). EMT-As are also referred to as paramedics or EMT-Ps in some EMS systems. The capabilities of each EMT level depend on the system, or region, in which they are operating. Ambulances are categorized as BLS or ALS. BLS ambulances are crewed by EMTs and involve basic or intermediate levels of care. ALS ambulances, by contrast, are crewed by paramedics and employ the highest level of prehospital care. In general, ambulances are staffed by 2 people.

All EMTs receive basic training in CPR and trauma care (including extrication, immobilization, and hemorrhage control). EMT-Bs, however, are generally limited to medical resources that are already accessible to the patient (prescription medications) and oxygen. The extent of assessment and treatment they could offer the patient in the case above (a stable patient with ongoing chest pain and dyspnea) would be to take vitals, provide oxygen as needed, and help the patient administer his prescribed nitroglycerin, aspirin, or inhaler (if available).

EMT-Is have additional training that encompasses IV insertion, a limited formulary, and usually EKG interpretation. The formulary at their disposal generally includes nitroglycerin, nebulized albuterol, IM epinephrine, and naloxone (basically medications that can be lifesaving and are known to have few adverse reactions). The formulary available to any EMT is based on the EMS region and its protocols under which they operate, with some being more flexible than others. For the patient in the case above, an EMT-I would be able to place an IV and administer nebulized albuterol, aspirin, and nitroglycerin (sublingual or transdermal) without needing to have access to the patient's home medications.

EMT-As, or paramedics, are trained in a wide range of procedures including ACLS, intubation, needle decompression, and, even in some cases, rapid sequence intubation (RSI). They are capable of administering ACLS medications and are generally the unit dispatched for unstable patients. If our patient above had become unresponsive, any EMT would be able to start compressions and attach the AED pads. Only an EMT-A would be able to give IV epinephrine and protect the patient's airway by intubating.

The field of EMS is young and remains disjointed, although many improvements have been made. The capabilities of the EMTs, the structure of the EMS system, and the resources available for either will vary based on the EMS region in which your practice is located. None of the above is a hard and fast rule; however, the general progression and structure should remain true.

TIPS TO REMEMBER

● Acknowledging and accepting the limitations of your EMS personnel, whether these are due to their skill levels or the environments in which they are working, will go far in maintaining a respectful working relationship.

● Bedside education regarding a patient just brought in is always welcome and encouraged especially when given to help rather than demean. A large portion of EMS personnel are volunteers, especially in more rural environments.

● Be considerate and thankful for the work of the EMTs. If you are busy, chances are they are as well.

● Always listen to the EMT's report because most of the time this is your only history. They have useful information that should not be dismissed (eg, a 12-lead EKG with a clear STEMI to show you). Try to avoid interrupting them.

● EMS care is still dependent on geographic location and subsequent resources available, although as it continues to establish itself, a more centralized system is emerging.

- DMC is an invaluable aspect of communication between the emergency department and EMS, allowing for improved patient care.
- There are different types of EMTs, each with a distinct role and set of capabilities based on level of training.
- EMTs function as an extension of the emergency department, providing life-saving and life-sustaining services with limited resources.

COMPREHENSION QUESTIONS

1. Which of the following is an example of DMC?
    A. A paramedic administering epinephrine in an asystolic patient
    B. A first responder obtaining a SAMPLE history
    C. An EMT requesting the appropriate facility for his patient
    D. An EMT instructed by the base station to administer IM epinephrine

2. What is the role of the first responder?
    A. Initiate immediate lifesaving interventions.
    B. Obtain incident and patient history.
    C. Relay pertinent information to the dispatcher and/or EMTs.
    D. All of the above.

Answers

1. **D.** This is the only scenario in which hospital-based personnel provide concurrent medical direction of patient care. Answer A would be a component of indirect medical control or physician input into the protocols that guide EMTs. The EMS Medical Director, of whom approximately 50% are EM physicians, heads the committee that proposes and finalizes the protocols.

2. **D.** First responders play many roles depending on the time it takes them to reach the scene.

SUGGESTED READINGS

Marx JA, Hockberger RS, Walls RM, eds. *Rosen's Emergency Medicine: Concepts and Clinical Practice.* 7th ed. Philadelphia: Mosby-Elsevier; 2010 [chapters 190–194] <http://www.mdconsult.com>.
Tintinalli JE, Kelen GD, Stapczynski JS, Ma OJ, Cline DM, eds. *Tintinalli's Emergency Medicine.* 7th ed. New York: McGraw-Hill; 2011 [chapters 1–5] <http://www.accessmedicine.com>.

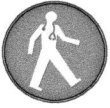

A 94-year-old Female With Altered Mental Status

Rebecka R. Lopez, MD and Jason A. Kegg, MD, FAAEM

CASE DESCRIPTION

A 94-year-old woman is brought to the ED by her daughter for confusion for the past 2 days. The patient is noted to be disoriented, tachypneic, and tachycardic. The patient's daughter denies a history of trauma or recent changes in medication. Initial workup of the patient reveals a negative head CT, normal EKG and cardiac enzymes, elevated WBC and creatinine, and a urinalysis suspicious for UTI. Urosepsis and acute kidney injury are diagnosed. Your ED is located in a 32-bed hospital without an intensive care unit (ICU).

1. Does this patient require a higher level of care than what your facility can accommodate? What if she deteriorates?

2. If you had to transfer this patient, how do you decide where she should go?

3. How should this patient be transferred: ground ambulance or air medical transport (AMT)?

Answers

1. An unstable, septic, geriatric patient will likely need continued monitoring and treatment in an ICU, especially if she begins to deteriorate.

2. Numerous factors go into this decision; however, the overlying theme is the closest facility that meets the patient's medical requirements. In this case, the patient should be transferred to the closest facility with an ICU.

3. An unstable patient requiring ICU care should be transported with EMTs trained in ACLS by the most effective and efficient manner. Depending on the transporter, there are usually many criteria that must be met in order to transfer a patient by AMT.

CASE REVIEW

The patient in the above case may not need to be transferred depending on how she responds to initial therapy. However, if she begins to deteriorate, begins requiring intensive medical care, or requires any additional services your facility cannot provide, she will need to be transferred. If a transfer is deemed necessary, the referring physician must contact the closest appropriate facility and arrange for a transfer as the patient requires more intensive medical care than can be provided at her current facility. After the patient has been stabilized to the best of the transferring facility's capabilities, the patient should be transferred with an ALS ground ambulance unless weather, traffic conditions, or transfer time indicate AMT would be more appropriate. If the patient requires vasoactive medications to maintain appropriate perfusion, she likely would benefit from advanced medical care during transport. Some patients require specialized nurses to travel with them for transport.

EMS TRANSFERS

When ambulances were first utilized, they were solely meant for transporting patients. Although the field of EMS has continued to expand its role in patient care, transporting patients still lies at its core. EMS transport now includes monitoring and treatment of critically ill patients while transporting them for more definitive care elsewhere.

The mode of transportation from the field, BLS, ALS, specialized ground ambulances, or AMT, is generally determined by the emergency dispatcher using a preset protocol based on the patient's presenting complaint, findings at the scene, and location of the nearest facility capable of treating the patient. Generally, most patients can be safely transported via ground ambulance to the nearest appropriate facility. There is still much debate concerning specific criteria for AMT. However, the basic all-encompassing criteria are a patient who (1) is unstable, (2) may require more advanced treatment during transport, and (3) will arrive at the appropriate facility within a meaningfully shorter time frame. Guidelines and protocols will differ among EMS systems and, although research has yet to determine the true lifesaving capacity of AMT, it remains a means of transporting seriously ill individuals to a resource-rich facility.

Determination of what facility the patient should be taken to depends on numerous factors including chief complaint (trauma, STEMI, obstetrics emergency, etc), acuity level, diversion status of the receiving facility, and even patient preference. Emergency Medical Treatment and Active Labor Act (EMTALA) requirements (Table 42-1) must also be met for the legal interfacility transfer of unstable patients.

Generally, interfacility transfers are initiated for patients requiring a higher level of care than that can be provided by the referring facility. These patients are generally transferred to medical centers that specialize in the care of certain types of patients (ie, trauma victims, burn victims, pregnant women, neonates, critically ill adults and children, heart attack and stroke victims, etc). Under EMTALA a receiving facility cannot refuse a transfer as long as it has the capacity (space, staffing, and equipment) to care for that patient. It is the responsibility of the referring facility to stabilize the patient to the best of its ability, explain risks and benefits

Table 42-1. EMTALA Requirements for an "Appropriate Transfer"

The patient has been treated at the transferring hospital, and stabilized to the best possible extent
The patient needs treatment at the receiving facility and the benefits of the transfer are greater than the risks, certified by a physician
The receiving hospital has been contacted, agrees to accept the transfer, and is capable of providing necessary care
The patient is accompanied by copies of his or her medical records from the transferring hospital
The patient is transferred with the qualified personnel and equipment

of the transfer to the patient and/or family member, and arrange the transfer. Direction of medical care during the transfer usually lies within the responsibilities of the accepting facility.

In a resource-poor region, the cost and time of transporting patients becomes a very important aspect of that patient's care. Some regions may not have access to more than a single ALS ambulance and some may have none. Utilizing resources efficiently is integral in transporting patients.

AMT has many other components that should be taken into consideration such as flying conditions, barometric effects on medical care, temperature regulation (especially in neonates and pediatric patients), and the overall safety of the crew. AMT is an integral component to EMS that, when used effectively and efficiently, can be a meaningful component of patient care.

TIPS TO REMEMBER

- Knowing the limits of the ED and its attached hospital is important for the emergency physician as a means of guiding appropriate patient care.
- Early determination of patients who will likely require transfer to a facility that can offer a higher and more appropriate level of care can help facilitate effective and efficient patient care.
- Protocols largely determine what means of transport are most appropriate for a patient. These protocols are an example of indirect medical control and they are created by the EMS medical director and assisting committees.
- AMT is not always the best means of transporting a patient, although it does provide an additional level of patient care that is invaluable.
- EMTALA dictates proper protocols for transferring patients with the main tenet to provide an appropriate level of medical care.

COMPREHENSION QUESTIONS

1. In what cases can an unstable patient be legally transferred to another facility?
   - A. The patient's insurance company refuses to pay for care received at the current facility.
   - B. The patient's medical needs exceed that of the current facility.
   - C. The consulting physician refuses to admit the patient at the current facility, although the patient's care lies within the means of that facility.
   - D. The systemic signs of inflammation (fever, leukocytosis, etc) are present.

2. Which of the following patients would likely *not* meet criteria for the use of AMT?
   - A. Victims of a MVC requiring immediate transport to the closest trauma center that is >2 hours away by road
   - B. Victims of a rock climbing accident with no nearby road access who have sustained multiple potentially lethal injuries
   - C. A woman who has received tPA for a suspected stroke with stable vital signs who needs transport to the nearest stroke center for continued monitoring and possible additional treatments
   - D. A G4P2 woman delivering twins at 27 weeks gestation in a hospital with no OB or pediatric coverage and the closest NICU is 3 hours away

Answers

1. B. This is the basis of an "appropriate transfer" as deemed by EMTALA.

2. C. This patient is stable. Assuming the nearest stroke center is within a reasonable distance, using AMT will not add any additional benefit over ground transport.

SUGGESTED READINGS

Marx JA, Hockberger RS, Walls RM, eds. *Rosen's Emergency Medicine: Concepts and Clinical Practice.* 7th ed. Philadelphia: Mosby-Elsevier; 2010 [chapters 190–194] <http://www.mdconsult.com>.

Tintinalli JE, Kelen GD, Stapczynski JS, Ma OJ, Cline DM, eds. *Tintinalli's Emergency Medicine.* 7th ed. New York: McGraw-Hill; 2011 [chapters 1–5] <http://www.accessmedicine.com>.

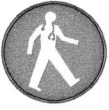

An Earthquake Strikes a Medium-sized City

Rebecka R. Lopez, MD and Jason A. Kegg, MD, FAAEM

CASE DESCRIPTION

On Monday at 9 AM a low-pitched rumble is heard in a medium-sized suburban city. As the large office buildings begin to sway, cereal boxes fall to the ground in the supermarkets; the strength of the earthquake is still to be determined. While most of the newer buildings have been built to withstand a 6.8-magnitude earthquake, many of the older buildings still lack the retrofitting to withstand much more than a 5.6. The shaking finally ceases after 20 seconds (a lifetime when it comes to earthquakes) and the damage begins to be assessed. Numerous buildings have sustained heavy structural damages including a small community hospital, an elementary school, and a supermarket. Many people are trapped within unstable structures. Expected wounds include, but are not limited to, lacerations, crush injuries, orthopedic injuries, and blunt trauma. The citywide disaster response plan is initiated.

1. How does patient care differ in response to a disaster? How does triage change?
2. Are children triaged differently in relation to a disaster?
3. Who is in charge of the disaster response?
4. How is the need for additional support determined?
5. Assuming a hospital has not been directly involved in the disaster at hand, how are its everyday operations affected by a disaster?

Answers

1. Patient care and triage take on a different look during disaster response. The number of patients is greatly increased, patients need to be continually reassessed, and the demand for resources far outweighs the supply. Patients in a disaster response are triaged on whether their lives can be saved with medical care.

2. Pediatric patients are triaged differently than adults based on their common complications and physiologic resilience.

3. The central leadership lies within the incident commander and physicians are considered resources. Although a large portion of a disaster response is medical care, it is not the only aspect that needs attention.

4. The general scale of the incident, including current casualties, resources utilized and available, and imminent threat of worsening casualties.

5. In response to a disaster, hospital resources are reallocated with stable patients being discharged, nurses being reassigned to handle the massive influx of patients expected, elective procedures cancelled and rescheduled, and an immediate inventory of available supplies assessed.

DISASTER PREPAREDNESS AND MANAGEMENT

Field Operations

A disaster, from an EMS perspective, is an event in which the demand for resources overwhelms the supply. This can describe many different situations. As much as the causes may differ (earthquakes, tornadoes, chemical spills, hospital power outages, fires, and bomb scares), disasters tend to have commonalities making disaster preparedness effective.

In order to more simply describe the functional impact of disasters and the requisite level of medical support needed, the potential injury-creating event (PICE) nomenclature has been instituted in many countries and EMS systems. A PICE is distinguished from a disaster due to the former's inherent ability to create injury. A tornado in the middle of an empty field is an example of a natural disaster but not a PICE. The PICE nomenclature utilizes a series of universal descriptors that allow for better communication and resource recruitment. It involves 3 different modifiers and a staging system from which the need for, and status of, outside assistance can be assessed. The first modifier discloses the potential for ongoing casualties (static vs dynamic); the second references if local resources have been overwhelmed and if distributing them differently will improve their status (disruptive) or if they need to be fully refilled (paralytic); the third reflects the extent of territory involved.

The stage of the PICE represents the chance that outside medical assistance will be required and is assigned as follows: Stage 0, no chance; Stage I, small chance, place assistance on alert; Stage II, moderate chance, place assistance on standby; Stage III, resources are overwhelmed and outside resources should be dispatched. While staging tends to result from the aforementioned modifiers (as seen in Table 43-1), the stage can be upgraded as needed. For instance, the 2001

Table 43-1. PICE Nomenclature

Modifiers	Static	Dynamic	Dynamic	Dynamic
	Controlled	Disruptive	Paralytic	Paralytic
	Local	Regional	National	International
Stage	Stage 0	Stage I	Stage II	Stage III

World Trade Center attack was a dynamic, local, paralytic PICE that, although it affected a small geographic area, was considered a Stage III PICE because the local and even state agencies were overwhelmed within minutes.

When a PICE is identified, organization of incident command, and its concurrent components, is of utmost importance. An incident command (or management) system provides for a centralized configuration that is amenable to working among multiple agencies and within numerous jurisdictions. There are 5 central pillars of an incident management system: (1) incident command; (2) operations; (3) planning; (4) logistics; and (5) finance. Each section has a chief with responsibilities within his or her own section and the responsibility for communication with the other chiefs as needed. This general structure allows for the ability to expand and collapse individual components when needed while continuing to serve as the central managing force.

Hospital-based Operations

While disaster response within the walls of a hospital may seem drastically different from those operations organized in the field, the basic structure remains the same. The Joint Commission requires all health care facilities to organize and implement a management system for disaster response that is usually headed by an Emergency Management Committee. This committee should always include a member of the emergency department. There are numerous additional components to the hospital-based response that are related to the daily functions at the hospital, such as bed status, ongoing inpatient care, pharmacy stock, and available staffing. The incident commander should be advised on the status of the hospital including involvement in the disaster itself (ie, structural damage), bed openings (especially ER and ICU beds), and anticipated needs in order to continue to direct resources. Every hospital has a defined surge capacity (what a hospital can handle above its usual day-to-day activities) that allows the hospital to handle the sudden influxes anticipated in the response. The role of the emergency department within the hospital during disaster response is to re-triage and treat patients.

TRIAGE STRATEGIES

Medical management in response to a PICE differs greatly from everyday medical care because the injuries tend to be numerous while the resources are scarce. Determination of which patients require medical care and then those who would actually benefit from medical intervention becomes a very important component to disaster medicine; hence, triage systems have been specifically designed to do just that. The simple triage and rapid treatment (START) and secondary assessment of victim endpoint (SAVE) triage strategies are the most widely used.

START is generally employed for a routine multiple-casualty PICE. It triages victims into categories of green, yellow, red, or dead. Green victims are classified as the "walking wounded" and do not require the limited resources available. The remaining victims are classified based on respiratory, perfusion, and neurological status (Figure 43-1) using an assessment that takes seconds. Yellow victims are those who may require intervention but at the time of triage have normal findings. Those classified as red have 1 or more of the following abnormal findings on assessment: tachypnea, lack of a radial pulse, cap refill >2 seconds, altered mental status, or unconsciousness. Victims are classified as deceased or nonsalvageable when no respiratory effort is present.

The pediatric version of the START system, known as JumpSTART, differs in that it allows for 5 rescue breaths prior to categorizing a victim as nonsalvageable (since most pediatric arrests are respiratory) and it allows for physiologic

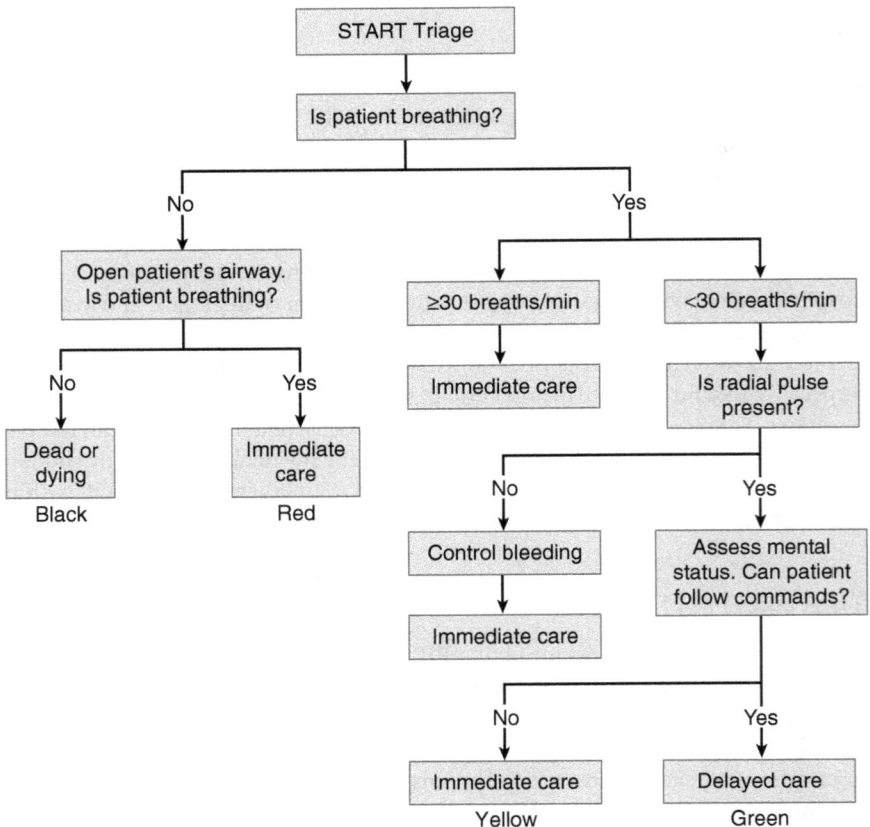

Figure 43-1. The START Triage System. (Reproduced, with permission, from Benson M, Koenig KL, Schultz CH. Disaster triage: START, then SAVE—a new method of dynamic triage for victims of a catastrophic earthquake. *Prehosp Disaster Med.* 1996;11(2):117–124.)

differences between children and adults. As victims are color-coded, they are taken to hospitals and reassessed and re-triaged by the hospital staff.

The SAVE triage protocol is an example of a triage system generally used in the most severe circumstances. Patients are triaged with SAVE after START in response to a PICE when definitive treatment is potentially days away or when demands have already far exceeded supplies (also known as catastrophic casualty management). SAVE triages victims into 3 categories: (1) patients deemed nonsalvageable no matter the intervention; (2) patients who will survive without available medical care; and (3) patients who will benefit from what minimal medical care is available. Anything considered more than basic medical care is reserved for those who are expected to improve. SAVE triage is used as a component of catastrophic casualty management because it incorporates resource availability and rations medical care, both of which are pertinent components of disaster medicine. The basic component of triage in disaster medicine is to do the greatest good for the greatest number of casualties.

TIPS TO REMEMBER

- Definitive care in disaster medicine differs greatly from everyday medical care in that it stratifies patient injuries primarily by resources required.
- There is a strategic protocolized response already set in place in the case of most disasters that has already been organized on local, regional, state, and national levels. Disaster response is a big part of EMS because it is field medicine on a large scale.
- START, JumpSTART, and SAVE triage systems help organize large numbers of patients into divisions of salvageable, nonsalvageable, and those not requiring immediate care.

COMPREHENSION QUESTIONS

1. What is the best position for a physician in response to a PICE?
    A. Triage
    B. Incident commander
    C. Hospital
    D. A or C

2. If a PICE has been described as Stage II, then outside assistance should be _____.
    A. Placed on alert
    B. Dispatched
    C. Unnecessary
    D. Placed on standby

3. Triage the following patients using the START triage mnemonic.

    A. Green

    B. Yellow

    C. Red

    D. Black

       i. A 34-year-old female. BP 120/80, P 110, R 24. She is alert and oriented but anxious. A 1-cm glass shard is imbedded in the globe of her left eye. Her right pupil is 5 mm and reactive to light but painful to her left eye. She has multiple full thickness facial lacerations. Neck has several lacerations, mainly on the left side. Carotids are 2+ and equal. No hematomas. Normal voice without stridor. Breath sounds are clear and equal. Numerous pieces of glass imbedded in the neck, face, and arms, with no obvious arterial bleeding.

       ii. A 26-year-old female. BP 98/80, HR 130 (femoral), RR 26. Awake and alert. She has numerous superficial lacerations to her face. PERRL. Airway patent and protected. Neck is supple, trachea midline. Breath sounds are clear and equal. Abdomen is firm and distended with a 14-cm metallic rod protruding from the midepigastrium. Extremities have numerous small shrapnel wounds and lacerations without deformity.

       iii. A 26-year-old female. BP 110/70, HR 100, RR 26. She has second-to third-degree buns involving her scalp, neck, back, and the back of both arms and legs (~50% total body surface area). Her face and chest have scattered first-degree burns. She is in no respiratory distress. Her neck is supple. Breath sounds clear and equal. Abdomen is soft, nontender. She has an obvious open fracture dislocation of her right ankle.

       iv. A 10-month-old male. HR 120, RR 0. He is limp and not alert. Pupils are equal, dilated, and minimally reactive. He is apneic, but a faint pulse is palpated. After repositioning his airway and administering 5 rescue breaths he remains apneic.

Answers

1. **D.** Generally wherever the incident commander determines the greatest need for an EM physician lies is where he or she will be placed. Triage and the physician's base hospital generally make the best use of an EM physician's skills.

2. **D.** Stage II describes a PICE in which there is a moderate chance that outside resources will be needed.

3. i. A.
   ii. B.
  iii. C.
   iv. D.

SUGGESTED READINGS

Marx JA, Hockberger RS, Walls RM, eds. *Rosen's Emergency Medicine: Concepts and Clinical Practice.* 7th ed. Philadelphia: Mosby-Elsevier; 2010 [chapters 190–194] <http://www.mdconsult.com>.
Tintinalli JE, Stapczynski JS, Ma OJ, Cline DM, Cydulka R, Meckler G, eds. *Tintinalli's Emergency Medicine: A Comprehensive Study Guide.* 7th ed. New York: McGraw-Hill; 2011 [chapters 1–2] <http://www.accessmedicine.com>.

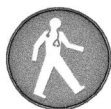

INDEX

Page numbers followed by *f* or *t* indicate figures or tables, respectively.

www.ingramcontent.com/pod-product-compliance
Lightning Source LLC
Chambersburg PA
CBHW060749220326
41598CB00022B/2377